£3

Introduction to Dental Anatomy

Churchill Livingstone Dental Series

ESSENTIALS OF ORAL BIOLOGY
D. Adams

ESSENTIALS OF DENTAL SURGERY AND PATHOLOGY, Third edition
R. A. Cawson

CLINICAL PHARMACOLOGY IN DENTISTRY, Second edition
R. A. Cawson and R. G. Spector

NOTES ON DENTAL MATERIALS, Fourth edition
E. C. Combe

DENTISTRY FOR THE ADOLESCENT,
J. A. Hargreaves

THE MANAGEMENT OF TRAUMATIZED ANTERIOR TEETH IN CHILDREN, Second edition
J. A. Hargreaves, J. W. Craig and H. L. Needleman

ESSENTIALS OF MEDICINE AND SURGERY FOR DENTAL STUDENTS, Third edition
A. C. Kennedy and L. H. Blumgart

THE IMPACTED WISDOM TOOTH, Second edition
H. C. Killey and L. W. Kay

THE PREVENTION OF COMPLICATIONS IN DENTAL SURGERY, Second edition
H. C. Killey and L. W. Kay

BENIGN CYSTIC LESIONS OF THE JAWS, THEIR DIAGNOSIS AND TREATMENT, Third edition
H. C. Killey, L. W. Kay and G. R. Seward

PRACTICAL DENTAL ANAESTHESIA
A. Kilpatrick

ANATOMY FOR STUDENTS OF DENTISTRY, Fourth edition
J. H. Scott and A. D. Dixon

PRINCIPLES OF PATHOLOGY FOR DENTAL STUDENTS, Fourth edition
J. B. Walter, M. C. Hamilton and M. S. Israel

BASIC AND APPLIED DENTAL BIOCHEMISTRY
R. A. D. Williams and J. C. Elliott

Introduction to Dental Anatomy

The Late **JAMES HENDERSON SCOTT**
Formerly Professor of Dental Anatomy
The Queen's University of Belfast

AND

Norman Barrington Bray Symons
M.Sc., B.D.S., F.F.D., R.C.S.I., F.D.S., R.C.S.Ed.
Professor of Oral Anatomy
University of Dundee

NINTH EDITION

CHURCHILL LIVINGSTONE
Edinburgh London Melbourne and New York 1982

CHURCHILL LIVINGSTONE

Medical Division of Longman Group Limited

Distributed in the United States of America by Churchill Livingstone Inc., 19 West 44th Street, New York, N.Y. 10036 and by associated companies, branches and representatives throughout the world.

First Edition 1952

Second Edition 1958

Third Edition 1961

Fourth Edition 1964

Fifth Edition 1967

Sixth Edition 1971

Seventh Edition 1974

Eighth Edition 1977

Reprinted 1979

Reprinted 1980

Spanish Edition 1980

Ninth Edition 1982

ISBN 0 443 02561 4

British Library Cataloguing in Publication Data
Scott, James Henderson
Introduction to dental anatomy.—9th ed.
1. Teeth
I. Title   II. Symons, Norman Barrington Bray
611′.314   QM311

Library of Congress Catalog Card Number 81-69412

Printed in Great Britain by Butler & Tanner Ltd, Frome, Somerset

DEDICATED TO THE MEMORY OF

Thomas Walmsley
M.D.

Professor of Anatomy
The Queen's University of Belfast
1919–1951

Preface to the Ninth Edition

In this edition the main change has been a considerable reduction in the amount of space devoted to the section on Comparative Dental Anatomy, including the deletion of the former Appendices 1 and 2. This curtailment should be more in keeping with the amount of teaching of the subject that is now given in most Dental Schools in this country. The teaching, however, of a basic amount is of value, not only because the dental student is thereby brought into contact with some of the most important biological concepts, but also because it serves to illuminate certain aspects of Human Dental Anatomy. For example, the importance of the relationship of the orientation of the enamel crystallites to the mineralising front is clearly demonstrated by the difference between the structure of reptilian and mammalian enamel. Nor is there any doubt that a knowledge of the structure and the growth of the rodent incisor is essential for the understanding of much of the experimental work that has been carried out on tooth eruption.

About thirty new illustrations have been added, the great majority of which are in the form of line diagrams; for I have long been of the opinion that much useful information can be readily transmitted by this means.

Some small additions and emendations have been made throughout the book.

I wish to express my thanks to the staff of Churchill Livingstone for their helpful cooperation in the production of the book. I am also indebted to Mrs C. M. Toner for help with the typescript, and to Mr Robert Smith and Mr A. G. Ness, for assistance with the photography.

Dundee, 1982 N. B. B. SYMONS

Extract from Preface to the First Edition

We have written this book in the hope that it will fill a gap among dental textbooks in a subject which in many ways occupies a central position in the dental curriculum. Dental Anatomy on the one hand looks backwards to General Anatomy, Physiology, Biochemistry and Histology for its basic knowledge and forwards to Dental Pathology, Surgery and Orthodontics for its clinical application. We believe that a textbook in this subject should not only give information on the structure and development of the dental tissues but should also attempt to correlate the tissues which make up a tooth with the functions in which the teeth, the mouth cavity and all its parts are concerned in the activities of the body.

Since teeth and their related parts have a phylogenetic history as well as an individual history and in that larger setting have illustrated in a remarkable manner the interaction of structure, form and function; we have given a considerable space to the treatment of Comparative Dental Anatomy. It is hoped that the method we have chosen in selecting certain aspects of a vast subject, which has ramifications in Zoology, Physical Anthropology and Palaeontology and provides the data for much of the current theory regarding human and mammalian evolution, will be more suitable than the mere cataloguing of dental formulae.

By including short references to clinical dentistry in some sections of the book we hope to leave the student safely upon the threshold of Dental Surgery and Pathology, and by covering some of the fundamental aspects of facial growth we hope to render a like service to Orthodontics.

We have been somewhat selective and dogmatic in those matters in which there is uncertainty and marked differences of opinion. Sometimes we have given our own ideas on these matters and sometimes the ideas we ourselves have chosen to give in our teaching. In order to correct as far as possible this bias we have incorporated a representative list of books and papers which we consider to be important, especially for post-graduate students who may wish to undertake a fuller study of the subject.

J. H. SCOTT, Belfast

September, 1952 N. B. B. SYMONS, Dundee

Contents

Appendices

SECTION I

The form and arrangement of the teeth

1. The Form and Relations of Human Teeth

Each tooth in man is composed of three calcified tissues, enamel, dentine, and cement, and one delicate specialised connective tissue, the pulp. Of the three calcified tissues the dentine forms the bulk of the tooth; but it is not normally exposed on the surface of the tooth, being covered in one region by the enamel and in another by the cement. Most centrally situated is the pulp tissue, surrounded by the dentine which forms the boundaries of the pulp cavity. The pulp tissue, forming the sensory and nutritive organ of the tooth, is therefore well protected by the more externally placed hard tissues (Fig. 1).

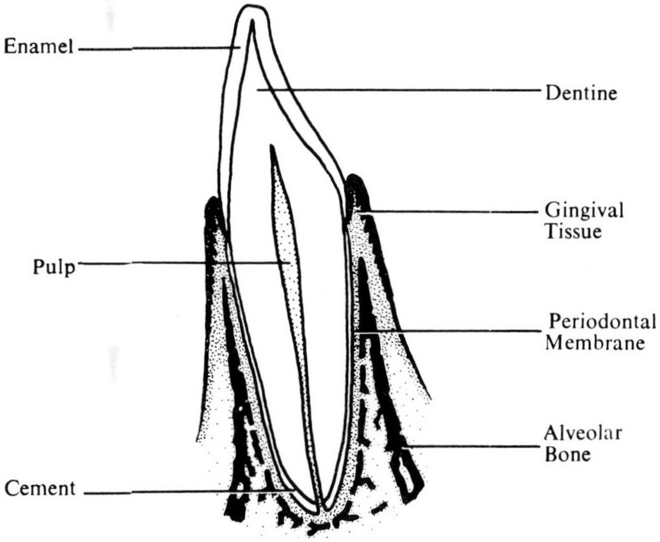

Fig. 1 Sagittal (labio-lingual) section of a permanent lower incisor and its supporting tissues.

Two of the calcified tissues, the dentine and the cement, are of mesodermal origin. The organic matrices of these two tissues are of a collagenous nature and similar, therefore, to that of bone, also a calcified tissue of mesodermal origin. Of the two cement is most similar to bone, both chemically and histologically. Dentine is a harder tissue than either cement or bone, having a greater proportion of inorganic material incorporated in it. It also shows considerable histological differences, especially in the presence of a system of minute tubules which everywhere permeate it and contain the protoplasmic extensions of the odontoblasts, a layer of specialised cells which line the surface of the pulp tissue.

Formation of dentine and cement can continue throughout life, so increasing their bulk. This, however, is confined to additions to one surface, in the case of the dentine its interior or pulpal surface, and in the case of the cement its external surface. Moreover, cement has the power of repairing any loss of its substance produced by resorption, by the deposition of fresh cement; dentine, on the other hand, is incapable of restoring any loss of its substance.

The enamel is of epithelial origin; it is a highly specialised tissue and is the hardest and most densely calcified tissue in the body. It is therefore well suited to take the heavy wear of mastication. Reflecting its different developmental origin the enamel has a non-collagenous organic matrix. Unlike dentine, cement, or bone the enamel does not show a continuous formation throughout life; once the thickness proper for the tooth has been produced no more is deposited.

Moreover, the enamel is unique amongst the calcified tissues in that when it reaches its functional state and is exposed in the mouth cavity it is completely cut off from any cellular elements. The enamel is therefore unlike the other three calcified tissues which have considerable, though varied, powers of reacting to injury by means of the cellular tissues which are related to them; the enamel does not possess this advantage. It should not be thought, however, that as a result the enamel is a completely inert unchanging mass, for it is now accepted that exchange and addition of ions can take place, at least from saliva, into the outer layers of the enamel by purely physico-chemical mechanisms.

The parts of the teeth. From the disposition of the enamel and the cement, two distinct parts may be recognised in each tooth. These are:

1. The crown, the part covered by enamel.
2. The root area, the part covered by cement.

For descriptive purposes one recognises on each tooth a 'neck' which is the part of the root area immediately adjacent to the crown. The line of junction of the crown and the root area is referred to as the cervical margin. This has a sinuous outline.

Each functioning tooth is implanted in a socket formed by the alveolar bone of the upper or lower jaw. The partition of alveolar bone between adjacent sockets is known as the interdental septum. The part of the tooth implanted in the bone is the root area, and it is attached to the alveolar bone by the periodontal membrane. The periodontal membrane is an exceedingly strong fibrous tissue which, though of no great width, has much more of the qualities of a ligament than a membrane. The dense bundles of collagenous fibres, which form the greater bulk of this tissue, are embedded at one end in the cement covering the root area of the tooth and at the other mostly in the alveolar bone.

The periodontal membrane together with the cement and the alveolar bone forms the main attachment apparatus of the tooth. By the nature of this arrangement the tooth, though firmly attached to the jaw, is yet permitted a certain amount of movement.

When the tooth is in position in the jaw, though the greater part of the enamel covered crown is exposed in the mouth cavity and the greater part of the cement is surrounded by the alveolar bone, yet there is a small area which neither appears in the mouth nor is related to the tooth socket (Fig. 1, 2). This part is in contact with the tissues of the gum (the gingiva); in a tooth which has newly erupted and become functional

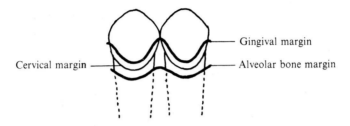

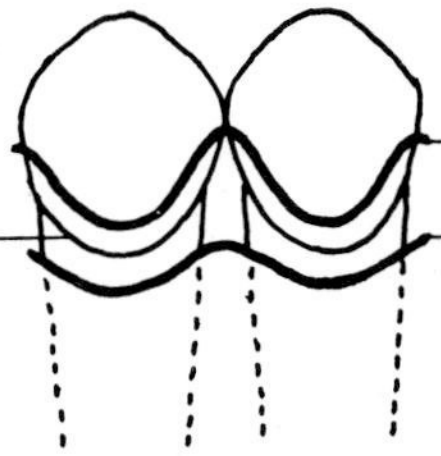

Fig. 2 Diagram illustrating the relationship of the margins of the gingivae and the alveolar bone to the teeth. The interval between these margins represents the area where the gingival tissues are in contact with the teeth. The interdental 'space' lies between the teeth and above the level of the alveolar bone.

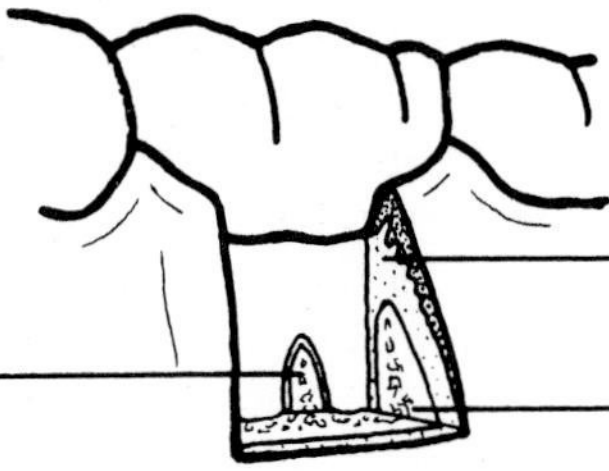

Fig. 3 Diagrammatic illustration of a lower molar with the surrounding tissues cut away on the buccal aspect to show the relationship of alveolar bone and gingival tissue to the tooth.

this includes the enamel-cement junction and a varying part of the tooth on either side of this junction (Fig. 3). The clinical crown of a tooth, therefore, is considered to be that part which projects into the mouth cavity. This does not always coincide in extent with the anatomical crown, the enamel covered part of the tooth. At first the clinical crown is less than the anatomical crown. Gradually, however, as frequently occurs with advancing years, this condition is altered by the rootward recession of the gingival tissues. Thus in old age the clinical crown may

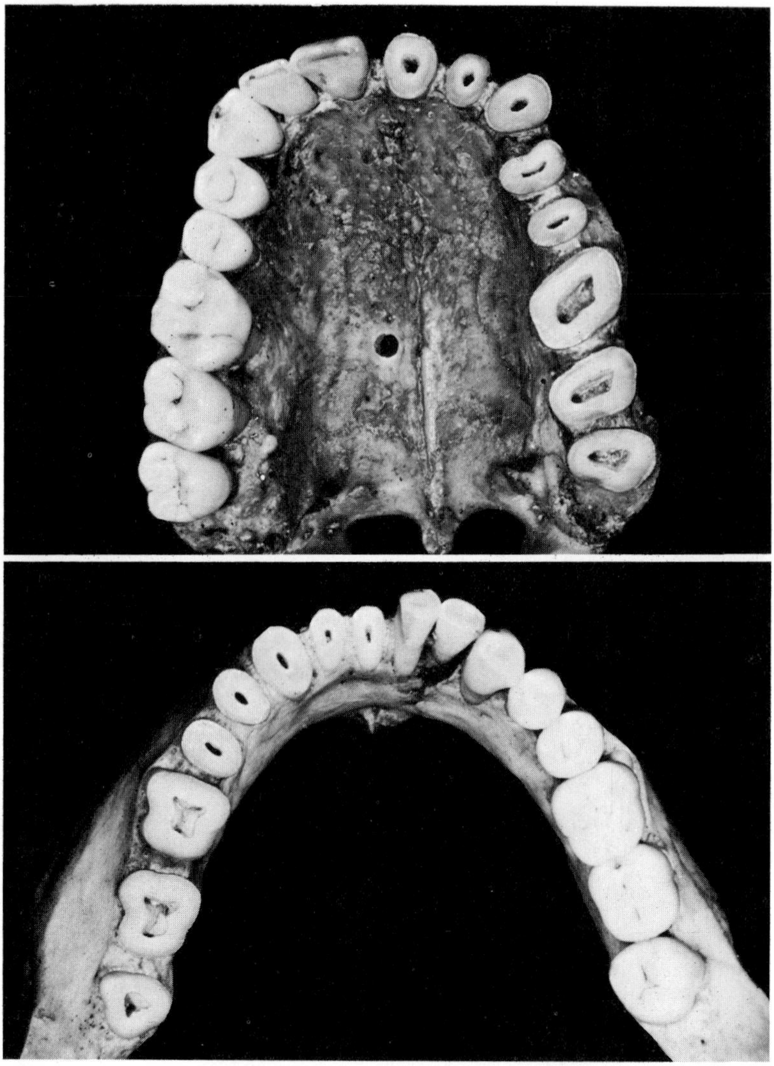

Fig. 4 Occlusal view of the upper and lower permanent dentitions. On one side the crowns of the teeth have been removed to show the shape of the teeth and the pulp chambers at the level of cervical region.

exceed the anatomical crown as part of the cement is exposed in the mouth (see p. 119).

The dentitions. In man there are two sets of teeth, the deciduous and the permanent dentitions. The deciduous dentition begins to appear in the mouth at about six months after birth and is complete at about two and a half years. From this time until about six years, when teeth of the permanent dentition first appear in the mouth, it is the functioning dentition. Usually the permanent dentition entirely replaces the deciduous dentition by about thirteen years and is itself complete towards the end of the second decade. The teeth making up each dentition are arranged in two arches, the dental arches or arcades, one in the lower jaw and one in the upper jaw. In each arch the teeth are arranged symmetrically on either side of the median plane (Fig. 4). The corresponding teeth on each side of the dental arches are mirror images, and in any individual are usually similar in size and form, but slight variations may occur, especially in the case of permanent upper lateral incisors and third molars.

Permanent dentition. The permanent dentition is made up of thirty-two teeth, sixteen in each jaw. The teeth in each half of each jaw are divided into four groups according to the form of the teeth:

1. An incisor group of two teeth.
2. One canine.
3. A premolar group of two teeth.
4. A molar group of three teeth.

This can be written in shorthand form as the dental formula:

$$I\frac{2}{2}\ C\frac{1}{1}\ P\frac{2}{2}\ M\frac{3}{3}$$

In the incisor, premolar, and molar segments in the upper jaw the teeth decrease in size in each group from before backward; in the lower jaw the incisor and premolar segments each show an increase in size from before backward, whereas the molars decrease in size.

The upper incisors and canines are larger than the corresponding lower teeth; the premolars of the upper and lower jaws are about equal in size, whereas the lower molars are usually larger than the corresponding upper teeth.

Deciduous dentition. Of the permanent teeth the incisors, canines, and premolars have deciduous (milk) predecessors which are shed as the permanent teeth erupt. The teeth which precede the permanent incisors and canines are also known as incisors and canines respectively, but the teeth which precede the premolars are deciduous molars, so the dental formula for the deciduous dentition is written:

$$I\frac{2}{2}\ C\frac{1}{1}\ DM\frac{2}{2}$$

There are twenty teeth in the deciduous dentition, ten in each jaw.

The permanent molars have no deciduous predecessors and they extend the dental arch at the back of the mouth as the jaws increase in size. The deciduous incisors, canines, and molars are usually replaced between seven and thirteen years; the three additional permanent molars appear in the mouth at about six, twelve, and eighteen years.

Surfaces of the teeth. Each tooth has four surfaces:

1. Mesial—nearest to the midline of the dental arch.

2. Distal—furthest from the midline of the dental arch.
3. Labial or buccal or vestibular—next to the lips or cheeks.
4. Lingual—next to the tongue. In the upper teeth this can be called the palatal surface.

These surfaces can be referred to collectively as the axial surfaces. In premolars and molars there is a fifth surface:

5. Occlusal—the crushing surface, by which these teeth in one jaw come into relation with those in the other jaw. In incisors and canines the place of the occlusal surface is taken by a cutting margin, the incisive edge, formed by the convergence of the labial and lingual surfaces. The occlusal surface is the cusp bearing surface.

Apart from the two end teeth in each dental arch which are the second deciduous molars at two and a half years, and then successively the first, second, and third permanent molars after their emergence into the mouth cavity, all the teeth in each arch are in contact with adjacent teeth through the most convex part of the mesial and distal surfaces of their crowns.

Together the mesial and distal surfaces may be referred to as interstitial or approximal surfaces. Clinically they are often known as proximal surfaces, but this term has the disadvantage of confusion with its anatomical usage.

The so-called contact 'points' on the interstitial surfaces are actually small circular or oval areas. In all directions from the contact areas the curving surfaces of the crowns diverge from each other forming spaces. Buccally, lingually, and incisally or occlusally these spaces are known as embrasures. The embrasures act as spillways for the food during mastication.

In the incisor region, and particularly in the lower arch, the contact areas are situated well towards the incisive edges. Passing backward along the dental arches the contact areas become placed progressively at a lower level on the crowns.

Rootwards from the contact area is the space bounded by the interstitial surfaces above the level of the alveolar bone (Fig. 2). This is called the interdental space and in life is occupied by a prolongation of gingival tissue, usually called the interdental papilla; this term however is inaccurate (see Fig. 259). The interdental gingival tissue is protected from the forces of mastication by the contact areas.

The buccal and lingual surfaces of the crowns of the premolars and molars are completely convex. In the incisors and canines the labial surface of the crown is completely convex; the lingual surface though largely concave shows a convexity near the cervical margin. These convexities protect the epithelial attachment of the gums by directing food particles on to the gum beyond and outside the site of the epithelial attachment.

The crowns of the teeth show a number of distinctive features, to the more important of which the following terms are given (Figs. 5, 6):

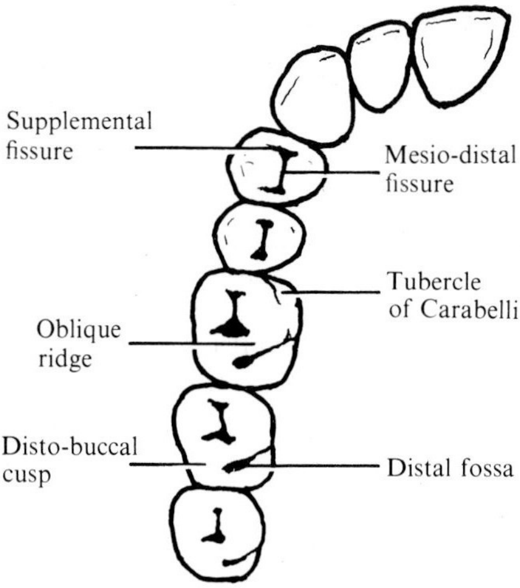

Fig. 5 Diagrammatic representation of the occlusal aspect of the upper right permanent teeth; a number of typical features are indicated.

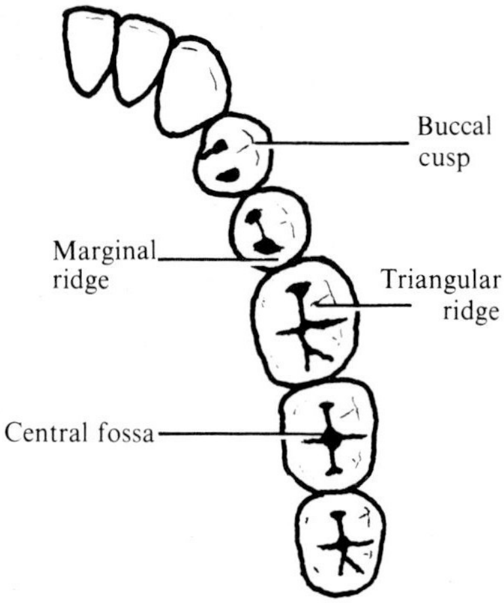

Fig. 6 Diagrammatic representation of the occlusal aspect of the lower right permanent teeth; a number of typical features are indicated.

cusp
cingulum
ridge
fissure or groove
fossa.

A cusp is any major elevation on the occlusal surface of a premolar or molar. In addition, the incisive edge of each canine is surmounted by a pointed cusp.

A cingulum is the convexity at the cervical third of the lingual aspect of the incisors and canines. In comparative dental anatomy the term has a much wider significance (see p. 405).

A ridge is any linear elevation. It may be marginal, or, if descending from the apex of a cusp towards the more central part of an occlusal surface it is known as a triangular ridge. This is on account of the shape of the slopes on either side of such a ridge. The junction of two triangular ridges produces a transverse ridge. On the upper molars one such ridge is called the oblique ridge because of its orientation.

A fissure or groove is a linear depression, found chiefly on occlusal surfaces, and separating the cuspal areas. A supplemental fissure or groove is a less strongly marked linear depression which may separate a marginal ridge from a cusp, or may partially subdivide the major cuspal areas. Fissures may be shallow and wide or deep and narrow. Their conformation may play an important role in the initiation and spread of dental caries.

A fossa is any major depression. On the occlusal surfaces of the molars the fissures run into the fossae.

The premolars and molars, which are sometimes spoken of collectively as the cheek teeth, each carry two or more cusps on the occlusal surfaces which are important in the establishment and maintenance of proper relationships between the upper and lower dentitions. Between the cusps of these teeth there is in each case a typical pattern of fissures (grooves) and fossae (Figs. 5, 6)..

The incisors, canines, and lower premolars normally have a single root; the upper premolars may have either one or two roots, though the second premolar is usually single rooted; the upper molars normally have three roots, whereas the lower molars normally have two roots. In the multi-rooted teeth there is an undivided part of the root

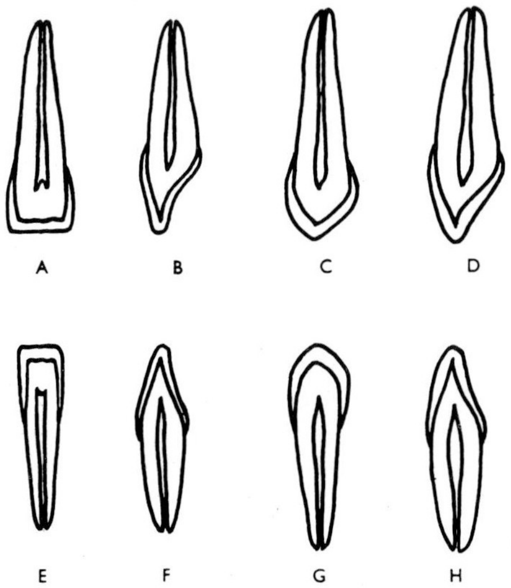

Fig. 7 Diagrammatic illustration of vertical sections through the anterior permanent teeth to show the form of the pulp cavities. (A) Mesio-distal section through upper central incisor. (B) Labio-lingual section through upper central incisor. (C) Mesio-distal section through upper canine. (D) Labio-lingual section through upper canine. (E) Mesio-distal section through lower incisor. (F) Labio-lingual section through lower incisor. (G) Mesio-distal section through lower canine. (H) Labio-lingual section through lower canine.

area between the cervical margin and the commencement of the roots proper.

Pulp cavity. The pulp cavity in each tooth consists of a pulp chamber in the crown and neck region and a root canal or canals depending upon the particular tooth. In a general way the pulp cavities follow the external contour of the teeth (Figs, 4, 7, 8, 9). Each root canal opens by an apical foramen or foramina at the apex of the root. The blood

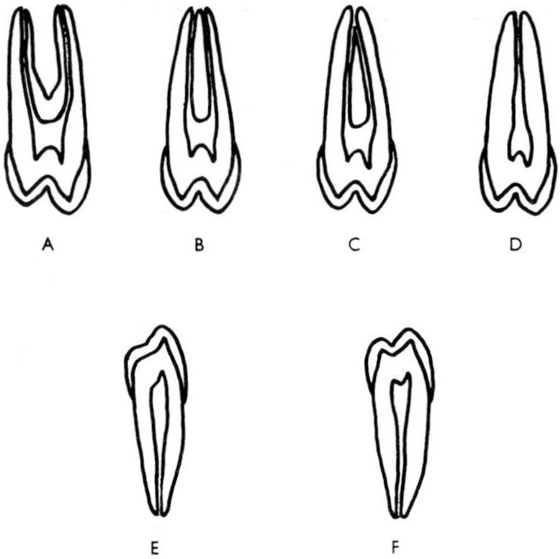

Fig. 8 Diagrammatic illustration of bucco-lingual sections through the premolars to show the form of the pulp cavities. (A), (B), and (C) Variations found in the pulp cavity of the upper first premolar. (B), (C), and (D) Variations found in the pulp cavity of the upper second premolar. (E) Pulp cavity in the lower first premolar. (F) Pulp cavity in the lower second premolar.

vessels, nerves, and lymphatics which supply the pulp tissue gain entrance to the tooth through the apical foramina. In single-rooted teeth, with the exception of some upper premolars, the pulp chamber merges imperceptibly into the root canal, which tapers very gradually to its opening at the root apex. In the upper second premolar the pulp chamber is often sharply defined from the root canal even when this is single. In molars the pulp chamber and root canals are readily distinguished as the narrow root canals open from the floor of a wide pulp chamber.

It should be noted that the standard descriptions of the pulp cavities are not always borne out in detail in individual teeth. The root canals may be quite as wide near the root apex as at their commencement, their outline may be very irregular, and complex branching may occur. Some of these branches may reach the surface of the root and are known as lateral canals (see section on the Pulp).

THE FORM, RELATIONS, AND CHRONOLOGY OF INDIVIDUAL PERMANENT TEETH

It should be realised that the form of each tooth can be considerably altered by wear, particularly the incisive edges of the anterior teeth and the occlusal surfaces of the cheek teeth. The descriptions given below are of teeth recently completed and so little affected by wear.

A. THE INCISORS

These teeth are adapted for incising or cutting the food. The upper incisors are carried by the premaxillary region of the jaw, the lower

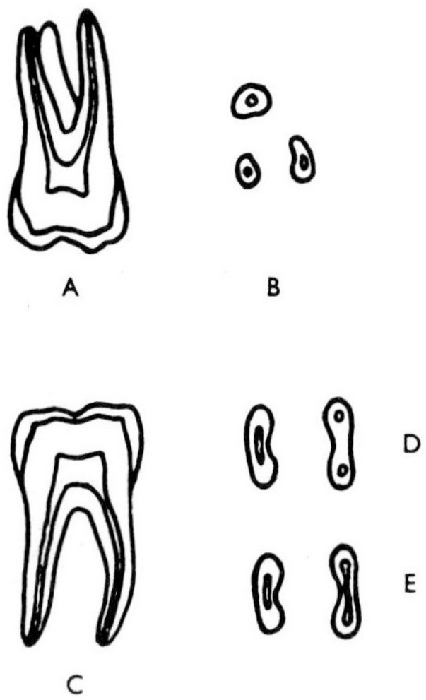

Fig. 9 Diagrammatic illustration of sections through typical permanent upper and lower molars to show the form of the pulp cavities. In each case the distal aspect is to the left of the diagram. (A) Mesio-distal section through an upper right permanent molar. (B) Transverse section through the roots of an upper right permanent molar. (C) Mesio-distal section through a lower right permanent molar. (D) and (E) Transverse sections through the roots of lower right permanent molars showing common variations in the form of the mesial root canals.

incisors are carried by the mandible and oppose them. In both jaws the tooth nearest to the midline of the dental arch is known as the central incisor and the second tooth as the lateral incisor. The incisive edge of newly erupted incisors shows three small tubercles which are, however, soon worn away with use (Fig. 12). The cervical margin of the crowns of the incisors is markedly sinuous, convex rootwards on the labial and lingual surfaces, and convex crownwards on the mesial and distal surfaces. The convexity on the mesial surface is so marked as to be almost V-shaped; on the distal surface the curvature is less pronounced.

In a certain number of European upper incisors and in a greater percentage in the teeth of Mongoloid, American Indian, and Eskimo races the lingual surfaces of the upper incisors show strongly developed mesial and distal marginal ridges on the lingual surface which involve both dentine and enamel. These have been called 'shovel-shaped' incisors.

The upper incisor region is a common site for supernumerary teeth

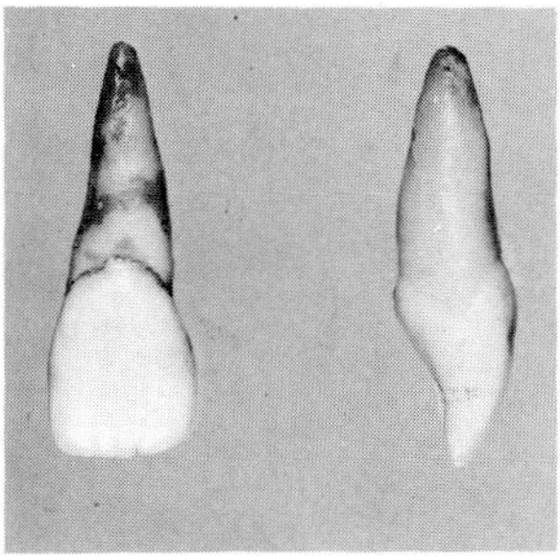

A B

Fig. 10 Upper left central incisor. (A) Labial aspect. (B) Mesial aspect.

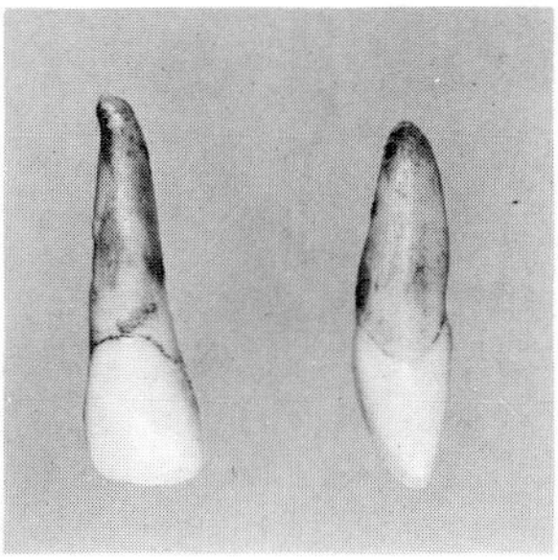

A B

Fig. 11 Upper right lateral incisor. (A) Labial aspect. (B) Mesial aspect.

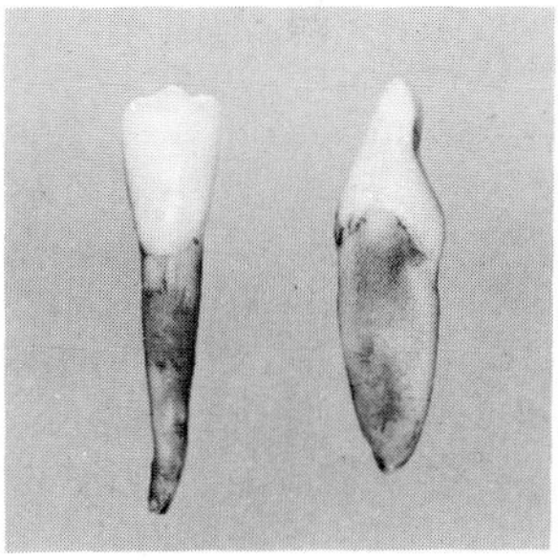

A B

Fig. 12 Lower right central incisor. Note the three small tubercles on the incisive edge of this specimen. These appear on all incisors when they are unworn. (A) Labial aspect. (B) Mesial aspect.

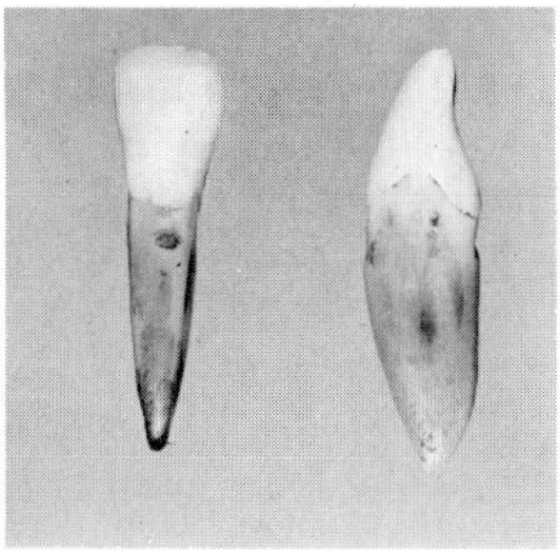

A B

Fig. 13 Lower left lateral incisor. (A) Labial aspect. (B) Distal aspect.

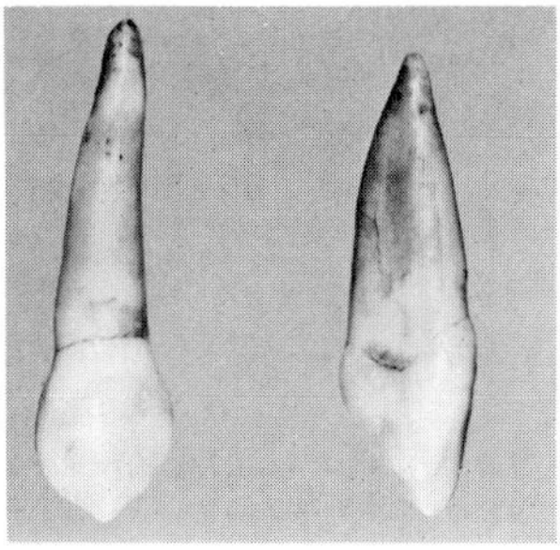

A B

Fig. 14 Upper left canine. (A) Labial aspect. (B) Mesial aspect.

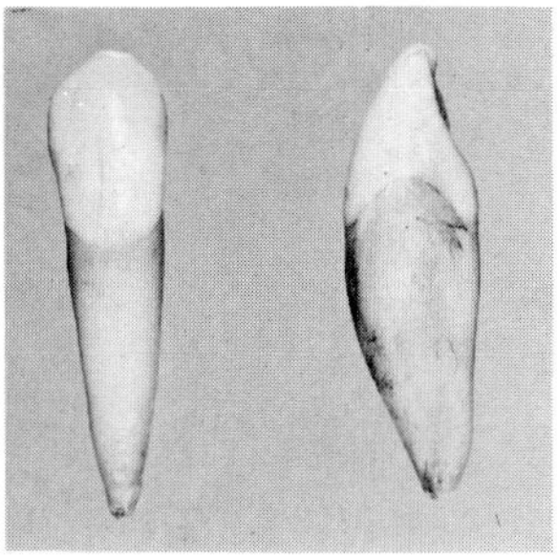

A B

Fig. 15 Lower right canine. (A) Labial aspect. (B) Mesial aspect.

which may lie between the teeth of the normal series or may be situated behind them on the palate.

Crowding of the lower incisors is common amongst all races, but particularly in Europeans.

Upper central incisor (Fig.10). The labial surface of the crown of this tooth is convex, though frequently it is flattened incisally. It may show two slight vertical grooves close to the incisive margin. The labial surface merges more gradually with the distal than with the mesial surface. The mesial outline of the labial surface is more straight than the distal. The lingual surface of the crown is concave, except towards the cervical margin where there is a well-marked bulge, the cingulum. The lingual surface is roughly triangular in outline and bounded mesially and distally by marginal ridges which run from the incisive edge to the cingulum.

Exaggeration of the marginal ridges produces the shovel-shaped incisor which is a characteristic of mongoloid dentitions. Between the marginal ridges and the cingulum lies the lingual concavity which may be partly divided by a slight central ridge into two shallow depressions. When viewed from the mesial or distal aspects the crown appears wedge-shaped. The mesial and distal surfaces are both inclined lingually. The angle formed by the incisive edge and the mesial surface is almost a right angle, whereas that formed by the distal surface and the incisive edge is more rounded.

The root is single, triangular in cross-section with rounded angles presenting labial, mesio-lingual, and disto-lingual surfaces which are not strongly demarcated. The root tapers gradually towards the apex. The pulp chamber is triangular in cross-section and from its roof two small projections are directed towards the mesial and distal angles of the incisive edge. Projections of the pulp chamber are known as cornua or horns of the pulp (Fig. 7). The root canal is circular in cross-section.

Calcification commences	3–4 months after birth
Completion of the crown	4–5 years
Appearance in the mouth cavity	7–8 years

Upper lateral incisor (Fig. 11). The general form is similar to that of the upper central incisor; the dimensions of the crown are much smaller though the root may be of almost equal length. Mesio-distally the crown is relatively as well as actually narrower. The pulp cavity is large in proportion to the size of the tooth. The following particular differences are shown by the upper lateral incisor: the angle formed by the incisive edge with the distal surface is more rounded; in front of the cingulum there is commonly a well-marked fossa or pit.

The lateral incisors are quite often congenitally absent or deformed, the most common deformity being that the teeth are conical or peg-shaped. In cases of cleft palate the lateral incisor, which is usually deformed, may be either on the mesial or distal side of the cleft, or it may be absent.

Calcification commences	10–12 months after birth

Completion of the crown	4–5 years
Appearance in the mouth cavity	8–9 years

Relations of upper incisors. The apices of the upper incisors are related to the floor of the front of the nasal cavities. The outer alveolar wall of their sockets is less thick than the inner wall. Their nerve supply is from the anterior superior alveolar (dental) branch of the infraorbital nerve; their supporting tissues (periodontal membrane, gum, and alveolar bone) are supplied by this nerve and also by the labial branch of the infraorbital nerve and by the naso-palatine nerve.

Lower central incisor (Fig. 12). This tooth is the smallest in the permanent dentition. It is long and narrow. The labial surface of the crown is convex, but shows a definite flattening in the incisal half. The lingual surface is concave except above the cervical margin where it is convex, though there is no well-marked cingulum as in the upper incisors. There are no definite marginal ridges on the lingual surface as in the upper incisors. The mesial and distal surfaces of the crown are triangular, so that from those aspects the crown appears wedge-shaped. Both mesial and distal surfaces form almost a right angle with the incisive edge.

The root is single, flattened on the mesial and distal surfaces, and is oval in cross-section. It is grooved longitudinally on the mesial and distal surfaces, the distal groove being more marked. Occasionally the root may show some degree of bifurcation. The pulp chamber has two cornua, directed towards the mesial and distal angles of the incisive edge. Both the pulp chamber and the root canal are narrow; there may sometimes be two root canals, placed buccally and lingually.

Calcification commences	3–4 months after birth
Completion of the crown	4–5 years
Appearance in the mouth cavity	6–7 years

Lower lateral incisor (Fig. 13). This tooth is slightly larger than the lower central incisor. The incisive edge is wider than that of the lower central incisor and so the crown is somewhat more fan-shaped. Usually the lingual surface shows more definite mesial and distal marginal ridges. Otherwise it is similar to the lower central incisor.

Calcification commences	3–4 months after birth
Completion of the crown	4–5 years
Appearance in the mouth cavity	7–8 years

Relations of lower incisors. The outer wall of their sockets is thinner than the inner wall. The apices of their roots lie above the level of the genial tubercles. The nerve supply of these teeth is from the incisive branch of the inferior alveolar (dental) nerve. Their supporting tissues are also supplied by the lingual nerve and by the mental branch of the inferior alveolar (dental) nerve.

B. THE CANINES

The name is derived from the Latin word for dog, *canis*, as the corresponding teeth are very prominent members of the dentition of these animals. They are also prominent in many other dentitions including the primates other than Man. In the human dentition, although these teeth have larger and stronger roots than those of other teeth, the crowns do not project to any marked degree beyond the level of the adjacent teeth. This permits of the wide range of side-to-side movement which is characteristic of the human dentition.

In all mammals the upper canine is the first tooth situated in the maxillary bone immediately behind the premaxillary suture which in man is obliterated during fetal life except on the hard palate; the lower canine is the tooth biting in front of the upper canine. In the human dentition the canines occupy a key position in the dental arch behind the incisors and in front of the multicuspid cheek teeth, but there is no natural space or diastema between them and the adjacent teeth as is common in many animals.

Upper canine (Fig. 14).The incisive edge is surmounted by a pointed cusp. The labial surface of the crown is convex and is ovoid in outline. It shows a poorly marked ridge which runs vertically from the apex of the cusp on the incisive edge towards the cervical margin. The lingual surface of the crown may be flat, convex, or slightly concave, but almost always shows a bulky cingulum. From the cingulum a vertical ridge runs to the apex of the cusp on the incisive edge, and on each side of this ridge is a hollow. The lingual surface is bounded mesially and distally by marginal ridges. The mesial slope of the incisive edge is shorter than the distal slope. The mesial surface of the crown is larger than the distal surface; both these surfaces are inclined lingually. At the junction of the distal surface and the incisive edge there is a marked convexity. The cervical margin is sinuous, but the crownward convexities found mesially and distally are not so marked as the corresponding ones in the incisors. The mesial convexity is more pronounced than that on the distal surface.

The root is single; in cross-section it is triangular, with rounded angles, and shows labial, mesio-lingual, and disto-lingual surfaces. The mesio-lingual and disto-lingual surfaces of the root are frequently grooved longitudinally. The pulp cavity is large and is oval in cross-section. There are no cornua, but the pulp chamber tapers towards the summit of the crown.

Calcification commences	4–5 months after birth
Completion of the crown	6–7 years
Appearance in the mouth cavity	11–12 years

Relations of upper canine. The outer wall of the canine socket is thinner than the inner wall. The root of the upper canine is embedded in the dense fronto-nasal bar of the maxilla between the front of the maxillary sinus and the lateral wall of the nasal aperture. The nerve supply to the upper canine is from the anterior superior alveolar (dental) nerve; the supporting tissues are supplied by this nerve, by the labial branch of the infraorbital nerve and by the anterior palatine nerve.

Lower canine (Fig. 15). The crown is narrower mesio-distally than is that of the upper canine, and the cusp surmounting the incisive edge is less pointed. The incisive edge is very markedly rounded at its junction with the distal surface. The labial surface is convex; it may show a vertical ridge as in the upper canine. The labial and mesial surface are quite clearly defined, being inclined acutely to each other, whereas the labial surface merges more gradually into the distal surface. The lingual surface does not show any well marked cingulum; it is similar to the lingual surface of the lower incisors except that a vertical ridge of enamel runs from the cusp on the incisive edge towards the cervical margin. On each side of the ridge there are hollows. There are mesial and distal marginal ridges. The mesial and distal surfaces of the crown are wedge-shaped but are longer than the corresponding surfaces of the upper canine. Both of these surfaces show a lingual inclination. The cervical margin is sinuous as in the incisors; the crownward convexity on the mesial surface is more marked than that on the distal surface. The lower canine differs from the upper canine in that the mesio-distal diameter of the crown is considerably less than the vertical height of the crown.

The root is normally single though very occasionally two roots occur. The root is oval in cross-section, flattened on the mesial and distal surfaces. The mesial and distal surfaces of the root are grooved longitudinally. The pulp cavity is narrower than in the upper canine but the pulp chamber shows the same tapering towards the summit of the crown. Two root canals may occasionally be present.

Calcification commences	4–5 months after birth
Completion of the crown	6–7 years
Appearance in the mouth cavity	9–10 years

Relations of lower canine. The outer wall of the socket of the lower canine is thinner than the inner. The nerve supply of the lower canine is from the incisive branch of the inferior alveolar (dental) nerve; its supporting tissues are supplied by the same nerve, by the lingual nerve, and by the mental branch of the inferior alveolar (dental) nerve.

C. THE PREMOLARS

The premolars are situated in front of the molars of the permanent dentition and replace the deciduous molars. Although used in crushing the food and having occlusal surfaces, their crowns are smaller and less complex than those of the molars. There are usually only two cusps, buccal and lingual in position, and of these the buccal is the larger. The lingual cusp is derived from the cingulum and the lower dentition shows a gradual transition from the canine with a cingulum through the first premolar with a small lingual cusp to the second premolar with a larger lingual cusp which may be divided into two. The cervical margin although sinuous is less so than in the incisors or canines, presenting rather shallow convexities facing rootwards on the buccal and lingual surfaces and crownwards on the mesial and distal surfaces. Seen from the buccal aspect the crowns of the premolars are ovoid. Although the premolars replace the deciduous molars they are completely different in form both in their crown and in their roots.

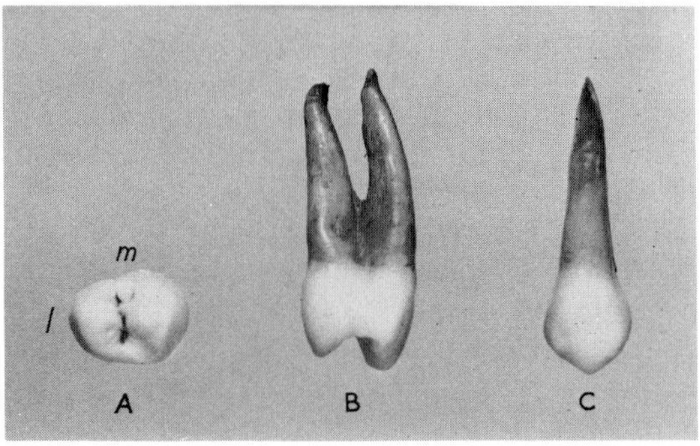

Fig. 16 Upper left first premolar. (A) Occlusal aspect. (B) Mesial aspect. (C) Buccal aspect. (*l*) lingual; (*m*) mesial.

Upper first premolar (Fig. 16). Viewed from the occlusal aspect the crown is ovoid in outline, being broader buccally than lingually. The mesio-distal dimension is much less than the bucco-lingual. The buccal, lingual and distal surfaces of the crown show varying degrees of convexity. The mesial surface, though convex near the occlusal surface, shows a concavity towards the cervical margin where it extends on to the mesial surface of the root area (Fig. 4). This concavity is sometimes called the canine fossa. Of the two cusps carried on the occlusal surface, the buccal is the larger. The lingual cusp is more pointed than the buccal. Both cusps show well-marked mesial and distal ridges. The mesial slope of the buccal cusp is longer than the distal slope (the reverse to the corresponding slopes in the upper canine). The apex of the lingual cusp is situated well anterior (mesial) to the mid-bucco-lingual diameter of the crown. The two cusps are separated by a well-marked central fissure running mesio-distally, but at the mesial and distal margins of the occlusal surface they are connected by low ridges. The fissure usually ends in two small fossae from each of which a groove turns buccally for a short distance, between the marginal ridges and the buccal cusp. A shallow extension of the central fissure usually turns over the mesial marginal ridge and appears for a short distance on the mesial surface.

There are usually two roots present, buccal and lingual in position, though sometimes the root may be single. When there is a single root, however, it presents distinct vertical grooves on the mesial and distal surfaces, the groove on the mesial surface being more marked. When two roots are found the undivided part of the root area between the crown and the roots proper shows mesial and distal grooving; the distance of the point of bifurcation from the cervical margin may vary considerably. Rarely three roots may be found, two of which are buccal and the third lingual in position. The pulp chamber is an elongated oval in cross-section, the long axis lying bucco-lingually. From the roof of the pulp chamber a cornu is directed towards the buccal cusp and another towards the lingual cusp. There are always two root canals completely separate if the tooth is double rooted, but when the root is single the two canals may join to form a single canal just below the apex of the root (Fig. 8). The rare three-rooted premolar has a separate canal in each root.

Calcification commences	$1\frac{1}{2}$–$1\frac{3}{4}$ years
Completion of the crown	5–6 years
Appearance in the mouth cavity	10–11 years

Upper second premolar (Fig. 17). The crown of the upper second premolar is similar in its general form to that of the upper first premolar. The occlusal surface is slightly smaller, more oval in outline, and its two cusps are more nearly equal in size. Both cusps show well-marked mesial and distal ridges. The apex of the lingual cusp is situated anterior (mesial) to the mid-bucco-lingual diameter of the crown as in the first premolar. The two cusps are connected by mesial and distal marginal ridges. The central fissure between the two cusps, though well marked,

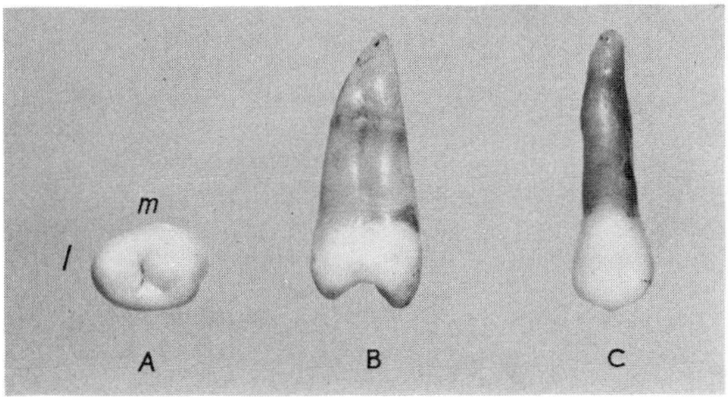

Fig. 17 Upper left second premolar. (A) Occlusal aspect. (B) Mesial aspect. (C) Buccal aspect. (*l*) lingual; (*m*) mesial.

is less extensive than that of the upper first premolar and is confined to the occlusal surface. Shallow grooves may be present which radiate irregularly from the central fissure. The buccal, lingual, and distal surfaces of the crown are similar in shape to the corresponding surfaces of the upper first premolar, but the mesial surface is also convex and does not present the concavity found on that surface in the upper first premolar.

The root is usually single and shows vertical grooves on the mesial and distal surfaces, but may occasionally be double. It is flattened mesially and distally. The pulp chamber is similar in form and presents the same cornua as that of the upper first premolar. There are usually two root canals, but sometimes when the root is single there may be only one root canal.

Calcification commences	2–2¼ years
Completion of the crown	6–7 years
Appearance in the mouth cavity	10–12 years

Relations of upper premolars. The outer wall of the sockets of both premolars is thinner than the inner wall. The apex of the root of the upper second premolar is usually related to the floor of the maxillary sinus, that of the upper first premolar only if the sinus is larger than normal. The nerve supply of the upper premolars is from the posterior superior alveolar (dental) nerve plexus, which is joined in front by a branch of the anterior superior alveolar (dental) nerve. The nerve plexus may also be joined by a middle superior alveolar (dental) nerve. Their supporting tissues are supplied from the same source and by the anterior palatine nerve.

Lower first premolar (Fig. 18). When viewed from the occlusal aspect the crown is roughly circular in outline, except mesio-lingually where it is flattened. There are two cusps, one buccal and one lingual. The buccal cusp is very much larger than the lingual cusp and dominates the occlusal surface; it has well-marked mesial and distal ridges. The two cusps are almost always connected by a central ridge of enamel on each side of which is a fossa. The distal fossa is larger than the mesial

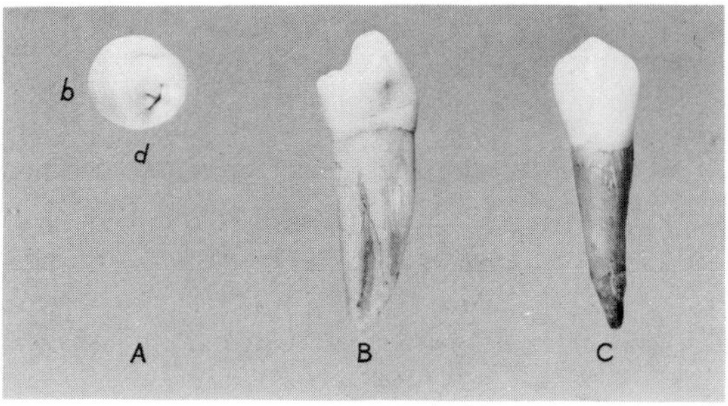

Fig. 18 Lower left first premolar. (A) Occlusal aspect. (B) Mesial aspect. (C) Buccal aspect. (*b*) buccal; (*d*) distal.

fossa. Mesial and distal marginal ridges are present connecting the two cusps and bounding the mesial and distal fossae respectively. Very frequently a fissure is present which runs from the mesial fossa over the mesial marginal ridge on to the mesio-lingual surface. The lingual cusp is very poorly developed and its apex is on a much lower level than that of the prominent buccal cusp. The crown is inclined lingually so that the apex of the buccal cusp is situated directly over the vertical axis of the root. The buccal surface of the crown is markedly convex, the lingual surface is convex mesio-distally, but only slightly so from occlusal surface to cervical margin. The mesial and distal surfaces in general are convex but slope towards the narrower root; they also converge towards the narrow lingual surface.

The root is single, oval in cross-section, but flattened on the mesial and distal surfaces. There is usually a vertical groove on the mesial and distal surfaces of which the mesial is the more marked. The mesial grooving is occasionally so marked as to suggest two roots fused distally and to produce an actual bifurcation close to the apex. The root is often curved distally towards the apex. The pulp chamber has usually only a single cornu directed towards the buccal cusp. There is normally a single root canal.

Calcification commences	$1\frac{3}{4}$–2 years
Completion of the crown	5–6 years
Appearance in the mouth cavity	10–12 years

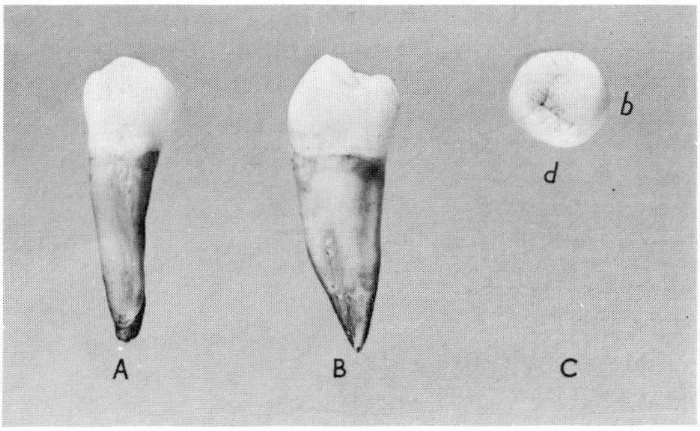

Fig. 19 Lower right second premolar. (A) Buccal aspect. (B) Mesial aspect. (C) Occlusal aspect. (*b*) buccal; (*d*) distal.

Lower second premolar (Fig. 19). The general form of the lower second premolar is somewhat similar to that of the first, but shows a number of distinctions. The crown is more subject to variation than that of the lower first premolar. The crown is larger and when viewed from the occlusal aspect is almost circular in outline. The two cusps are more nearly equal in size. The buccal cusp is less pointed than in the lower first premolar and shows well-marked mesial and distal ridges. On the lingual cusp these are less well defined. The two cusps are commonly united by a central ridge on each side of which is a fossa, mesial and distal. The distal fossa is larger than the mesial fossa. Well formed mesial and distal marginal ridges connect the cusps and bound the mesial and distal fossae respectively. Very frequently the central ridge is absent and the cusps are separated by a fissure running mesio-distally between the two fossae. Sometimes the central ridge though present is poorly formed and is crossed by the fissure. The apex of the lingual cusp is well in front of the mid-bucco-lingual diameter of the crown. The lingual cusp is sometimes divided into two subsidiary cusps of which the mesial is the larger; the distal division varies greatly in size; it is sometimes little more than an elevation of the distal marginal ridge. When there are two lingual cusps the crown is sometimes broader lingually than buccally. The mesial and distal surfaces converge towards the narrower root. The lingual surface is broader than in the first premolar.

The root is single, oval in cross-section, and somewhat flattened mesially and distally, and may show vertical grooves on these surfaces. It is often curved in a distal direction towards the apex. The pulp chamber has two cornua, one directed towards each cusp; when the lingual cusp is divided into two there may be three cornua. The root canal is single.

Calcification commences	$2\frac{1}{4}$–$2\frac{1}{2}$ years
Completion of the crown	6–7 years
Appearance in the mouth cavity	11–12 years

Relations of lower premolars. The outer wall of the sockets of the lower premolars is thinner than the inner wall. The apices of their roots lie above the mylohyoid line. The nerve supply to the lower premolars is from the inferior alveolar (dental) nerve or its incisive branch. Their supporting tissues are supplied by these nerves, by the lingual nerve and by the mental branch of the inferior alveolar (dental) nerve.

D. THE MOLARS

These teeth are adapted for crushing and grinding the food. They are multicuspid and multirooted with large occlusal surfaces carrying three to five cusps and a complex pattern of grooves or fissures. In the upper dentition the molars decrease in size from before backwards chiefly as a result of a reduction in the size of the disto-lingual cusp which may be entirely absent in third molars. In the lower jaw the first molar is the largest but the third molars may be either larger or smaller than the second molars. Permanent molars have no deciduous predecessors. The cervical margin is much less sinuous than in the more anterior teeth. Upper molars have three roots; lower molars two. The roots tend to become shorter, closer together and show a greater backward inclination towards the back of the series.

Upper first molar (Fig. 20). Viewed from the occlusal surface the crown is rhombic in outline; the mesio-lingual and disto-buccal angles are obtuse. There are four cusps known according to their positions as mesio-buccal, mesio-lingual, disto-buccal and disto-lingual; of these the mesio-lingual is the largest. The buccal cusps are more pointed than the lingual cusps. All the cusps show mesial and distal ridges though often the disto-lingual cusp is so rounded that these are barely distinguishable on it. Mesial and distal marginal ridges connect the mesial and distal cusps respectively. The mesio-lingual cusp is joined to the disto-buccal cusp by an oblique ridge which divides the occlusal surface into two areas of which the mesial is the larger. Each area contains a fossa. From the mesial fossa buccal and mesial fissures pass between the buccal and mesial cusps respectively; the buccally directed one continues on to the buccal surface. From the small distal fossa a well-marked fissure runs parallel to the oblique ridge, separates the lingual cusps, and turns on to the lingual surface of the crown. A fifth cusp, or at least a small elevation, is commonly found (in about 60 per cent of cases) on the lingual side of the mesio-lingual cusp about half-way between its apex and the cervical margin. It is known as the tubercle of Carabelli. The buccal, lingual, and distal surfaces of the crown are convex; the mesial surface is almost flat. The lingual surface is markedly convex. The apices of the lingual cusps are situated nearer the mid-mesio-distal diameter of the crown than those of the buccal cusps.

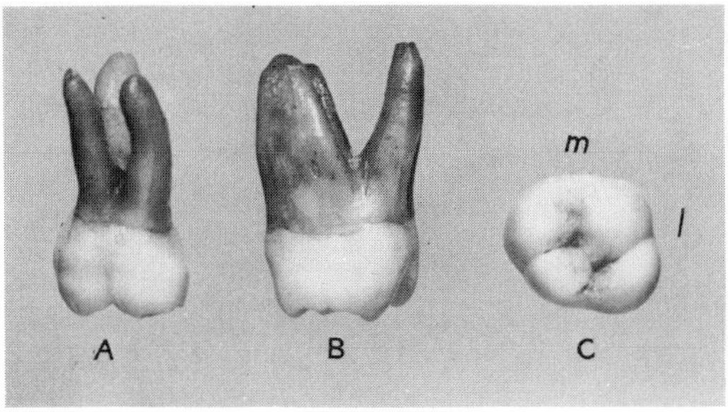

Fig. 20A, B and C Upper right first molar. (A) Buccal aspect (B) Mesial aspect. (C) Occlusal aspect. (*l*) lingual; (*m*) mesial.

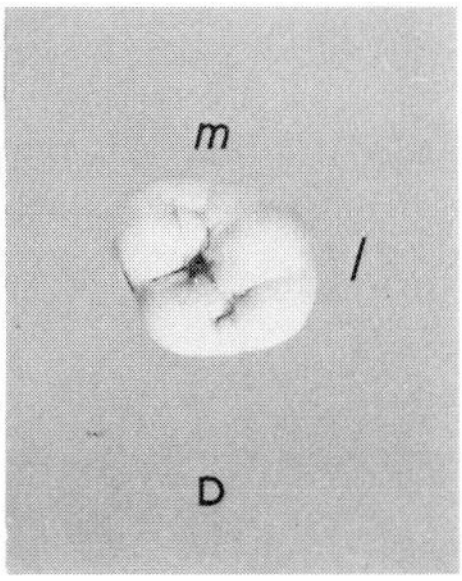

Fig. 20D Upper right second molar, occlusal aspect. (*l*) lingual; (*m*) distal.

There are three roots, mesio-buccal, disto-buccal, and lingual (palatal) in position. The roots do not arise immediately at the neck of the tooth but are united to the crown by a common undivided part. The buccal roots are flattened on their mesial and distal surfaces; the mesio-buccal root is broader and is usually slightly longer than the disto-buccal. The lingual root is longer and stronger than either of the buccal roots, it is conical in form and diverges widely from the other roots. The pulp chamber is box-shaped, and from its roof cornua are directed towards the cusps (Fig. 9). The opening into the disto-buccal root canal is much closer to a line drawn between the openings into the mesio-buccal and lingual root canals than might be expected (Fig. 4).

Calcification commences	At or shortly before birth
Completion of the crown	$2\frac{1}{2}$–3 years
Appearance in the mouth cavity	6–7 years

Upper second molar (Fig. 20D). The form of the upper second molar is generally similar to that of the first. The mesio-distal diameter of the crown, however, is usually slightly smaller and the rhomboidal outline of the occlusal surface is more marked. Both the disto-lingual and distobuccal cusps are reduced in size. Occasionally the disto-lingual cusp may be replaced by two or more small cusps along the marginal ridge or it may be absent. If the cusp is entirely absent the distal margin of the occlusal surface is replaced by the oblique ridge joining the mesio-lingual and disto-buccal cusps, giving the occlusal surface of the tooth a triangular outline.

The lingual root is less divergent and sometimes it may be united to one of the buccal roots. The root canals in this case may remain distinct.

Calcification commences	$2\frac{1}{2}$–3 years
Completion of the crown	7–8 years
Appearance in the mouth cavity	12–13 years

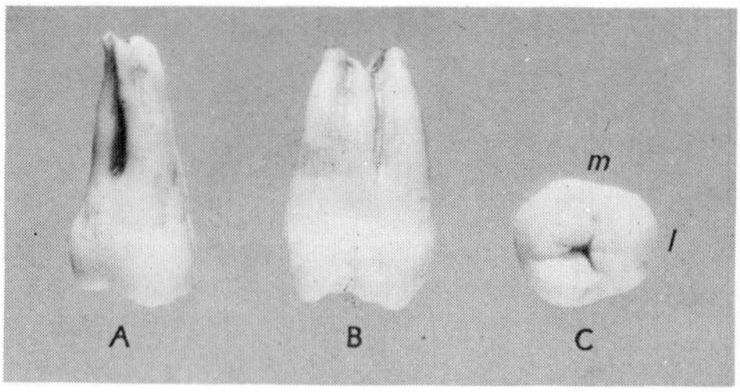

Fig. 21 Upper right third molar. (A) Buccal aspect. (B) Mesial aspect. (C) Occlusal aspect. (*l*) lingual; (*m*) mesial.

Upper third molar (Fig. 21). This is similar in form to the second molar, though it is smaller. It is even more liable to variations often amounting to actual anomalies. Very frequently the occlusal surface is triangular in outline and shows only three cusps, the disto-lingual cusp and distal fossa being absent. The distal surface is more convex than that of the first and second molars (Fig. 4).

The roots are often fused together and then form a single tapering mass.

Calcification commences	7–9 years
Completion of the crown	12–16 years
Appearance in the mouth cavity	17–21 years

Relations of upper molars. The outer wall of the sockets of the upper molars is thinner than the inner wall. The roots of the upper molars are in close relationship to the floor of the maxillary sinus. Sometimes the sinus may even dip down between the roots of individual molars. The nerve supply to the upper molars is from the posterior superior alveolar (dental) nerve plexus. Their supporting tissues are supplied from this source and by the anterior palatine nerve and sometimes from the buccal nerve.

Lower first molar (Fig. 22). When viewed from the occlusal aspect

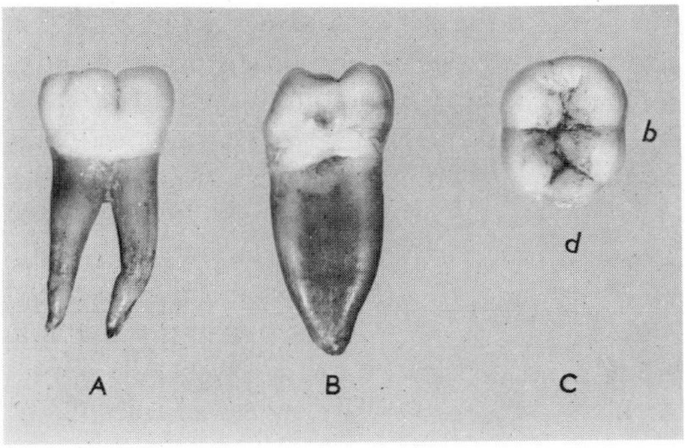

Fig. 22A, B and C Lower right first molar. The occlusal surface of this tooth shows the *Dryopithecus* pattern. (A) Buccal aspect. (B) Mesial aspect. (C) Occlusal aspect. (*b*) buccal; (*d*) distal.

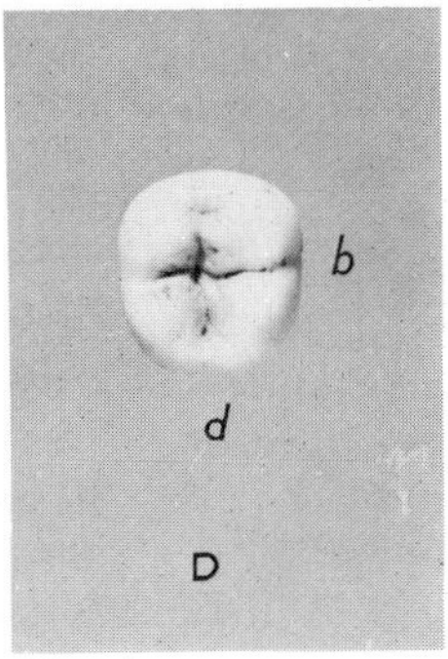

Fig. 22D Lower right second molar, occlusal aspect. (*b*) buccal; (*d*) distal.

the crown is roughly oblong, being longer mesio-distally than bucco-lingually. The buccal part of the crown is, however, longer mesio-distally than the lingual half, and the mesial part is broader bucco-lingually than the distal half. There are five cusps. The four principal cusps are named mesio-buccal, mesio-lingual, disto-buccal, and disto-lingual from their respective positions. The fifth cusp is named distal as it is situated between and somewhat distal to the disto-buccal and disto-lingual cusps. The four principal cusps show mesial and distal ridges, which are most marked in the pointed lingual cusps. The distal cusp is usually so rounded that the comparable ridges are not easily distinguishable. The mesial cusps are connected by a mesial marginal ridge, and the disto-lingual and distal cusps by a distal marginal ridge.

The four principal cusps are separated by a cruciate pattern of fissures which radiate from a central fossa. The posterior (distal) fissure bifurcates and separates the distal cusp from the disto-buccal and disto-lingual cusps. One arm of the bifurcation turns on to the buccal surface, the other arm proceeds more directly distally and may turn on to the distal surface. Thus from the buccal aspect the crown presents three elevations, the mesio-buccal, disto-buccal, and distal cusps. The buccal arm of the cruciate fissure system passes between the mesio-buccal and disto-buccal cusps on to the buccal surface, where it frequently terminates in a small pit. The lingual arm of the cruciate fissure system passes between the two lingual cusps and may extend on to the lingual surface. The three distal cusps are smaller than the two mesial cusps and are on a lower level. The lingual cusps are more pointed than the buccal cusps. The two mesial cusps approximate on the occlusal surface to form a low transverse ridge. In front of this ridge there is usually a small mesial fossa which is the anterior (mesial) termination of the mesio-distal limb of the cruciate fissure system.

When five cusps are present and the mesio-lingual cusp is in contact with the disto-buccal cusp at the floor of the central fossa, the lower molar is said to show the primitive *Dryopithecus* pattern which is constant in all the lower molars of anthropoid apes and in the *Dyropithecus* group of extinct anthropoids. It is present in nearly 90 per cent of cases in the lower first permanent molars, in about 5 per cent of third molars but is uncommon in second molars of European people (Fig. 22C).

An accessory cusp, the 'paramolar' cusp, is rarely present on the buccal surface of first molars. It is much less common on second and third molars.

The buccal, lingual, mesial, and distal surfaces of the crown are all convex, the buccal surface markedly so. The apices of the two buccal cusps are situated nearer the mid-mesio-distal diameter of the crown than those of the lingual cusps. This is the reverse condition to that in the upper molars.

There are two roots, one mesial and one distal. The roots do not arise immediately at the neck of the tooth but are united to the crown by a common undivided part. The buccal and lingual surfaces of this undivided trunk show vertical grooving directed towards the bifurcation of the roots. The roots are broad and are flattened mesially and distally, the mesial root more so than the distal root. The mesial root is curved backward and shows a broad well-marked vertical groove on its distal surface. The distal root is not so large and shows a similar but narrower groove on the mesial surface. The distal root may show little if any back-

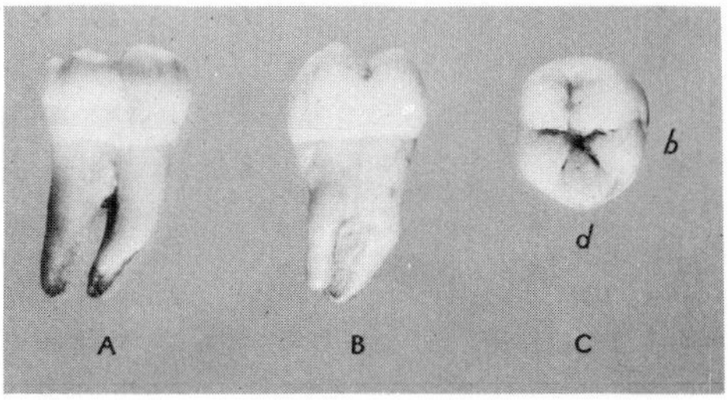

Fig. 23 Lower right third molar. (A) Buccal aspect. (B) Mesial aspect. (C) Occlusal aspect. (*b*) buccal; (*d*) distal.

ward curvature. The mesial root also shows a broad but shallow vertical groove on its mesial surface. The pulp chamber is box-shaped with its long axis mesio-distal in direction, and from it cornua are directed towards the principal cusps. There are usually two root canals in the mesial root, but these are often connected by a thin ribbon of pulp tissue (Fig. 6). There is normally one root canal in the distal root.

Calcification commences	At or shortly before birth
Completion of the crown	$2\frac{1}{2}$–3 years
Appearance in the mouth cavity	6–7 years

Lower second molar (Fig. 22D). In its general form the lower second molar is similar to the first. Usually, however, it has only four cusps, the distal cusp being absent. In this tooth the disto-buccal and disto-lingual cusps are connected by a distal marginal ridge. The disto-buccal cusp is relatively larger and placed farther distally than in the first molar. The posterior (distal) fissure does not show any bifurcation and the total fissure pattern is more definitely cross-shaped; the buccal and lingual arms meet the mesio-distal limb of the fissure system at right angles. In a small percentage of cases a well-defined distal cusp is present, and the occlusal surface is then the same as in the first molar.

Both roots are usually curved backwards and are not so widely separated as in the first molar; sometimes they may be fused.

Calcification commences	$2\frac{1}{2}$–3 years
Completion of the crown	7 –8 years
Appearance in the mouth cavity	11 –13 years

Lower third molar (Fig. 23). This may show an occlusal pattern of either the four or five cusped variety. It frequently shows, however, considerable variations in the details of this pattern so that the relative proportions of the cusps are abnormal; this is particularly found in the five-cusped variety. The distal surface is markedly convex. Some third molars occur in which the crown is larger than those of second molars.

The roots are curved in a backward direction. They are often fused and are generally smaller than in the second molar. The roots may be grooved, or even perforated, by the inferior dental nerve.

Calcification commences	8–10 years
Completion of the crown	12–16 years
Appearance in the mouth cavity	17–21 years

Relations of lower molars. The inner wall of the socket of the third lower molar is thinner than the outer wall, which is strengthened by the external oblique ridge of the mandible. This is often also the case in the second molar and may sometimes apply to the first molar. The apices of the roots of the third molars and sometimes of the second lie below the level of the mylohyoid ridge. The nerve supply to these teeth is from the inferior alveolar (dental) nerve. Their supporting tissues are supplied by this nerve and by the lingual and buccal nerves. The apices of the roots of the lower molars are usually in close relationship to the inferior alveolar (dental) nerve (Fig. 242). Occasionally the roots of the third molar may even be perforated by the nerve.

TOOTH SOCKETS

The sockets of the permanent teeth occupy the alveolar processes of the jaws and conform closely in size and shape to the roots of the implanted teeth.

Upper jaw

Central incisors. The mouth of the socket is rounded and the socket cavity cone-shaped. The interdental septum between the central incisor of each side is divided by the intermaxillary suture and the incisive canal lies behind and between the two sockets. The labial alveolar wall of the socket is often very thin.

Lateral incisors. The mouth of the socket is more oval in shape with a greater labio-lingual diameter; the socket cavity is cone-shaped and usually less deep than that of the central incisors.

Canines. The mouth of the socket is oval with the labio-lingual diameter slightly greater than the mesio-distal. The socket is deep, cone-shaped and tends to incline backwards; the interdental septa between the canines and lateral incisors may be of considerable thickness. The labial alveolar wall is often very thin.

Premolars. The mouths of the sockets are oval and usually show a slight constriction near the middle of the longer bucco-lingual diameter. In the socket of the first premolar a well-marked vertical ridge runs down the mesial wall and if the root of the tooth is bifurcated this ridge becomes a partition dividing part of the socket into a buccal and a lingual compartment. In the socket of the second premolar the vertical ridge is situated on the distal wall.

Molars. If all the molar teeth are three-rooted the sockets for the teeth are in general similar in form with, however, a tendency for the three compartments to be closer together in the case of the second and especially of the third molars. The roots of the third molar are frequently united and if so the socket is usually a single cone-shaped cavity wider in front than behind. The compartments for the palatal roots usually show rounded openings and taper towards the roof. The lingual alveolar plate is often very thin. The mouth of the mesio-buccal compartment is usually oval-shaped and its mesial and distal walls somewhat flattened. It lies anterior as well as buccal to the palatal compartment. The opening of the disto-buccal compartment is rounded and it is conical in form. The interradicular septa which separate the three compartments are thick and show the openings of numerous small foramina for blood vessels. The roofs of one or more of the compartments may be deficient and communicate with the floor of the maxillary air sinus.

Lower jaw

Incisors. The mouths of the sockets are oval with a greater labio-lingual diameter; the mesial and distal walls are flattened and the interdental septa are thin and sharp. The socket for the second incisor is somewhat larger than that for the first. The labial alveolar walls of the sockets are often very thin.

Canines. The mouth of the socket is oval with the long labio-lingual diameter somewhat obliquely placed and wider labially than lingually. The socket is cone-shaped.

Premolars. The mouths of the sockets are oval with a longer bucco-lingual diameter; the cavities are cone-shaped. The interdental septum between the premolar sockets is thicker than those between the anterior teeth.

Molars. The mouth of the mesial compartment of the socket for the first molar is oval-shaped with a constriction near the middle of the longer bucco-lingual diameter; the mesial and distal walls are flattened and show vertical ridges. The distal compartment is more truly oval and the cavity is more cone-shaped. The sockets for the second and third molars may be similar to that for the first but owing to a tendency for the roots to fuse they often show a single compartment with vertical buccal and lingual ridges; such cavities are wider in front than behind. The margins of the interradicular septa show numerous small foramina for blood vessels. Both the buccal and lingual alveolar walls of the sockets are usually robust.

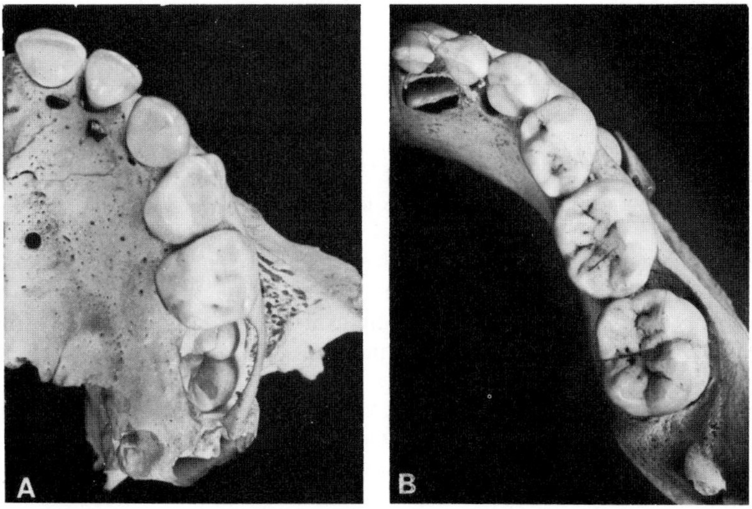

Fig. 24 Occlusal view of the deciduous teeth. (A) Left half of the upper arch. (B) Right half of the lower arch. In both jaws the permanent first molar can be seen. In the lower jaw the roofs of the crypts for this tooth and for the permanent central incisor have been resorbed. (*By courtesy of Dr R. Sprinz.*)

THE DECIDUOUS TEETH

General differences between deciduous and permanent teeth. The deciduous teeth differ in a general way from the permanent teeth in the following respects:

1. Size. The deciduous incisors and canines are smaller in all dimensions than their permanent successors; and the deciduous molars are smaller than the permanent molars. The mesio-distal length of the deciduous molars is, however, greater than that of the succeeding premolars

(Fig. 135). The extra space made available by this difference is made use of in occlusal adjustments which take place during the period of tooth replacement.

2. Form. The crowns of the deciduous teeth are more bulbous than those of permanent teeth; the cusps are more pointed and less rounded when the teeth first erupt; the contact points involve a smaller surface of contact between the teeth. The crowns of the incisors and canines are relatively broader mesio-distally than those of the corresponding permanent teeth.

3. Colour. The deciduous teeth are, as a rule, whiter in colour in the mouth cavity than the permanent teeth; their enamel is less transparent.

4. Enamel margin. In deciduous teeth the enamel-cement junction is less sinuous and the enamel ends more abruptly. In the first deciduous molars especially the crown shows a well-marked bulge at the mesio-buccal region close to the cervical margin.

5. Roots. The roots of the deciduous teeth are shorter and less robust than are those of the permanent dentition, though relative to the size of the crowns they are longer. In the deciduous molars the undivided part of the root area is much less extensive than in the permanent molars, and the roots diverge widely and abruptly from the short trunk. The roots are fully formed about one year after eruption, but root resorption commences one or two years before the teeth are shed.

6. Pulp cavities. These are, relative to the size of the teeth, larger than those of the permanent teeth, and therefore the bulk of the surrounding dentine is proportionally less than in the permanent teeth.

7. Permeability of enamel. The enamel of deciduous teeth remains permeable until root resorption commences, when the degree of permeability is greatly reduced.

8. Attrition. The deciduous teeth show a degree of attrition which is relatively greater than that shown by the permanent teeth.

The colour of the teeth and the amount of attrition both depend upon the same factor, the level of mineralisation of the enamel. More highly mineralised enamel is harder and so is more slowly worn away than less highly mineralised enamel. Highly mineralised enamel is very translucent and so the colour of the underlying dentine can shine through the enamel and impart a yellowish tinge to the tooth.

A. DECIDUOUS INCISORS

Apart from general differences in size and colour, etc., the deciduous incisors are similar to their permanent successors. The crowns are, however, more bulbous.

Calcification of the deciduous incisors commences between the fourth and fifth month of fetal life. At birth the crowns of the teeth are two-thirds calcified; the crowns are fully calcified about two months after birth; the teeth appear in the mouth six to nine months after birth and the roots are complete about a year later.

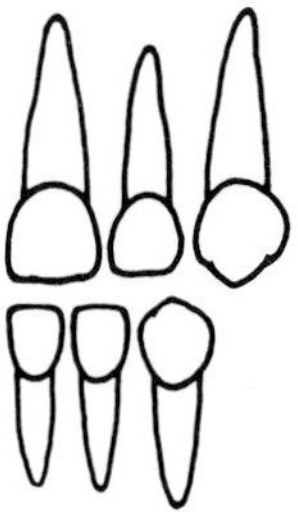

Fig. 25 Diagrammatic illustration of the upper and lower left deciduous incisors and canines seen from the labial aspect.

B. DECIDUOUS CANINES

The crowns of the deciduous canines are much more bulbous than are those of the permanent teeth and have well-marked mesial and distal convexities. When newly erupted the tip of the cusp is pointed particularly in the upper tooth, but it soon becomes blunted with wear. In the upper canine the mesial slope of the incisive edge is longer than the distal slope.

Calcification of the deciduous canines commences in the fifth month of fetal life. At birth the crown is one-third, calcified; the crowns are fully calcified at about nine months after birth; the teeth appear in the mouth at sixteen to eighteen months and the roots are complete about a year later.

C. DECIDUOUS MOLARS

Upper first molar. Seen from the occlusal aspect the crown is irregularly quadrilateral (trapezoid); the buccal side is longer than the lingual, and the mesio-lingual angle is obtuse. There are two cusps, buccal and lingual, separated by a broad but rather shallow central fossa. The buccal cusp is in the form of an elongated ridge which may be partially divided into two or three lobes. The buccal and lingual cusps are connected by poorly defined mesial and distal marginal ridges which bound the central fossa. The buccal surface of the crown shows a well-marked bulge towards the cervical margin below the mesio-buccal root. There are three roots, mesio-buccal, disto-buccal and lingual (palatal) in position.

Upper second molar. Apart from the general differences between deciduous and permanent teeth and the wide divergence of the roots, this tooth is very similar in form to the first permanent upper molar; it has the same number and arrangement of cusps and roots. The mesio-lingual cusp is the largest and is connected to the disto-buccal cusp by an oblique ridge dividing the occlusal surface into a larger mesial fossa and a smaller distal fossa as in the first permanent molar. The tubercle or cusp of Carabelli is frequently present.

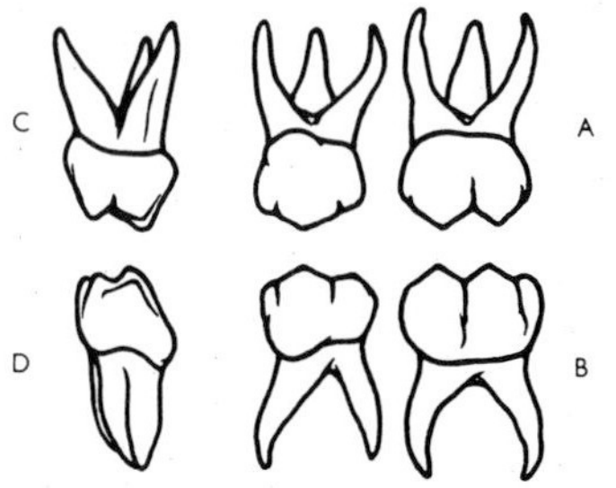

Fig. 26 Diagrammatic illustration of the deciduous molars of the left side. (A) the upper molars and (B) the lower molars, both seen from the buccal aspect. (C) the mesial aspect of the upper first molar. (D) the mesial aspect of the lower first molar.

Lower first molar. The occlusal surface is elongated in the mesio-distal direction. It carries four cusps, two buccal and two lingual; of these the most prominent is the mesio-lingual. Frequently the buccal cusps are poorly developed. There is a mesial and a distal marginal ridge. The mesio-lingual angle of the crown is very markedly obtuse. The mesio-buccal and mesio-lingual cusps are connected by a transverse ridge which divides the occlusal surface into a small mesial and a large distal fossa. The distal fossa is bounded by this ridge, the four cusps, and the distal marginal ridge. The mesial fossa lies between the mesio-buccal and mesio-lingual cusps and the mesial marginal ridge which sweeps in a pronounced mesially directed convexity between the two cusps. The buccal surface of the crown shows a well-marked bulge towards the cervical margin above the mesial root. There are two roots, mesial and distal in position.

Lower second molar. This tooth, apart from the general differences between deciduous and permanent teeth, is similar in form to the first permanent lower molar; it has the same number and arrangement of cusps and roots. The central fossa is, however, relatively more extensive, and the fissure arrangement does not usually show the *Dryopithecus* pattern (see p. 26).

Calcification commences in the deciduous molars during the fifth to sixth months of fetal life. At birth the occlusal surfaces of the first molars are calcified; the individual cusps of the second molars are calcified and may be joined to one another to form a calcified ring; the centre of the occlusal surfaces being as yet uncalcified. The crowns of the first deciduous molars are fully calcified by the sixth month after birth and those of the second molars by the end of the first year. The first deciduous molars appear in the mouth at twelve to fourteen months: the second deciduous molars appear in the mouth at twenty-four to thirty months. The roots of the deciduous molars are complete about one year later.

Certain characters of the deciduous dentition such as the higher more pointed cusps, the deeper fossae on the occlusal surfaces of the molars, the form of the crown of the newly erupted canine and the associated space (diastema), are held to be primitive in nature. It should be remembered, however, that:

1. The permanent molars which are characteristically human in form are almost certainly members of the same tooth family as the deciduous molars; that is, they are deciduous teeth, without permanent successors, which erupt at the back of the arch as room is made available by growth of the mandible and maxilla.

2. Spacing between the deciduous incisors and canines is possibly a growth phenomenon and need have no evolutionary or morphological significance whatever.

THE DENTAL ARCHES

Each dental arch conforms to a catenary curve. The shape of the dental arches reflects that of the dental laminae which in turn is related

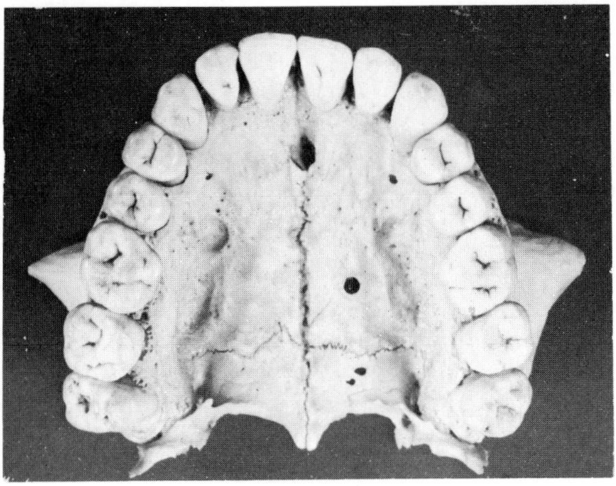

Fig. 27 Occlusal view of the permanent upper teeth in a well-formed arch. (*By courtesy of Dr R. Sprinz.*)

to that of Meckel's cartilage and the lower margin of the nasal capsule. The lower arch is somewhat smaller than the upper so that the incisive edges of the upper incisors and canines and the buccal cusps of the upper cheek teeth fall slightly outside those of the lower teeth. The incisors and canines are sometimes described as forming the anterior (labial) segment of each arch; the premolars and molars (or deciduous molars) form the posterior or buccal segments (Fig. 27). The anterior segment may be curved or flattened and the buccal segments may be straight or show a slight buccal convexity. The canine may appear to belong more to the posterior than to the anterior segment or vice versa, or it may form a prominent buttress between the two segments giving the arch a somewhat rectangular shape.

In both arches the incisive edges of the incisors and canines are in line with the buccal cusps of the cheek teeth. The lingual cusps of the cheek teeth tend to decrease in size towards the front and are represented in the teeth of the anterior segment by the cingulum. In the human dentition the teeth in each arch form a continuous series, there being no large, constant gaps or diastemata. Each tooth or dental unit is attached to its neighbour by the transeptal fibres of the periodontal membrane (Fig. 235).

Neither the upper nor the lower arch conforms to a flat plane; the lower teeth taken together follow the curvature of the segment of a sphere; that is the so-called compensating occlusal curvature is concave. As the curvature is concave in the lower arch it is convex in the upper, so as to maintain the occlusal relations of the teeth. The expression of this curvature in the arrangement of the cheek teeth as seen from the buccal aspect is known as the curve of Spee (Fig. 28); in the coronal plane the arrangement of the occlusal surfaces of the cheek teeth so that the upper molars face somewhat buccally and the lowers somewhat lingually is known as the curve of Monson (Fig. 275). The curvature of the arches is correlated to the curved path of the mandibular condyles on the articular surfaces of the glenoid fossa and articular eminence during mastication.

FUNCTION AND DENTAL ARCH FORM

The teeth in each arch are constantly exposed to the considerable stresses of mastication. These stresses tend to drive each tooth vertically into its socket or to displace it in a lateral direction. Both these effects are prevented by those principal fibres of the periodontal membrane, which attach the tooth to the alveolar bone, and by the transeptal fibres which unite the teeth to one another. However, in certain teeth the tendency to lateral displacement is exaggerated by the obliquity of their implantation in the alveolar process. Normally this is countered by certain factors which are either to be found in the form and arrangement of the teeth themselves, or else lie external to the teeth as the muscles of the cheeks, lips, and tongue, and the density and degree of development of the alveolar bone.

If these balancing factors, either intrinsic or extrinsic, are disturbed or removed or are inadequate, then the normal arrangement of the teeth in the arch is upset. The loss of a tooth, by eliminating the support which members of an arch give to each other, frequently leads to tilting or actual bodily drifting of adjacent teeth; this is an example of the elimination of one of the intrinsic factors. Incompetent lip action may allow incisor teeth to take up abnormal positions or there may be destruction or atrophy of part of the bony socket; in these cases the extrinsic factors are inadequate.

It is worth noting that the teeth of the deciduous dentition are not so readily displaced from the normal arch arrangement as those of the

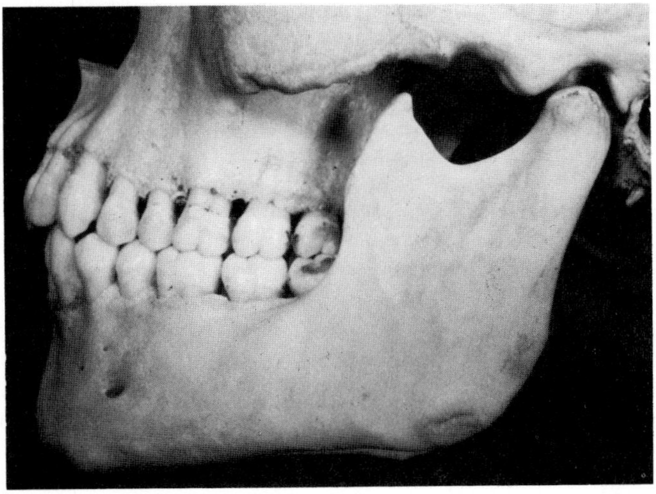

Fig. 28 Lateral view of the permanent teeth with good occlusion. (*By courtesy of Dr R. Sprinz.*)

permanent dentition. The greater stability of the deciduous compared with the permanent arches is due in part to the vertical implantation of the deciduous teeth. This is illustrated by the frequent existence of spacing between the teeth of the deciduous dentition without any tilting of the adjacent teeth (Fig. 24A).

In a functional analysis the permanent dental arch may be divided on each side into two segments, an anterior or labial made up of the incisors, and a posterior or buccal composed of the premolars and molars. The canine tooth is common to both segments. Morphologically the crown of the canine shows this; the mesial surface is similar in height to the interstitial surfaces of the incisors, whereas the distal surface is like the premolars in this respect.

In the lower buccal segments the molar teeth show a lingual inclination whereas in the upper buccal segments they have a buccal inclination. In the former the inclination is to some extent limited to the crowns of the teeth which are inclined inwardly on the roots; in the latter the large palatal root tends to prevent further outward tilting (Fig. 32). Displacement from the arch is also partly prevented in the former case by the tongue and in the latter by the buccinator muscle.

In both upper and lower buccal segments the teeth in general have a mesial inclination. This is often little shown by the premolars but is marked in the case of the molars. The result is a tendency for the buccal segments to be driven mesially during their functional activity, the canines being thrust in a mesio-labial direction. This tendency to mesial displacement of the buccal segments has been thought to be part of the mechanism responsible for 'the mesial drift of the teeth' (see p. 128).

The upper incisors show both a mesial and a labial inclination, with a consequent tendency to be displaced in these directions. The mesial inclination of one upper anterior segment is met by the opposing mesial inclination of the anterior segment of the other side. The effect is, however, carried on each side to the canine and this tends to be displaced from the arch in a disto-labial direction. The resultant of this and the mesio-labial thrust from the buccal segment is that the canine is liable to be displaced labially. This is checked by the action of the buccinator muscle, which exerts a retaining action on the arch and particularly in the area where its fibres, many of them after decussating, are passing into the lips. Moreover the canine is stabilised by its large, firmly implanted root. The shape of the canine root is also a factor in resisting this dislodgement from the arch. In cross-section it is generally somewhat triangular showing labial, mesio-lingual, and disto-lingual surfaces. This gives a very large area of attachment for the periodontal fibres on the lingual aspect.

The effect of the labial inclination of the upper incisors is increased by the way they meet the lower incisors in occlusion; the lower incisors striking obliquely against the lingual surfaces of the upper teeth (Fig. 32). Labial displacement of the upper incisors is prevented in part by the action of the orbicularis oris muscle, by the transeptal fibres which unite the incisor teeth to one another and to the firmly anchored canines, and also by the shape of their roots. In cross section these are similar to the root of the upper canine with a greater area for attachment of the periodontal membrane on the lingual side.

The upper arch is supported lingually by the teeth of the lower arch and buccally by the muscles of the cheeks and lips. The lower arch is supported buccally by the teeth of the upper arch and lingually by the tongue. In addition, lingual displacement of the lower arch is rendered unlikely, especially in the anterior segments, by the very arrangement of the teeth. The more the teeth are thrust together the firmer the arch becomes—that is, the principle of the 'contained arch'.

It should be appreciated that in the foregoing account the relationship of masticatory function and the form of the dental arcades has been treated very generally. Each tooth should be considered to some extent separately, for not only may there be individual variations in the implantation of a particular tooth, but the direction of the stress falling on each tooth is rendered complex by the meeting of the inclined planes of the cusps, ridges, and surfaces of the teeth.

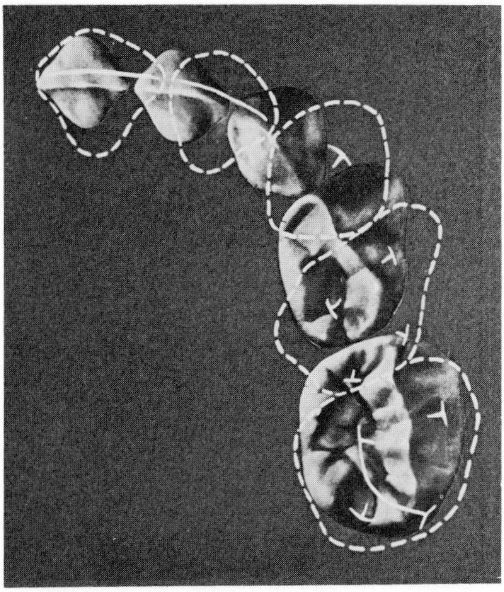

Fig. 29 Three years of age. Ideal occlusion. Diagram of the occlusal surfaces of lower deciduous teeth with the outline of the opposing teeth, points of cusps, etc. (*By courtesy of Prof S. Friel.*)

In a certain number of children abnormal muscle action may occur, such as tongue thrusting, or habits such as thumb sucking may be established. This can lead to severe derangement of the normal arch form, particularly in the anterior segments.

OCCLUSION

When the jaws are closed and the heads of the condyles are in the resting position in the glenoid fossae, the cusps, fossae, and incisive edges of the individual teeth of the upper and lower arches come into contact with one another; the sum of these relations make up the occlusion of the dentition (Figs. 28, 29, 30, 31). If the dentition is normal in its development and form, there is normal occlusion; if not, the occlusion is abnormal and a condition of malocclusion exists. The detailed analysis of the various relations which make up normal occlusion during the various stages of development of the dentitions belongs to the subject of Orthodontics. Here only a general statement of the more important relations is given.

1. The buccal cusps and incisive edges of the upper teeth occlude outside of (buccal or labial to) those of the lower teeth (Fig. 32).
2. The lower canines always close in front of (mesial to) the upper canines (Fig. 28). This is true in all mammals with canine teeth. Sometimes, however (as in the lemurs), the lower canines have a similar form

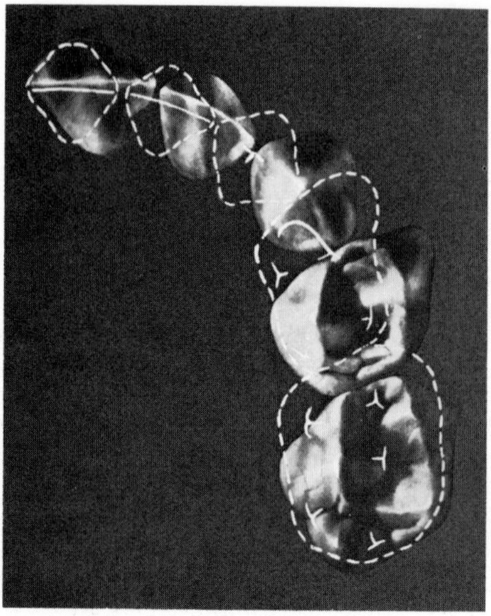

Fig. 30 Three years of age. Ideal occlusion. Diagram of the occlusal surfaces of upper deciduous teeth with the outline of the opposing teeth, points of cusps, etc. (*By courtesy of Professor S. Friel.*)

and function to the incisors and the first premolars take on the form and function of canines. In such cases, however, the canine-like teeth close behind the upper canines.

3. In the stage of full development of both the deciduous and permanent dentitions the mesio-lingual cusps of the upper molars occlude with the central fossae of the corresponding lower teeth. At the same time the apices of the mesio-buccal cusps of the upper teeth occlude outside, but opposite the buccal groove between the mesio-buccal and disto-buccal cusps of the lower teeth (Fig. 28).

4. Each tooth in the upper dental arch is opposed not only by the corresponding tooth in the lower arch, but also by the tooth immediately distal. This arrangement is necessitated by the much greater mesio-distal width of the upper central incisor compared with that of the lower central incisor. The sole exception to this in the permanent dentition is the upper third molar which occludes only with the lower third molar, and in the deciduous dentition the upper second molar which occludes only with the lower second molar.

Normal occlusion of the teeth is not to be considered simply as a series of articular relationships between the upper and lower teeth but as a developing dynamic process involving the development and eruption of the individual teeth, the growth and structure of the jaws and of the mandibular joint, the arrangement of the supporting parodontal tissues, and the balanced functional activity of the muscles of mastica-

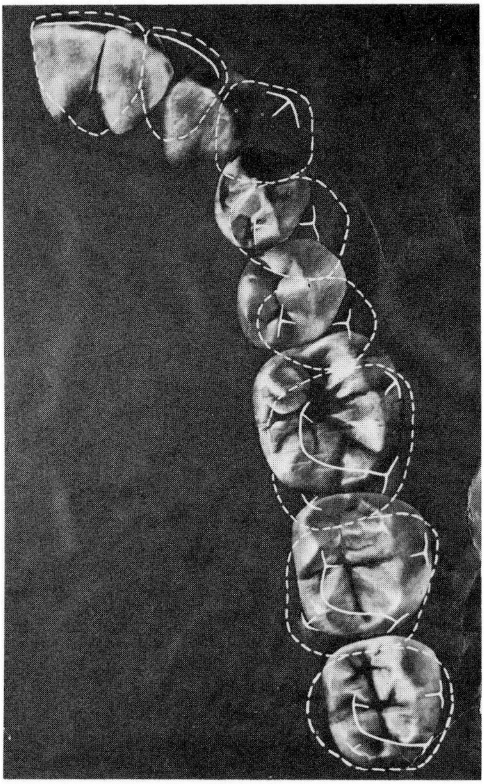

Fig. 31 Adult. Ideal occlusion. Diagram of the occlusal surfaces of the lower permanent teeth with the outline of the opposing teeth, points of cusps, etc. (*By courtesy of Prof S. Friel.*)

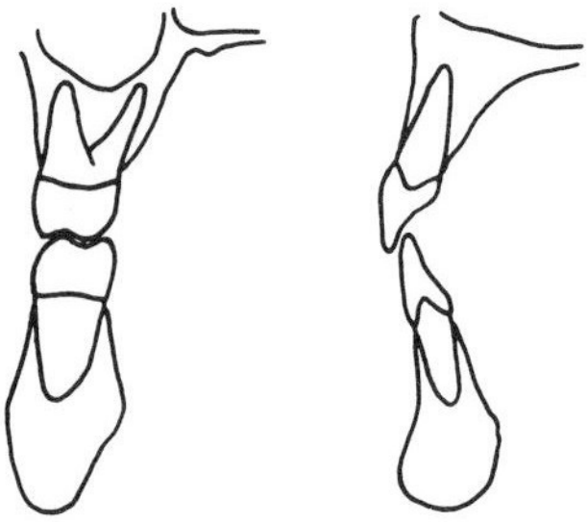

Fig. 32 Diagrammatic illustration of bucco-lingual and labio-lingual sections through the molar and incisor regions respectively showing the occlusal relationships of the upper and lower teeth.

tion, the lips, the cheeks, and the tongue. The functional coordination of all these elements is controlled by a system of reflex nerve arcs involving the V, VII, IX and XII cranial nerves and what may be called a diffuse 'masticating centre' or group of centres in the brain stem and upper part of the spinal cord. It may be said that the greater part of dental practice is concerned with maintaining, repairing, and replacing the various elements of the occlusal apparatus.

Functional changes. The size of the cusps of the cheek teeth (premolars and molars), and the extent to which the upper buccal cusps overlap the buccal surfaces of the lower teeth, and the upper incisors and canines overlap the lower canines and incisors, vary from dentition to dentition. In any individual the amount of the overlap varies with age and the extent to which the teeth are used. The extent to which the upper incisors overlap the lower incisors in the vertical plane is known as the overbite; in the anteroposterior direction the extent of the overlap is known as the overjet (Fig. 33).

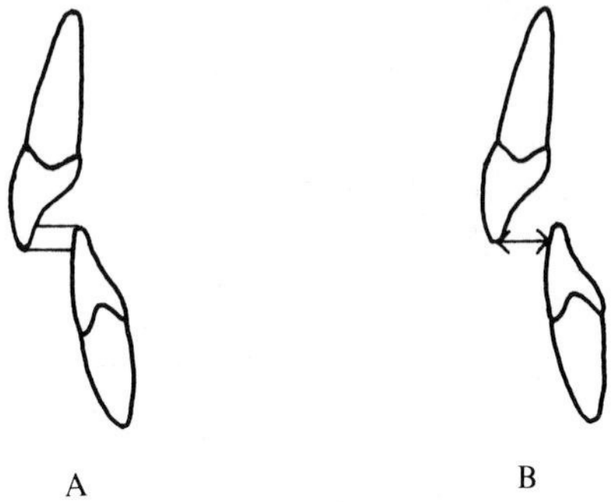

Fig. 33 Diagram illustrating details of incisor relationship. In A the amount of overbite is represented by the vertical distance between the horizontal lines related to the incisive edges. In B the amount of overjet is represented by the length of the arrowed line.

With increasing age it is normal for the cusps to become worn, so that the covering enamel is lost and the dentine exposed. In middle-aged individuals, especially in primitive races in which the food requires much chewing and is frequently mixed with gritty material, the cheek teeth often show flattened occlusal surfaces with no cusps or with the cusps greatly reduced. The teeth most likely to show excessive wear are the first and second molars; the third molars which erupt later are often comparatively unworn. In the lower jaw the buccal cusps wear down more rapidly than the lingual cusps; in the upper jaw the lingual cusps show the greater degree of wear.

With use and age the contact points between adjacent teeth also change their nature. In newly erupted teeth the contact points are limited in size and are circular or slightly oval in form. The teeth wear by rubbing against one another as they move slightly in their sockets during mastication, and the contact areas become more extensive and form flattened surfaces of contact. Normally the size of the tooth crowns exposed in the mouth (clinical crowns) remains fairly constant. As tooth substance is lost at the occlusal surfaces and incisive edges, the crowns are reduced in size. This process may be compensated for by a recession of the gums. If, however, wear is excessive, the occlusal surfaces may come close to the gum surface. The degree of wear of the occlusal surfaces may differ on the two sides of the mouth.

In a well formed and functionally efficient dental apparatus there is a structural relationship between the form of the arches, the size and occlusal relations of the cusps, the size of the roots, the form of the glenoid fossae and the degree of development of the articular eminences. The functional relationship established during childhood and adolescence by the development of the occlusal relations of the arches is maintained in adult life by the pattern of use of the muscles of mastication.

RACIAL DIFFERENCES IN TEETH AND DENTITIONS

Most human populations are of very mixed origins, but at present some communities exist which have probably remained isolated and inbreeding for a considerable period of time. Such isolation of communities was probably much more common in prehistoric times and played an important part in human evolution, allowing variations of form and function to become established in population groups to an extent that later mixing with other groups did not entirely eliminate, so that such variations may still appear in individual families and isolated cases even in mixed urban populations.

The Australian Aborigines and the Eskimos have the largest teeth; the smallest teeth are found among Bushmen of south Africa and the Lapps (see Appendix 1). A characteristic feature of the Lapp dentition is the small size of the crowns of the teeth associated with relatively long and well-developed roots. The difference between the massive dento-facial skeleton of the Eskimo and the Lapp is marked. Both live under somewhat similar conditions and on a similar diet. They afford an interesting example of the interaction of genetic and functional factors in dento-facial morphology. As root formation continues after tooth eruption, this feature may depend to some extent upon masticatory function.

In the Bantu races of Africa the lower molars often increase in size from before backward, so that the third molar may be the largest of the series. This condition is sometimes also found in Eskimo dentitions. Bantu upper first premolars usually have two roots and may have three roots as in *Sinanthropus* and living anthropoid apes. Alveolar prognathism is common in the incisor region of Bantu, Negro, and Australian dentitions and is associated with a reduction in the degree of incisor crowding.

The *Dryopithecus* pattern of five cusps with contact between the mesio-lingual and disto-buccal cusps in the lower molar teeth is found most frequently in the West African Negro (99 per cent in first molars, 17 per cent in second molars, and 20 per cent in third molars) and the Australian Aboriginal (100 per cent, 5 per cent and 14 per cent respectively). In Mongoloid and White races it is very uncommon to find it in teeth other than the first permanent molars. Non-European populations show less reduction in the number of cusps in upper molars, lower second premolars, and lower second molars.

Mongoloid dentitions (Eskimos, American Indians and Chinese) show the following characteristics:

1. A high prevalence of shovel-shaped incisors.
2. A low prevalence of Carabelli's tubercle on the first permanent molars.
3. A tendency for the development of enamel pearls on the occlusal surfaces of molars and premolars and on the lingual surfaces of canines, especially among Eskimos.
4. The mandibular third molars are frequently absent.
5. Lower second molars with five cusps are frequent.

Negro dentitions show the following characteristics:

1. Shovel-shaped incisors are uncommon.
2. Carabelli's tubercle is infrequent on first permanent molars.
3. Enamel pearls are uncommon.
4. Mandibular third molars are rarely absent.
5. Supernumerary teeth, especially premolars, are common.
6. Dento-alveolar prognathism is a characteristic feature.
7. Lower second molars with five cusps are frequent.

The dentitions of White races show the following characteristics:

1. Shovel-shaped incisors are very uncommon.
2. The tubercle of Carabelli is much more frequent than in Mongoloid or Negro races.
3. Enamel pearls are not common.
4. Mandibular third molars are less frequently absent than among Mongoloid races but more often absent than among Negroes.
5. Lower second molars with five cusps are much less frequent than among Mongoloid or Negro races.

TEETH AND GENETICS

Characters such as size, shape and fissure pattern of teeth are genetically determined. These features are the expression of the developmental history of the enamel organ and its extension, Hertwig's sheath (p. 78). The absence of certain teeth, especially the upper lateral and lower central incisors, lower second premolars and the third molars, is often inherited; sometimes the inheritance is associated with dominant genes, at other times with recessive or sex-linked genes. Supernumerary teeth are both hereditary and racial, and are most frequent in the order: negroid, mongoloid and caucasoid races. Extra premolars are especially frequent among negroid peoples.

The order and time of tooth eruption has a genetic basis although other factors such as ductless gland disorders and ill-health are also involved. If retardation of tooth eruption occurs, it is usually progressive, that is, the permanent teeth are more retarded than deciduous teeth.

In the human dentition the most stable teeth in the permanent dentition and the ones which show the minimum of genetic and racial variabilities are the canines, central incisors and first molars; the most variable teeth are the upper lateral incisors, the second premolars and the second and third molars.

Features involving the morphology of individual teeth, and which are genetically determined, include the tubercle of Carabelli, the paramolar cusps on the buccal surfaces of molar teeth, shovel-shaped incisors, and the *Dryopithecus* pattern of lower molar teeth. Certain forms of malocclusions of the teeth and abnormal relationships between the upper and lower jaws are inherited, including the famous Hapsburg jaw. In the latter the mandible is overdeveloped and protrudes beyond the upper jaw so that the lower incisors bite in front of the upper teeth. Interesting patterns of dentofacial relationships are shown in crossing various breeds of dogs, while such stable breeds as the bulldog, boxer and pekinese show gross malocclusion of the teeth.

THE SUPPORTING STRUCTURES OF THE TEETH

The tissues immediately surrounding and investing the tooth: the gums (gingivae), the periodontal membrane, the cement and the alveolar bone make up a structural and functional unit often referred to as the periodontium (Fig. 1). Elsewhere in the text the structure and development of each of the parts making up the periodontium are described.

In a normal, functional dentition each tooth is attached to the walls of its socket by the principal fibres of the periodontal membrane passing between the cement of the tooth and the wall of the socket (lamina dura) as bundles of collagenous fibres. The rim of the socket of each tooth (the alveolar crest) falls some distance short of the enamel-cement junction of the tooth. To that part of the cement which projects beyond this level are attached the transeptal fibres uniting each tooth to its neighbours across the interdental septa of the alveolar bone, the alveolar crest fibres, and the gingival fibres which pass into and support the gum surrounding the tooth. The gum is firmly attached to the tooth and alveolar bone through these collagenous fibres and is therefore structurally a mucoperiosteum. It is also attached to the enamel adjacent to the enamel-cement junction through the epithelial attachment. This is composed of epithelium derived from the reduced enamel epithelium, which cover the enamel surface prior to the emergence of the tooth into the mouth cavity, and the epithelium of the oral mucous membrane (Fig. 100).

The bone of the alveolar crest plays a vital role in supporting the gingivae. If for any reason it is destroyed the adjacent gum tissue loses its main means of support and gradually becomes separated from the tooth. The chief purpose of periodontal treatment in such cases is to restore the normal relationship and attachment between the gum tissue and the bone, although this may involve alterations in the relationship between the gingival tissue and the tooth.

The epithelial attachment is also an important and vulnerable site in the periodontium. The attachment of the epithelium to the adjacent enamel is not strong and is readily damaged by adverse mechanical forces such as impacted masses of food debris around the necks of the teeth. As a result pockets are formed, first as minute tears in the epithelium of the marginal gingiva and later as extensions between the epithelium and the enamel. These pockets readily become sites of acute or chronic inflammatory changes which involve the subepithelial tissues (lamina propria) of the gum and later the adjacent alveolar bone.

In a normal tooth the epithelial attachment ends at the enamel cement junction (Fig. 102) but with age or as a result of adjacent inflammatory changes the epithelium tends to migrate along the surface of the cement towards the apical region of the tooth. This process occurs at the expense of the attachment of the gingival fibres, the transeptal fibres and, if extensive, of the oblique fibres of the periodontal membrane and is an important factor, along with the destruction of the adjacent alveolar bone, in the progressive loosening of the teeth which is characteristic of long-standing gingival disease.

In a normal dentition with a healthy periodontium the response to increased functional stress is a strengthening of all the component parts. The alveolar bone becomes denser, its cortical layer thicker, its cancellous structure more closely knit, the collagenous fibre bundles of the periodontal membrane including the transeptal and gingival fibres become thicker and stronger, the cement to which they are attached thicker by further surface deposition and the overlying gingival epithelium tends towards keratinisation and a thickening of its superficial layers. Excessive stress, however, which may result from psychosomatic phenomena such as tooth grinding during sleep may, if long continued, cause a breakdown in the periodontium especially if there is an associated neglect of oral hygiene.

BIBLIOGRAPHY

Brothwell, D. R. (1963). *Dental Anthropology*. Oxford: Pergamon Press.

Burdi, A. R. (1968). Morphogenesis of dental arch shape in human embryos. *J. dent. Res.* **47**, 50.

Foster, T. D. & Hamilton, M. C. (1969). Occlusion in the primary dentition. *Brit. dent. J.* **126**, 76.

Kraus, B. S., Jordan, R. E. & Abrams, L. (1969). *Dental Anatomy and Occlusion*. Baltimore: Williams & Wilkins.

Krogman, W. M. (1960). Oral structures genetically and anthropologically considered. *Ann. N.Y. Acad. Sci.* **85**, 17.

Lasker, G. W. (1950). Genetic analysis of racial traits of the teeth. *Cold Spr. Harb. Symp. quant. Biol.* **15**, 191.

MacConaill, M. A. & Scher, E. (1949). The ideal form of the human dental arcade. *Dent. Rec.* **69**, 285.

Moorrees, C. F. A. (1957). *The Aleut Dentition*. Cambridge, Mass.: Harvard University Press.

Picton, D. C. A. (1962). Tilting movements of teeth during biting. *Arch. oral Biol.* **7**, 151.

Tratman, E. K. (1950). A comparison of the teeth of people (Indo-European racial stock with the Mongoloid racial stock). *Dent. Rec.* **70**, 31 and 63.

Wheeler, R. C. (1974). *Textbook of Dental Anatomy and Physiology*. 5th *ed.* London: Saunders.

SECTION II

The development and growth of the face, teeth and jaws

2. The Development of the Face and the Oral Cavity

Before taking up the developmental history of the teeth and jaws it is advisable to revise the development of the face even though this study may have been covered in the general anatomy course.

The primitive mouth cavity. When the human embryo is about three to four weeks old (3 mm C.R. stage) the primitive mouth cavity (stomodeum) is a narrow slit-like space lined by ectoderm. It is bounded above by the under surface of the brain capsule, and below by the upper surface of the pericardial sac, within which lies the developing heart. The developing mandibular processes (the first of the visceral or branchial arches) form a rim-like elevation bounding the cavity at the

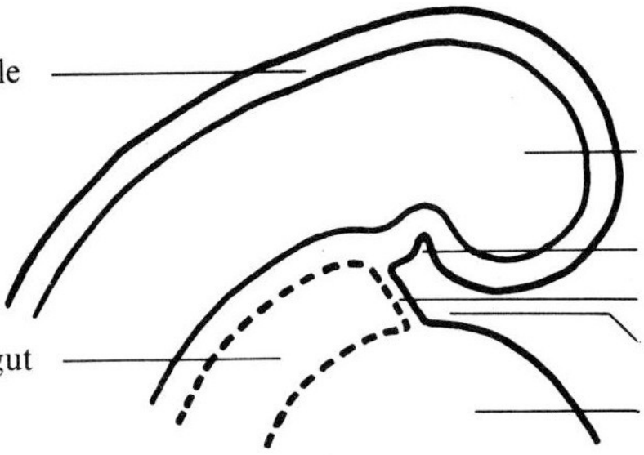

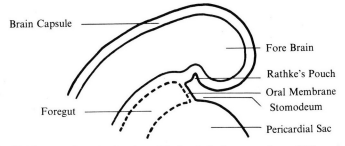

Fig. 34 Diagram of a sagittal section of the head of a human embryo of 2·5 mm (approx. $3\frac{1}{2}$ weeks).

sides. At the back of the cavity is the thin oral membrane forming a septum which at this stage separates the primitive mouth cavity from the pharynx (the anterior end of the foregut). The membrane slopes upward and backward so that the roof of the primitive mouth is more extensive than the floor (Fig. 34). Immediately in front of the place of attachment of the oral membrane to the roof of the mouth and in front of the terminal end of the notocord there is a slit-like ectodermal pouch of the mouth cavity passing upward towards the base of the brain. This is Rathke's pouch, from which develops the anterior part of the pituitary gland. The posterior part of the gland develops as a downgrowth from the hypothalmic region of the developing brain. The anterior part soon loses its connection with the primitive oral cavity, but cysts may develop along its original site and be found in the roof of the pharynx or within the body of the sphenoid bone.

Already at this stage the oral membrane becomes sieve-like and soon

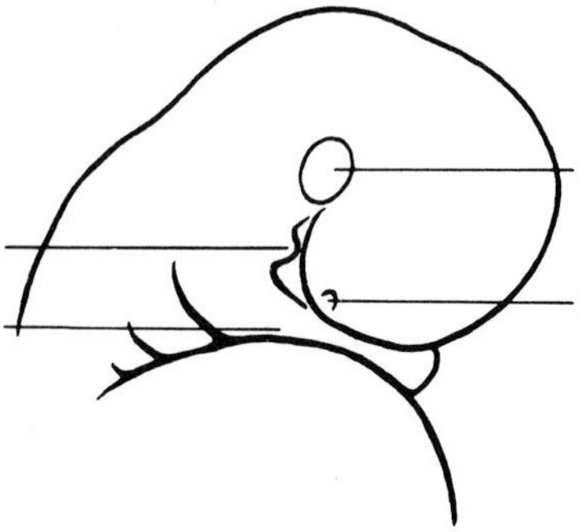

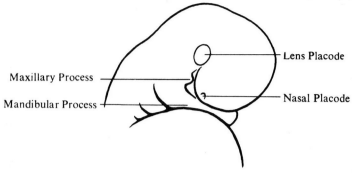

Fig. 35 Diagrammatic illustration of the head of a human embryo of 6 mm (fifth week).

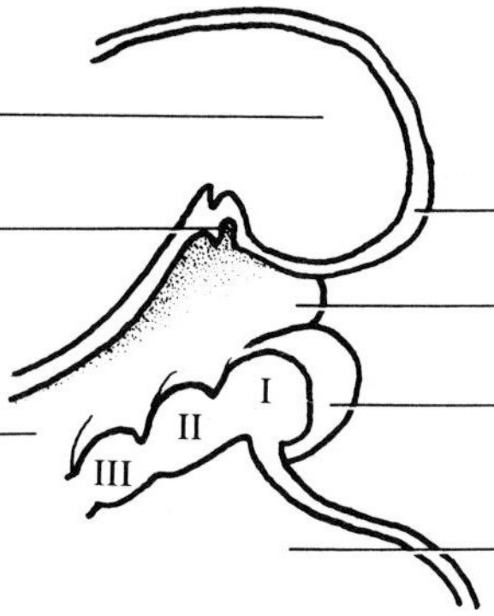

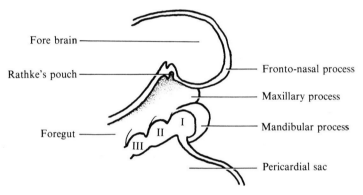

Fig. 36 Diagram of a sagittal section of the head of a human embryo of about five weeks. The oral membrane has disappeared and the united first three branchial arches form the floor of the stomodeum having grown between it and the pericardial sac.

commences to break up, so that the primitive mouth cavity becomes directly continuous with the pharynx.

The mandibular and maxillary processes. As the developing mandibular processes grow ventrally on each side of the head until they meet one another in the midline, they come to form the lower boundary of the mouth opening, intervening between it and the pericardial sac (Figs. 35, 36). Behind, at the angle of the mouth opening, is the bud-like maxillary process, which is derived from the upper surface of the back part of the mandibular process (Fig. 35). As development continues, the maxillary process on each side grows forward beneath the brain capsule and comes more and more to form the upper margin of the mouth opening, which then ends behind at the angle between the mandibular and maxillary processes (Fig. 37). The forward growth of the mandibular and maxillary processes is essentially an extension of mesodermal tissue beneath the covering ectoderm.

The united mandibular processes together with the second and third branchial arches form the floor of the primitive mouth cavity (Fig. 36). A thickening of mesoderm in front of the fore-brain gives rise to the fronto-nasal process.

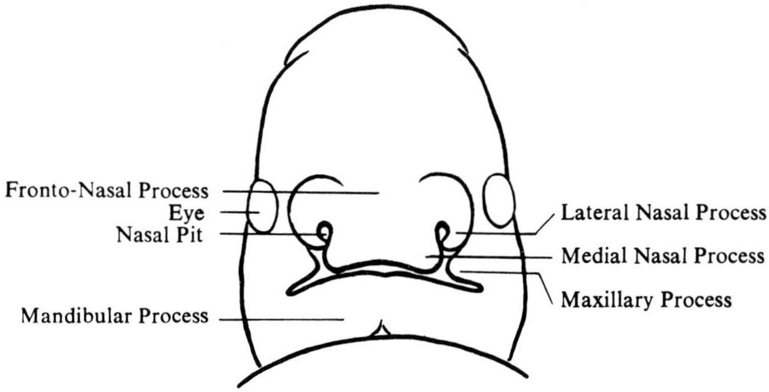

Fig. 37 Diagrammatic illustration of the head of a human embryo of 10 mm (approx. five weeks).

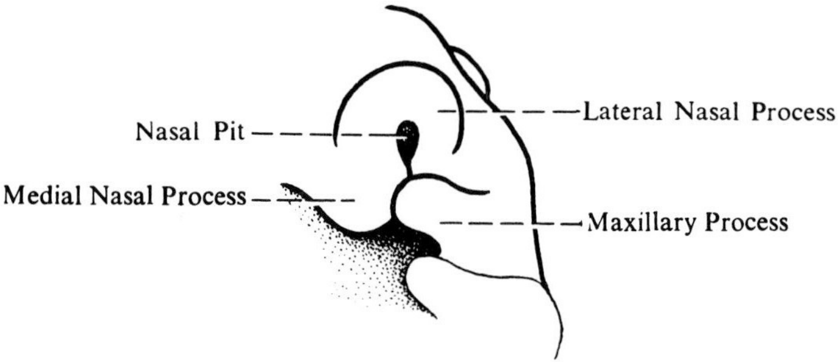

Fig. 38 Diagrammatic illustration of the region of junction (the primary palate) of the maxillary process with the medial and lateral nasal processes.

When the embryo is about four to five weeks old (6 mm C.R. stage) the epithelium covering the brain capsule has thickened in two places on each side of the head. The more ventral of these thickenings is the nasal placode, which forms the olfactory epithelium of the nose; the more dorsal is the lens placode, from which develops the lens of the eye (Fig. 35). Although the lens develops from the surface epithelium it later sinks to a deeper level.

At first the developing eyes are situated at the side of the head (Fig. 37). Later they move towards the middle line. In some cases this migration fails to take place and the condition of hypertelorism results, characterised by an excessive width across the bridge of the nose.

Between the developing eye and ear regions on each side of the face there is an upward migration of maxillary process mesoderm. In this region develop the ramus of the mandible, the zygomatic arch, the tympanic ring, the muscles of mastication and the greater wing of the sphenoid.

The fronto-nasal process and the nasal cavities. By the time the embryo is about five weeks old (10 mm C.R. stage) the nasal placode has become depressed below the surface of the developing face and lies at the bottom of a nasal pit, which is surrounded above and at the sides by an elevated rim of tissue forming the medial and lateral nasal processes. Below, the nasal pit is connected to the stomatodaeum by a narrow furrow (Fig. 37). The area between the nasal pits and including the medial and lateral nasal processes of each side constitutes a ventral extensions of the fronto-nasal process, which at this stage forms part of the upper margin of the mouth opening.

Meanwhile, the growing maxillary process has come forward beneath the developing eye and lies against the lateral nasal process so that maxillary mesoderm comes into continuity with that of the fronto-nasal process. The maxillary process mesoderm divides into two streams one of which passes forward below the lateral and medial nasal processes, forming a shelf of tissue, the primary palate (Figs. 38, 40); the other ascends between the lateral nasal process and the developing eye. The primary palate completely shuts off each nasal pit from the mouth opening. With further growth this shelf of maxillary mesoderm meets the corresponding mesoderm of the opposite side of the face in the middle line. In this way the fronto-nasal process mesoderm becomes shut off

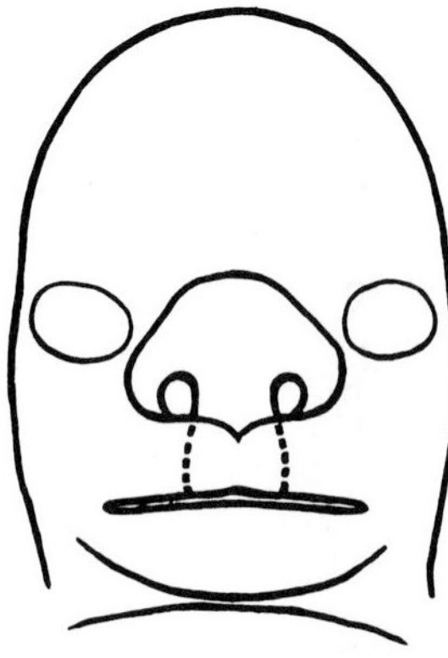

Fig. 39 Diagrammatic illustration of the head of a human embryo of 20 mm (seven weeks). The part of the fronto-nasal process which is buried deep to the maxillary processes is shown in broken line.

from forming any part of the upper margin of the opening into the mouth cavity. (Fig. 39).

An alternative theory postulates union of maxillary and fronto-nasal mesoderm without, however, any migration of the maxillary mesoderm towards the middle line. This would permit the fronto-nasal process to contribute to the formation of the upper lip, as well as the incisor alveolar region and palate anterior to the incisive foramen.

The nasal pit on each side, which up to this stage has been a cul-de-sac, gains an opening into the stomodeum behind and above the primary palate on each side of the fronto-nasal process (primary nasal septum) by the disintegration of the tissue between the bottom of the pit and the stomodeum. In this manner the primary nasal cavities are formed (Fig. 40). Between the fronto-nasal process (primary nasal septum) and the maxillary processes (primary palate) lie the posterior openings (posterior nares) of the primary nasal cavities.

Septal process. When the embryo is about six weeks old the maxillary process forming the side wall of the upper part of the primitive mouth cavity, or oro-nasal cavity, begins to develop two inwardly directed processes. The uppermost of these (the septal process) grows towards the middle line of the roof of the mouth cavity beneath its epithelial lining so that the mesodermal tissue, forming the brain capsule, becomes shut off from the roof of the primitive mouth cavity everywhere, except in the region of the olfactory epithelium, by a layer of maxillary process mesoderm. The processes of each side carry with them branches of the maxillary nerve, the naso-palatine nerves and a vascular plexus derived from the maxillary artery. Hence in the adult the mucous membrane lining the nasal cavities is supplied by branches of the maxillary division of the trigeminal nerve except in the olfactory area and in the region of the primary nasal septum, which is, as we have seen, derived from the fronto-nasal process.

The nasal septum. After the septal processes of each side meet in the middle line they have brought into existence a bed of mesodermal tissue in the roof of the oro-nasal cavity. The cavity extends upwards and backwards into this tissue on either side of the middle line, leaving a

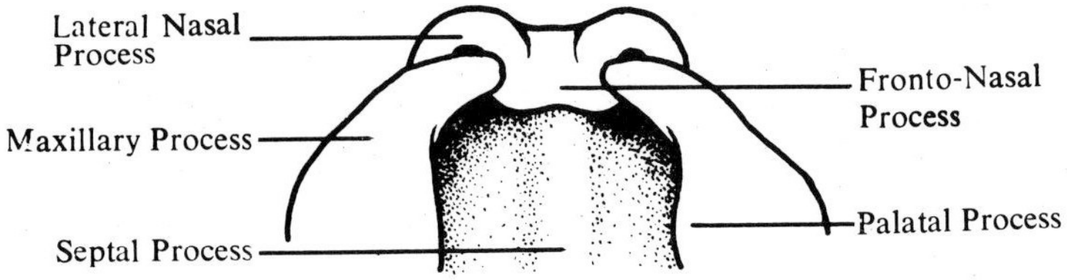

Fig. 40 Diagrammatic illustration of the head of a human embryo of about six weeks seen from the primary mouth cavity. The primary nasal cavities are connected to the primary mouth cavity above the region of fusion of each maxillary process with the nasal processes (the primary palate).

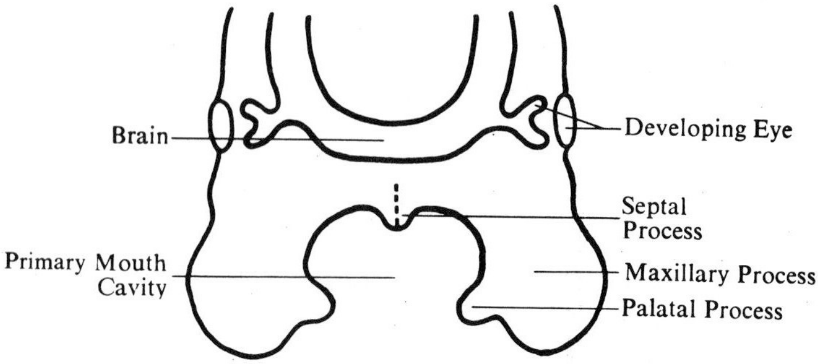

Fig. 41 Diagrammatic illustration of a coronal section through the head of a human embryo to show the septal and palatal processes of the maxillary processes.

ridge of undisturbed tissue between them. This is the primordium of the secondary portion of the nasal septum which is continuous in front with the primary nasal septum. In this manner the definitive nasal septum is made up of two parts: an anterior more primitive part derived from the fronto-nasal process and a posterior larger secondary part derived from the maxillary process. At this stage the latter part of the septum has a free lower margin in contact with the dorsal surface of the tongue (Fig. 42). With descent of the tongue and development of the naso-pharynx the septum continues to grow downwards and backwards.

Within the growing nasal septum and on each side of the septal cartilage develops the epithelial lined organ of Jacobson. In many animals these are well developed in the adult and have their openings in close relationship to a patent incisive canal. They are probably related to the senses of smell and taste.

The palate. The second inwardly directed extension of each maxillary process is formed at a lower level than the septal process and at first forms a downward hanging fold, the palatal fold, on either side of the developing tongue, which at this stage almost fills the primitive mouth cavity (Fig. 42). With growth in size of the mouth cavity, especially in vertical height, the tongue sinks downward and the two palatal folds are enabled to meet one another, and the lower edge of the developing nasal septum, above the dorsum of the tongue (Fig. 43). Elevation and fusion of the palatal folds occur in the human fetus between the eighth and eleventh weeks. There is first union between the epithelium covering the three processes (Fig. 44). Later the epithelium disintegrates and the mesodermal tissues of each process come into continuity. Remains of the epithelial tissue often form a series of small cysts along the sites of union, and from these oral cysts may develop in adult life. In this manner the primitive mouth cavity becomes divided into three parts, a right and left nasal cavity on each side of the nasal septum above the developing palate, and a mouth cavity proper below the palate.

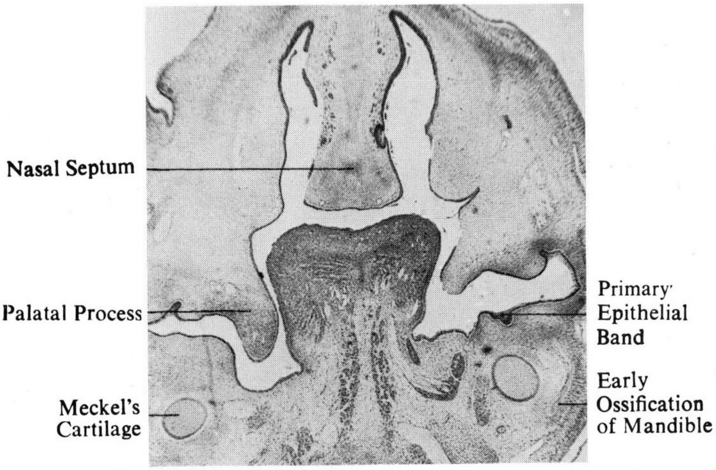

Fig. 42 Coronal section of the head of a human embryo of 22 mm C.R. length (about seven weeks). The palatal processes lie vertically on each side of the tongue. × 20.

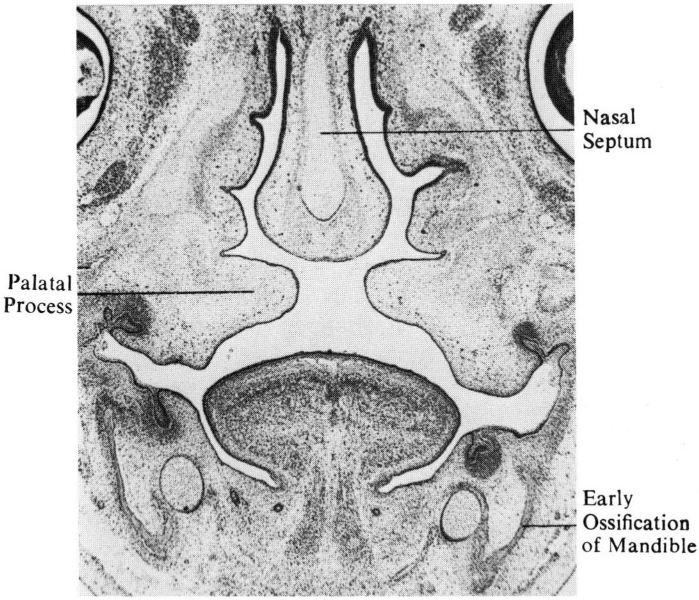

Fig. 43 Coronal section of the head of a human embryo of 27 mm C.R. length (about eight weeks). The palatal processes have become horizontally directed and would soon fuse with each other and with the nasal septum. × 20.

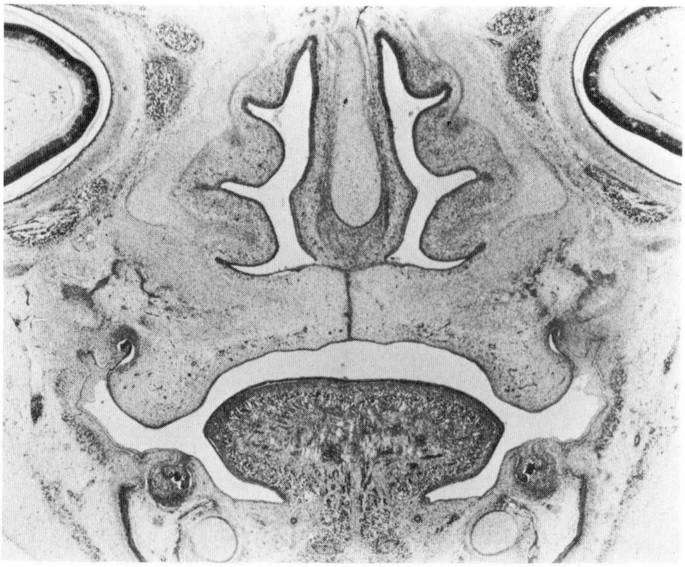

Fig. 44 Coronal section of the head of a human fetus of 31 mm C.R. length. The nasal septum and palatal processes have come into contact but are unfused as their epithelial covering still separates them. × 18. (*By courtesy of R. Latham.*)

Later the united palatal folds are invaded by bone in front (hard palate) and by muscle behind (soft palate). The bone extends from the premaxillary, maxillary, and palatine centres of ossification to form the hard palate (see pp. 96–101). The muscle tissue is derived from two sources: the tensor palati muscles from the mandibular arches, the remaining muscles of the soft palate from the fourth visceral arches, which also give origin to the upper pharyngeal muscles. The different origin of the muscles explains the difference in their nerve supply; the tensor palati by the mandibular division of the trigeminal nerve, which is the nerve of the mandibular arch, the other muscles by the cerebral part of the accessory nerve through the pharyngeal branch of the vagus.

The facial skeleton. Before the appearance of centres of ossification and also during the early stages of bone formation, the skeleton of the face is formed by cartilage. Meckel's cartilage develops within the mandibular arch (Figs. 42, 45) and extends from the developing cranial base in the region of the otic capsule to the middle line in the future chin region, where it meets the cartilage of the opposite side. The cartilage of the nasal capsule develops in the maxillary process tissue and extends forward into the fronto-nasal process. Behind it is continuous with the cartilage of the cranial base, which develops beneath the brain and its membranes (Fig. 45). Within the united primary and secondary parts of the nasal septum it forms the septal cartilage (Fig. 43). The lateral parts of the nasal capsule lie in the side walls of the nasal cavities, its

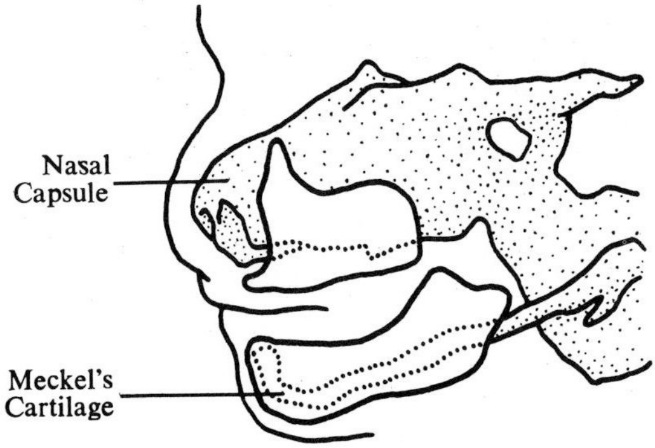

Fig. 45 Diagram illustrating the relationship of the maxilla and mandible to the earlier formed cartilaginous skeleton, the chondrocranium, at about eleven weeks. The cartilage is shown in stipple.

lower free end on each side turning inward as the cartilaginous skeleton of the developing inferior turbinate process (Figs. 43, 46).

At a later stage in development the maxillary, premaxillary and lacrimal bones develop on the outer side of the cartilage of the nasal capsule, the palatine bone develops on its inner aspect. The mandible develops on the outer side of Meckel's cartilage, and the vomer develops in relation to the lower edge of the septal cartilage (Fig. 118). The facial part (lateral mass) of the ethmoid bone with its turbinate processes replaces the cartilage of the upper part of the side wall of the nasal capsule, and the separate inferior turbinate bones (inferior conchae) replace the lower part of the cartilage. The perpendicular plate of the ethmoid, which is a cranial bone, invades the septal cartilage from above and behind. Between the area of formation of the lateral mass of the ethmoid and of the inferior turbinate the cartilage of the nasal capsule atrophies (Fig. 46). It is in this region that the developing maxillary sinus first comes into direct relationship with the growing maxilla about the middle of fetal life. Part of the cartilage of the nasal capsule persists to form the front part of the nasal septum and the alar cartilages of the nose. Remains of the cartilage may, however, persist and in some cases becomes the sites of origin of facial chrondrosarcoma.

Part of Meckel's cartilage is incorporated in the growing mandible, part of it forms the spheno-mandibular and spheno-malleolar ligaments, and its proximal end ossifies to form the malleus of the middle ear.

The tongue. The tongue develops in two parts: (*a*) The anterior part arises from the mandibular arches as paired eminences within the mouth cavity, and from a midline structure, the tuberculum impar, in the floor of the mouth between the first (mandibular) and second (hyoid) visceral arches; (*b*) the posterior part is derived from the third visceral arches; this grows forward over the second arches, to become

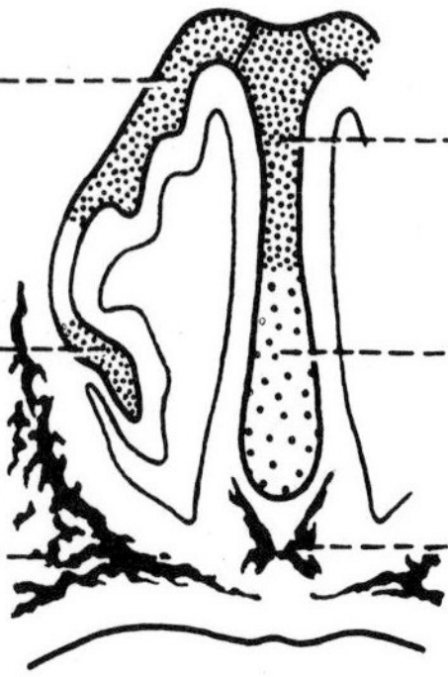

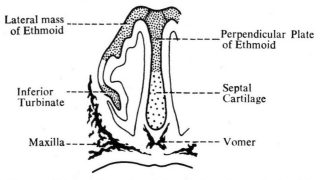

Fig. 46 Diagram of the nasal capsule and the membrane bones developed in relation to it. Area of the nasal capsule replaced by bone shown in heavy stippling; area of the nasal capsule persisting as cartilage shown in light stippling; area of the nasal capsule which disappears, unshaded.

continuous with the anterior part of the tongue, the sulcus terminalis in the adult marking the site of union of the two parts (Fig. 47). Primarily the united central part of the second arches takes part in the formation of the early tongue eminence but it is later excluded from the surface by the forward growth of third arch material. At this early stage a median swelling, the hypobranchial eminence, lies behind the second arch. From the back of the hypobranchial eminence is derived the epiglottis.

During its early development the tongue lies partly in the nasal cavities (Fig. 42). Later it descends from this position in part as a result of a more vertically directed growth of the mandible and in part as a result of the opening out of the cranial base angle. The descent of the tongue permits the palatal folds to unite above its dorsum (Fig. 44).

The anterior part of the tongue has for its sensory nerve supply the lingual nerve (branch of the trigeminal) and the chorda tympani nerve (branch of the facial nerve of the second visceral arch), whereas the sensory nerve supply of the posterior part of the tongue is from the glossopharyngeal nerve, the nerve of the third visceral arch. The foramen caecum on the dorsum of the tongue between the anterior and posterior parts indicates in the adult the site of a downgrowth of the epithelium of the floor of the mouth, which gives origin to the thyroid ductless gland. Remains of this epithelium may later give rise to cysts in the tongue or in the upper part of the neck. The muscles of the tongue appear between the sixth and eighth week of fetal life. They are derived from the upper somites of the neck region and have as their motor nerve supply the twelfth cranial (hypoglossal) nerve.

In the groove between the developing tongue and the lower jaw the sublingual and submandibular salivary glands develop as downgrowths of the oral epithelium. The greater part of the submandibular duct is developed by a cutting off of a segment of the original floor of the oral

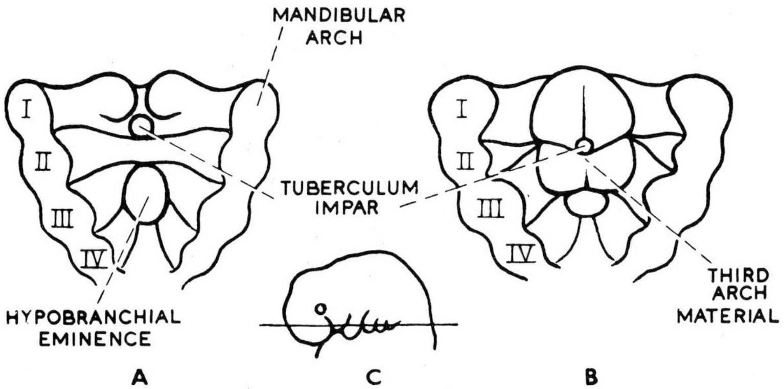

Fig. 47 Diagram to show the development of the tongue. (A) Floor of the mouth at 9 mm C.R. length. Anterior part of the tongue appearing as paired lateral swellings from the mandibular arch. (B) Floor of the mouth at later stage when third arch material has moved forward over the second arch to form the posterior (pharyngeal) part of the tongue. (C) Figure showing the plane of section of (A) and (B). (*Modified from Hamilton, Boyd, & Mossman.*)

cavity. This explains the opening of some of the sublingual ducts into the submandibular duct.

On the dorsum of the tongue develop the various lingual papillae, and in relation to its posterior (pharyngeal) part areas of lymphoid tissue. Lymphoid tissue develops also in the forward and upward extensions of the third arch mesoderm in the region of the tonsils and nasopharynx (adenoids).

The cheeks and parotid gland. The cheeks consist of tissue derived from both mandibular and maxillary processes. On either side of the mouth in the cheek region a lateral outpouching of the mouth cavity passes outward for some distance between the maxillary process above (upper jaw) and the mandibular process below (lower jaw). The outer limit of this pouch on either side is where the oral epithelium passes from the maxillary to the mandibular process and lines the inner surface of the cheek (Fig. 43). Later the vertical height of this part of the mouth cavity (the vestibule) is further increased (see p. 68). At the back of this lateral oral pouch on each side of the mouth cavity the parotid salivary gland develops as an outgrowth of oral epithelium. This at first passes outward and then turns backward superficial to the developing ramus of the mandible and the masseter muscle to reach the retro-mandibular region, where it develops in relation to the upper part of the external carotid artery, the posterior facial vein, and the facial nerve so that these structures become secondarily enclosed in gland substance. The opening of the duct into the vestibule of the mouth cavity is at first opposite the developing first upper deciduous molar. By three to four years of age it lies opposite the crown of the erupted second deciduous molar, by twelve years of age it is opposite the crown of the first permanent molar, and in the adult it is opposite the second permanent molar.

Early in their development the cheeks and lips are invaded by muscle tissue derived from the second (hyoid) visceral arch. This muscle tissue forms the buccinator muscle in the cheeks and the other muscles which make up the complex musculature of the lips. Its nerve supply is that of the second visceral arch, the seventh cranial (facial) nerve. As the buccinator muscle sheet grows backward, it surrounds the duct of the growing parotid gland, which comes to pierce the muscle. At the back of the mouth cavity the buccinator becomes united to the superior constrictor muscle of the pharynx at the pterygo-mandibular raphe.

Facial deformities. In the classical view of the formation of the face and oral cavity the various embryological processes or folds taking part are thought of as being covered by epithelium which must break down before full union of the processes can take place. It has become generally accepted that the embryonic folds are not completely separate from each other but are ridges or elevations of tissue corresponding to underlying mesodermal growth centres and are delineated from each other by grooves or depressions between these growth centres. Fusion of these areas is achieved by a gradual smoothing out and disappearance of the grooves or furrows between them. The one exception is in the division of the original mouth cavity or stomodeum into oral cavity and nasal cavities where epithelial covered processes, the palatal processes, come into contact with each other and the septal process. The covering epithelium of these three processes must break down after the processes have made contact in order to allow of a true fusion by the underlying mesoderm. The difference explains why epithelial remnants are to be found without exception along the mid-line of the palate in the fetus but not at the junction of the mandibular processes or at the junction of the maxillary process with the fronto-nasal process.

Failure of union of the palatal processes produces varying degrees of cleft palate which may range from a bifid uvula to a complete cleft of the palate which is generally associated with harelip. In some cases one palatal process may unite with the septal process so that one nasal cavity communicates with the oral cavity and the other does not.

It should be appreciated that the formation of the palate is brought about early in intra-uterine life by soft tissue processes and that the ossification which produces the hard palate only subsequently invades the area from the maxillary, premaxillary and palatal centres. This means that the bony clefts which are found in the full-term fetus are secondary features determined by the earlier failure of growth of certain embryological processes. Similarly the position of the lateral incisor tooth in the jaw relative to a palatal cleft is determined by the position of the budding of this tooth, if it is formed in the circumstances, relative to the original cleft between the embryological processes.

Much work has been carried out on the genesis of cleft palate and it is clear that normal union of the palatal processes falls into two stages. Firstly the elevation of the palatal folds from their early vertical position on either side of the tongue to a horizontal position above the tongue where they can meet, and secondly the disintegration of the covering epithelium so that the underlying mesoderm can meet and fuse.

Failure of closure of the palate has been ascribed to a delay in the movement of the palatal processes from their earlier vertical position to their definitive horizontal position. Interference with this movement could be due to the mechanical obstruction of the tongue or alternatively to insufficient growth of the palatal processes. It has certainly been observed in *in vitro* studies with rats and mice that the palatal folds have a potentiality for fusion which is not reached until a particular period in intrauterine life and remains for a limited period of 12–14 hours. The change in the position of the palatal folds from vertical to horizontal is rapid taking about three hours in mice, and only about another six hours for fusion. Insufficient growth within the palatal processes themselves could lead to failure of their elevation and it has been shown that in cortisone induced clefts in rodents there is a diminution in the number of cells in the palatal folds and an associated reduction in the quantity of sulphated acid mucopolysaccharides. These substances due to their water absorptive powers and their viscosity could produce dimension and form changes in such a structure. Other workers have shown an increased amount of elastic tissue in the palatal folds around the time of closure and have suggested that the elasticity of these fibres may be responsible for their elevation.

It has often been stated that space is made available above the tongue for the horizontal positioning of the palatal shelves by the descent of the tongue associated with rapid growth of the lower jaw and neck region. However, it has been shown that any space in the mouth cavity seen in histological sections at this stage is an artifact and that the tongue grows at the same rate at this time as the lower jaw. It is proposed instead that contraction of the muscles of the tongue leads to a slight depression of its dorsal surface which triggers off an interchange in position between tongue and palatal processes. The semi-gelatinous nature of these structures allows the palatal shelves to take up a horizontal position above the tongue and the tongue flows laterally into the area vacated by the palatal processes. Spontaneous muscular movements have been found to be significantly reduced in embryos from mice which have been treated with anti-inflammatory steroids, notably cortisone. This concept, however, does not exclude the need for some force within the palatal processes to produce their movement.

In normal palatal formation the meeting of the palatal processes is accompanied by a temporary union of the covering epithelial layers followed by a breakdown of this epithelium and by fusion of the underlying mesoderm. The presence of lysosome-like bodies has been demonstrated in the epithelial cells and these are probably responsible for the breakdown of the epithelium. It has been suggested that the breakdown of the basal lamina between epithelium and the connective tissue is of particular importance in permitting the fusion of the mesodermal tissues of the palate. The appearance of cytoplasmic prolongations of the basal epithelial cells which penetrate the basal lamina has been described. However, it is difficult to decide whether these prolongations cause the loss of integrity of the basal lamina or whether they follow as a result of this loss.

All the available evidence from studies of palatal union suggests that the sequence of events is an autolytic breakdown of the epithelial cells followed secondarily by a penetration of the mesodermal connective tissue cells rather than an active invasion of the epithelium by the mesodermal cells.

It has been observed that cleft palate is associated with an increased degree of flexion of the cranial base. This suggests that cleft palate may be associated with a range of dimensional and morphological alterations in growth of the head which may be genetically determined.

The condition of bilateral hare-lip is the result of the persistence of the original grooves between the lower part of the fronto-nasal process and the maxillary processes. It is usually associated with cleft palate.

In cases of unilateral harelip there is failure of growth between the fronto-nasal process and the maxillary process on the affected side. Failure of union between the mandibular processes is very uncommon but when present produces complete or partial clefts of the lower jaw and lip in the middle line. Clefts running from the upper lip to the inner corner of the eye result from failure of growth of the whole of the maxillary process of one or both sides of the face, the resulting cleft separating the maxillary and fronto-nasal processes; clefts running from the angle of the mouth towards the ear are the result of abnormal separation between the mandibular and maxillary processes.

A different type of facial cleft may be produced during early development by the occurrence of a localised zone of necrosis which is due to the failure of capillary formation in the marginal areas of the distribution of the arteries supplying the face. This has been called 'fetal dysplasia of Streeter.' These clefts may have no relation to the sites of fusion of the facial processes. They are often associated with amniotic adhesions.

The tongue may show certain developmental abnormalities. It may be excessively large (macroglossia) or very small (microglossia). In the latter case the tongue deformity is often associated with an underdevelopment of the whole mandibular arch region. In newborn infants the fraenum may be abnormally large and may limit movement of the tongue. This condition usually rectifies itself later and surgery is rarely necessary.

BIBLIOGRAPHY

Baratz, R. S. & Zenati, N. A. (1979). The content of water, protein, DNA, RNA and sugar in fetal rat palatal processes during reorientation and fusion. *Arch. oral Biol.* **24,** 607.

DeAngelis, V. & Nalbandian, J. (1968). Ultrastructure of mouse and rat palatal processes prior to and during secondary palate formation. *Archs. oral Biol.* **13**, 601.

Farbman, A. I. (1969). The epithelium-connective tissue interface during closure of the secondary palate in rodent embryos. *J. dent. Res.* **48**, 617.

Ferguson, M. W. J. (1978). Palatal shelf elevation in the Wistar rat fetus. *J. Anat. Lond.* **125**, 555.

Hamilton, W. J., Boyd, J. D. & Mossman, H. W. (1972). *Human Embryology*. 4th ed. Cambridge: Heffer.

Humphrey, T. (1969). The relationship between human fetal mouth opening reflexes and closure of the palate. *Amer. J. Anat.* **125**, 317.

Kraus, B. S., Kitamura, H., & Latham, R. A. (1966). *Atlas of Development Anatomy of the Face*. London: Harper & Row.

Mott, W. J., Toto, P. D. & Hilgers, D. C. (1969). Labeling index and cellular density in palatine shelves of cleft-palate mice. *J. dent. Res.* **48**, 263.

Pruzansky, S. (1961). *Congenital anomalies of the face and associated structures.* Springfield: Thomas.

Sperber, G. H. (1976). *Cranio-facial Embryology*. 2nd. ed. Bristol: Wright.

Streeter, G. L. (1942–51). Developmental horizons in human embryos. *Contr. Embryol. Carneg. Instn.* Vols. 30–34.

Walker, B. E. & Quarles, J. (1975). Effects of anti-inflammatory steroids on mouse embryonic movements during palatal development. *J. dent. Res.* **54**, 1200.

Warbrick, J. G. (1960). The early development of the nasal cavity and upper lip in the human embryo. *J. Anat., Lond.* **94**, 351.

Wood, P. J. & Kraus, B. S. (1962). Prenatal development of the human palate. *Arch. oral Biol.* **7**, 137.

Wragg, L. E., Diewert, V. M. & Klein, M. (1972). Spatial relations in the oral cavity and the mechanism of secondary palate closure in the rat. *Arch. oral Biol.* **17**, 683.

3. The Early Development of the Teeth

When the development of the teeth is about to commence, the mouth cavity is lined by an epithelium which consists of a layer of low columnar cells. In some regions, particularly over the potential tooth-bearing area, there is a more superficial part formed by flattened cells two or three layers thick. The basal cells of the epithelium rest on a basal lamina and are separated by it from the underlying mesodermal tissue of the maxillary and mandibular processes.

At this stage neither the upper nor lower jaw (maxillary and mandibular processes) shows separate lip or gum regions, and it is only gradually that these parts become distinguishable (Fig. 48). The separation of lips

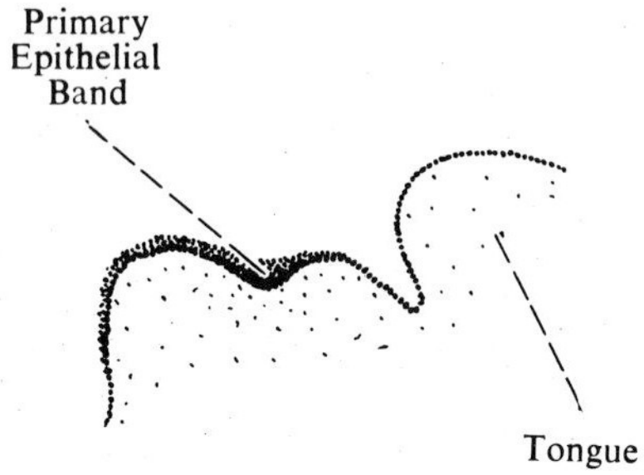

Fig. 48 Diagrammatic illustration of a sagittal section through the anterior part of the lower jaw showing the formation of the primary epithelial band.

and cheeks from the gums is closely associated with the initial development of the teeth.

As the primordia of the teeth appear and develop the cells of the oral epithelium which are superficial to the basal columnar layer become thickened in the region of the lips, cheeks, vestibule of the mouth, and the site of origin of the dental lamina (Fig. 49).

Primary epithelial band. The first indication that tooth formation is soon to begin is a localised proliferation of the oral epithelium which occurs in the lateral region of both maxillary and mandibular processes at about the 12 mm C.R. stage (sixth week of embryonic life). This proliferation soon become continuous across the middle line at the front of the mouth and forms a horseshoe-shaped structure which projects from the deep surface of the oral epithelium into the underlying mesoderm in each of the developing jaws. This structure is the primary epithelial band (Fig. 48). The band of the maxillary process (upper jaw) is situated somewhat more buccally than the band of the mandibular process (lower jaw) (Fig. 42).

Vestibular band and dental lamina. During the seventh week each primary epithelial band begins to divide on its deep aspect into two processes (Fig. 49). The outer or more buccal of these is known as the vestibular band (lip-furrow band) since it first marks off the region of the

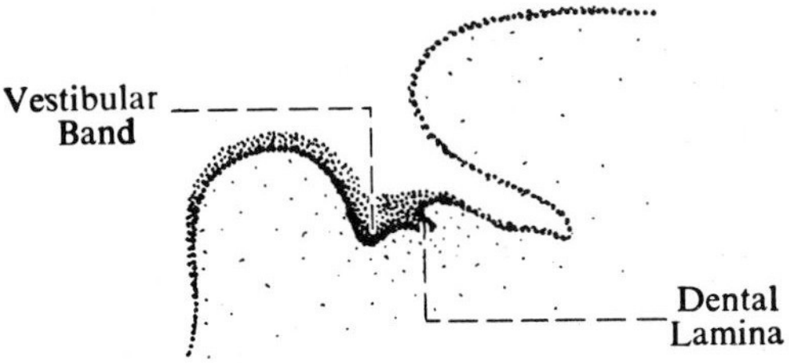

Fig. 49 Diagrammatic illustration of a sagittal section through the anterior part of the lower jaw showing the early appearance of the vestibular band and the dental lamina.

lips and cheeks from the gums and later produces a true separation of these parts. It is, even at this stage, a somewhat thicker process than the inner, the dental lamina, which is intimately concerned in the development of the teeth. With continued growth the dental lamina penetrates more deeply into the tissues of each jaw. At the front of the mouth this growth is in a lingual direction, so that the dental lamina diverges from the vestibular process and forms a continuous shelf-like projection of epithelium; further back in the mouth it remains more vertical.

THE EARLY DEVELOPMENT OF THE TOOTH GERMS

Enamel organs. Shortly after its initiation, the dental lamina of each jaw shows at intervals along its length small rounded swellings which

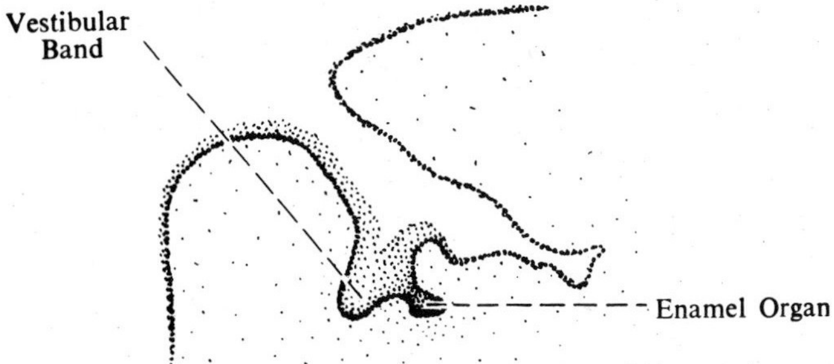

Fig. 50 Diagrammatic illustration of a sagittal section through the anterior part of the lower jaw showing the vestibular band and the dental lamina after the first appearance of an enamel organ.

involve the whole thickness of the lamina, and almost its whole depth from its free edge to its base where the lamina is attached to the mouth epithelium (Fig. 50). These epithelial swellings of the lamina are the enamel organs of deciduous teeth (Figs. 51, 52). On each side of each jaw four enamel organs develop; for the two deciduous incisors, the deciduous canine, and for the first deciduous molar. As the dental lamina grows backward behind the level of the opening of the parotid duct, enamel organs develop along this posterior segment in a manner

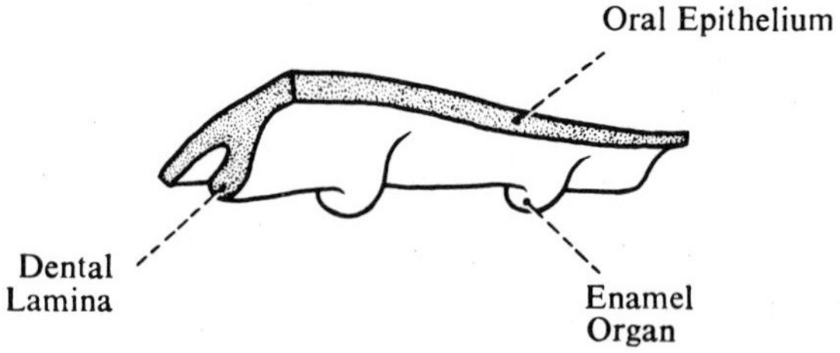

Fig. 51 Diagrammatic illustration of a strip of oral epithelium with part of the lower dental lamina to show the arrangement of the enamel organs of the deciduous teeth after their first appearance.

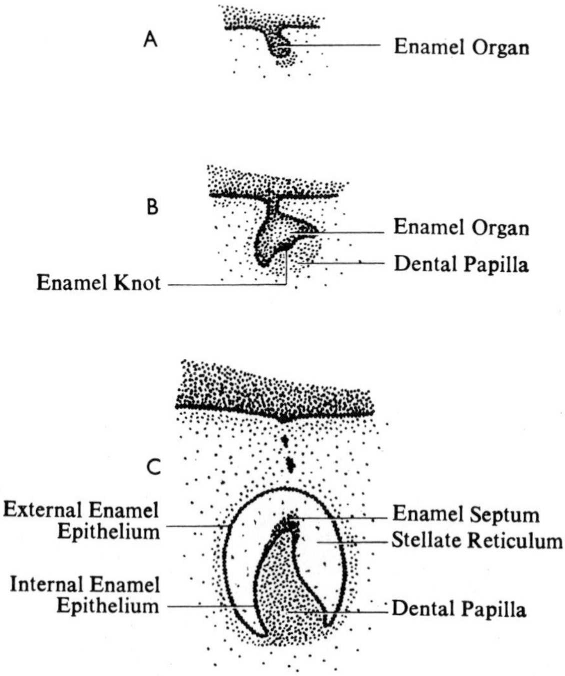

Fig. 52 Diagram to show the development of the tooth germ. (A) The primary enamel organ. (B) The enamel organ at the cap stage. (C) The enamel organ at the bell stage.

similar to their development along the anterior segment; the first of these is for the second deciduous molar, which is followed by those for the permanent molars. These with the four earlier appearing enamel organs constitute the primary enamel organs.

There is a considerable interval between the time of the formation of the enamel organs for the other deciduous teeth and that of the second deciduous molar; the latter does not begin to develop until the 40 mm C.R. stage (about ten weeks). The earliest indication of the enamel organ for the first permanent molar appears about the 100 mm C.R. stage (about 16 weeks). The enamel organs for the second and third permanent molars do not appear until after birth. From about the tenth week the enamel organs and the dental lamina conform to a catenary curve.

When first formed there is considerable spacing between adjacent enamel organs. With growth of the tooth germs the spacing between them becomes reduced.

Contrary to the classical description, the deciduous enamel organs do not first appear on the buccal side of the lamina above its free growing edge, nor do the primordia of the successional permanent teeth develop from the remaining free part of the lamina. There is at this early stage no indication whatever of the primordia of the successional permanent teeth. The primordia of the successional permanent teeth develop later by a process of budding off from the lingual side of each deciduous enamel organ.

Dental papilla. In relation to each of the developing deciduous enamel organs, the adjacent mesodermal tissue shows a distinct proliferation which forms a dense mass of cellular tissue. From this tissue develops the dental papilla (primitive pulp) and the follicular sac for each of the developing tooth germs. The term tooth germ or tooth bud is used to describe both the ectodermal and mesodermal constituents (enamel organ, dental papilla and dental follicle) which together are concerned in the development of a tooth (Figs. 52, 53).

The deeper surface of each enamel organ is known as the papillary surface since it is related to the mesodermal condensation which forms the dental papilla. The papillary surface is at first slightly convex, but soon becomes concave in outline (the cap stage of the enamel organ) and commences to enclose the mesodermal tissue of the dental papilla. In this manner each enamel organ acquires a growing rim which in all its circumference continues to grow deeper into the tissues. The growing dental papilla is at this stage partly enclosed within the ever-deepening concavity of the enamel organ and partly free of contact with the enamel organ (Fig. 53).

In the early stages of its growth each deciduous enamel organ shows at the centre of its concavity a slight projection of epithelium which partly divides the enclosed part of the dental papilla into buccal and lingual parts. This is the enamel knot. The enamel knot is, however,

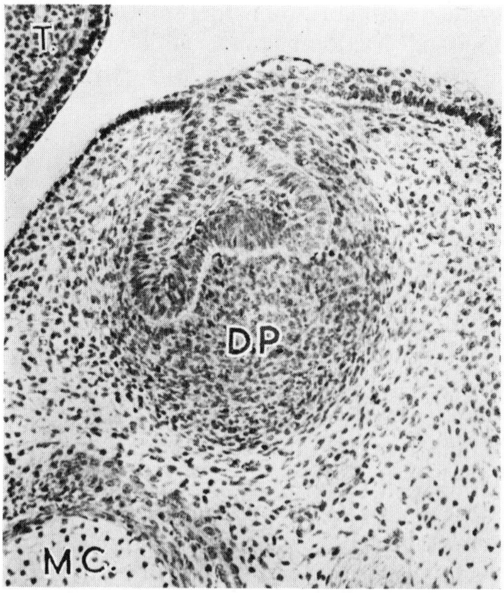

Fig. 53 Developing tooth germ. Enamel organ at the early cap stage with enamel knot still present. External to the superficial surface of the enamel organ is the cellular condensation, continuous with that of the dental papilla, which gives rise to the dental follicle. (D.P.) dental papilla; (M.C.) Meckel's cartilage; (T.) tongue. Coronal section of the lower first deciduous molar of a human embryo of 27 mm. C.R. length (approx. 8 weeks). × 135.

a transitory structure which soon becomes taken up into the substance of the enamel organ (Figs. 52, 53).

From the cap stage the enamel organ continues to increase in size and to alter in shape. Continued growth gradually transforms the enamel organ from a cap-shaped structure into a bell-shaped one, so that the dental papilla in the hollow of the enamel organ is surrounded on all sides by epithelium except at its base where it is continuous with the mesodermal tissue of the developing dental follicle (Figs. 52, 54).

Formation of vestibule. During the early development of the enamel organs changes take place in the arrangement of the vestibular band and the dental lamina. The vestibular band increases in bulk and forms a much broader process than the dental lamina, and its central cells are much larger (Fig. 54). In the region of the lower first deciduous molar tooth germ and backward from it, however, the vestibular band appears as a very shallow and rather inconspicuous structure, and not closely related to the dental lamina as elsewhere in the mouth cavity. Indeed, here it seems to have a different place of origin from the oral epithelium (Figs. 64, 75). At about the time when the enamel organs reach the late cap stage, a vertical cleft-like space comes into existence in the central part of the vestibular band which separates off in some degree the lips and cheeks from the gums, and so deepens the vestibular region of the mouth cavity (Fig. 54). At the back of the mouth the vestibular band related to the upper jaw grows backward for a time into the mesoderm as a solid epithelial process.

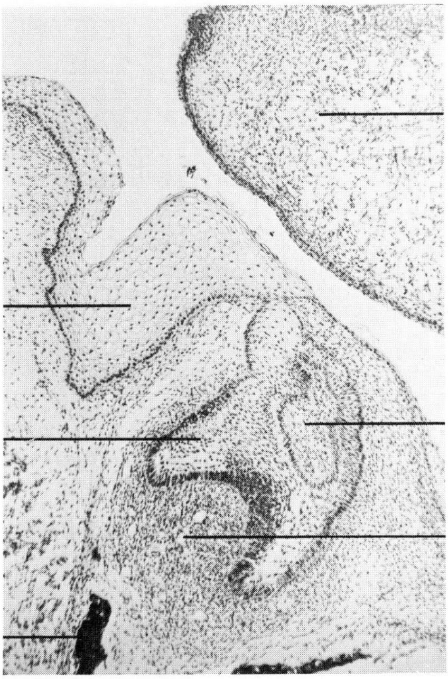

Fig. 54 The vestibular band and developing tooth germ. Shedding of the central cells of the vestibular band has taken place. The tooth germ of the deciduous lower first molar shows a well-marked enamel niche. Coronal section of human fetus of 55 mm C.R. length (Twelfth week). × 70.

Changes in the dental lamina. As the enamel organs pass in their development from their first appearance as rounded swellings of the dental lamina to the cap stage, so the dental lamina connecting them to the oral epithelium becomes lengthened. By the time the early bell stage of the enamel organ is reached the dental lamina related to each enamel organ begins to appear as if divided into two parts, lingual and buccal in position, bounding with the enamel organ an area filled with mesodermal tissue (Fig. 54). Actually the two laminae (inner and outer cords of Bolk) are not completely separate, as the buccal lamina is a smaller sheet of epithelium inclined towards the lingual lamina (the true dental lamina), so that the mesoderm-filled area bounded by the two laminae and the enamel organ is strictly a funnel-shaped depression or niche. Depending on the inclination of the buccal lamina to the dental lamina, so the opening of this niche is directed either mesially or distally (Fig. 55).

There is also a more shallow area bounded by the two laminae and the enamel organ on the other, mesial or distal, aspect of the buccal lamina from the deep enamel niche and this is sometimes referred to as an enamel niche. Thus one can speak of both a mesial and a distal enamel niche in relation to each enamel organ. With further growth of the enamel organ the enamel niche becomes relatively smaller, and

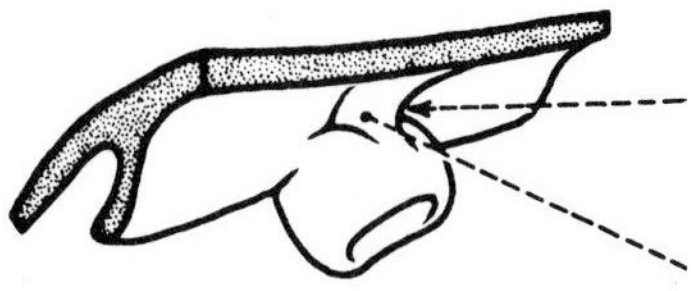

Fig. 55 Diagram illustrating the relationships of an enamel organ at the early bell stage to dental lamina and buccal lamina and the formation of an enamel niche.

as the buccal lamina gradually loses its attachment to the enamel organ it eventually disappears. The significance of the niche is uncertain. It may be an indication of a dual origin of the mammalian enamel organ from two reptile enamel organs.

Soon after the commencement of dentine and enamel formation in the deciduous tooth germs, all parts of the dental lamina connecting these tooth germs to the oral epithelium and to each other begin to show signs of degeneration, eventually becoming broken up to form a network of strands and clumps of epithelial cells around and above the deciduous enamel organs (Fig. 89).

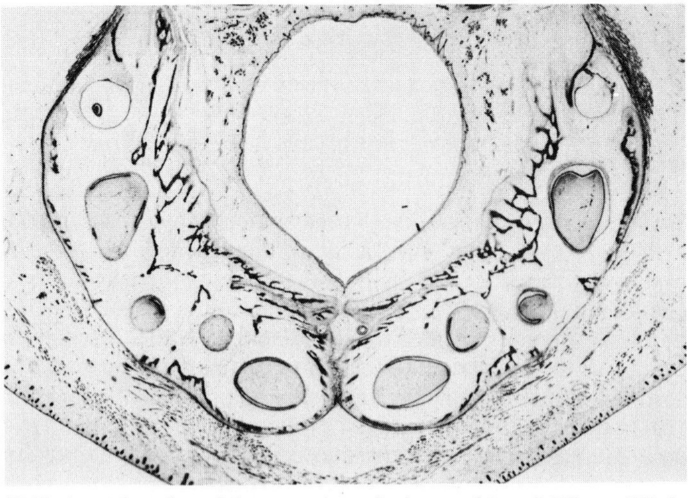

Fig. 56 Horizontal section of the upper jaw of a human fetus of 110 mm C.R. length (approx. 16 weeks). The tooth germs for all the deciduous teeth are present, also the backward extension of the dental lamina posterior to the deciduous tooth germs on both sides. The lateral incisor is already lingually positioned relative to the central incisor and canine tooth germs. Note the structure of the bone at this stage and the incisive canal. × 7.

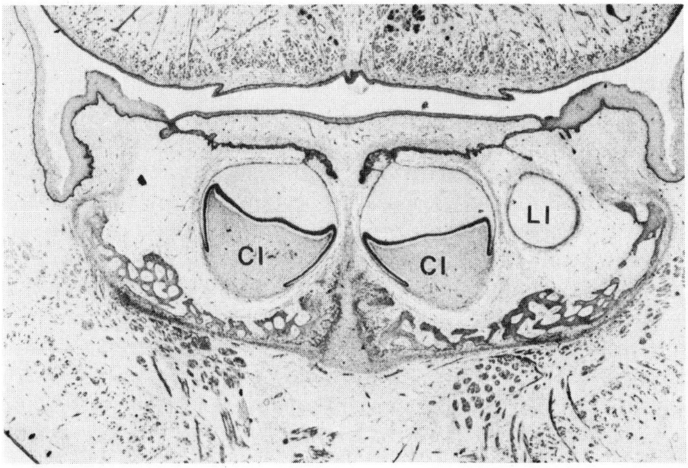

Fig. 57 Coronal section of the anterior part of the lower jaw and tongue of a human fetus of 110 mm C.R. length. The section cuts through the tooth germs of both deciduous central incisors and on one side through the enamel organ of the deciduous lateral incisor. The enamel organs have reached the full bell stage. The dental lamina is also shown and the lamina for both permanent central incisors. CI, deciduous central incisor; LI, deciduous lateral incisor. × 14.

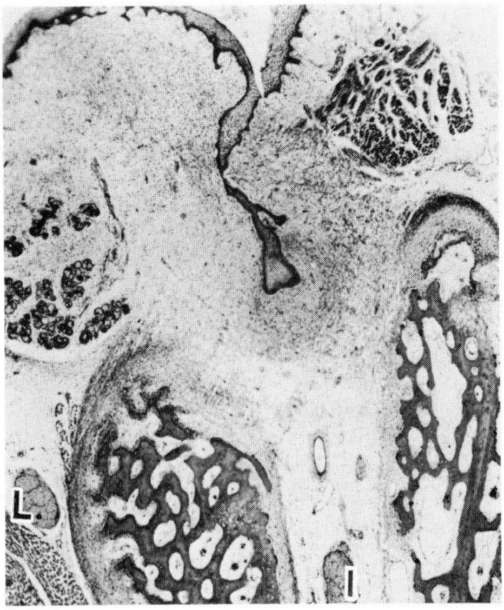

Fig. 58 Developing tooth germ for the lower first permanent molar. Arising from the buccal side of the dental lamina is the small process which represents the tooth-gland lamina. I, inferior dental nerve; L, lingual nerve. Human fetus of 110 mm C.R. length (approx. 16 weeks). × 25.

Tooth-gland lamina. In relation to the deciduous canines and to each of the deciduous and permanent molars an additional small epithelial process appears during the cap stage of the enamel organ. This is seen as a small bud or lamina on the buccal side of the tooth germ, but its exact position of origin varies with the tooth. In the case of the canines and the upper first deciduous molar it arises from the oral epithelium close to the origin of the dental lamina and, in a coronal section, is easily mistaken for the vestibular process (Figs. 83, 84). The lamina related to the upper first deciduous molar may sometimes bifurcate and then somewhat resembles an enamel organ at the cap stage. In relation to the second deciduous molars and the first permanent molars it arises from the buccal aspect of the dental lamina (Fig. 58). The lamina is more remote from the lower first deciduous molar arising directly from the oral epithelium between the dental lamina and the shallow vestibular process. It has also been supposed that this epithelial process, which is quite distinct from the buccal lamina forming the enamel niche, represents the vestige of a predeciduous dentition; the view of Bolk, however, that it is equivalent to the tooth-gland lamina found in a similar position in reptiles is possibly the correct one.

Dental lamina for permanent molars. Behind the deciduous tooth germs the dental lamina continues to proliferate backward into the tissues on each side of both jaws from its free margin. This part of the dental lamina appears as an epithelial process without any direct attachment to the oral epithelium and only connected to it through the more anterior part of the dental lamina (Figs. 56, 60). From this part of the dental lamina the enamel organs for the three permanent molars appear in succession. These arise in the same way and go through the same cap-shaped and bell-shaped stages as the enamel organs of the deciduous teeth (Figs. 58, 60). When the dental lamina in relation to the developing deciduous teeth breaks down, this posterior extension of the dental lamina loses even its indirect connection to the oral epithelium.

Successional permanent teeth. The enamel organs for the other permanent teeth (those with deciduous predecessors) arise in a quite different way. During the fourth month of fetal development (55–100 mm C.R. length) a small process of epithelium begins to appear on the lingual aspect of each enamel organ, not far removed from the attachment of the dental lamina to the enamel organ. This is the lamina for the successional permanent tooth (Figs. 57, 59, 64). From this lamina an enamel organ develops and passes through the stages as already described for the enamel organ of a deciduous tooth, though much later in time.

During the development of the permanent molars, which have no deciduous predecessors, an epithelial lamina arises on the lingual side of each enamel organ. This does not give rise to any enamel organ, but its position and time of appearance (after the full differentiation of the

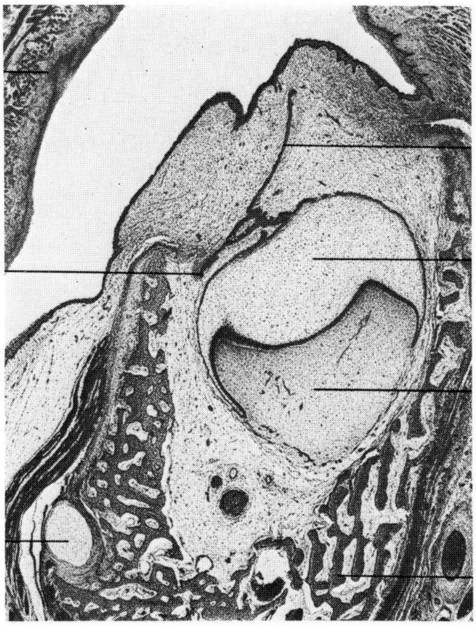

Fig. 59 Developing tooth germ. Enamel organ at the advanced bell stage. Coronal section of the lower jaw of a human fetus of 120 mm C.R. length. × 20.

enamel organ) are suggestive of its similarity to the lamina which arising in relation to each deciduous enamel organ gives rise to the successional permanent tooth. This fact, associated with the observation that the permanent molars arise in series with the deciduous teeth from the original dental lamina, supports the contention that the permanent molars are not strictly part of the permanent dentition but belong developmentally to the deciduous series.

Differentiation of enamel organ. From the beginning the cells forming the outer layer of the enamel organ appear different from those in the interior. The external cells are of a low columnar type since they are continuous with the basal layer of cells of the oral epithelium, and like the basal layer of the oral epithelium, they rest on a basal lamina which separates them from the adjacent mesoderm. The deeper cells of the enamel organ are roundish and closely packed together. As the enamel organ becomes concave on the surface in relation to the dental papilla, *i.e.*, as it enters the early cap stage, the cells of the outer layer on the papillary surface become taller (Fig. 53). From this stage the part of the outer layer of the enamel organ on its convex surface is known as the external enamel (or dental) epithelium, and the part lining its concave papillary surface is known as the internal enamel (or dental) epithelium. At the rim of the enamel organ the external and internal enamel epithelia are continuous. This region, which is a site of active cellular proliferation, is usually called the cervical loop of the enamel organ (Figs. 52, 63).

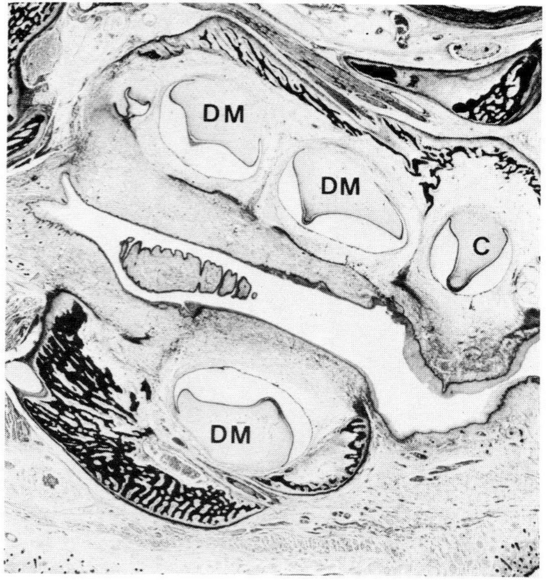

Fig. 60 Sagittal section of human fetus of 135 mm C.R. length. In this section in the lower jaw the developing first deciduous molar is shown, in the upper jaw the developing deciduous canine, both deciduous molars and the first permanent molar. Beneath the upper deciduous molars the dental lamina may be traced, and in relation to the first permanent molar its backward extension which gives origin to the second and third permanent molars C, deciduous canine; DM, deciduous molar. ×6.

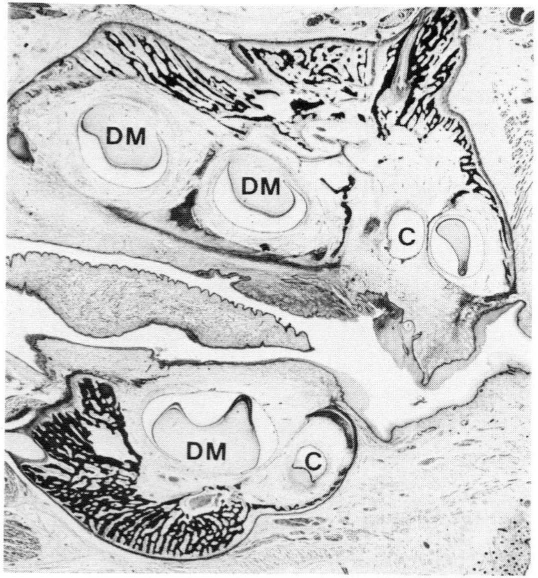

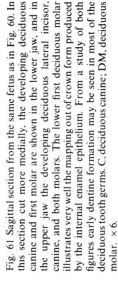

Fig. 61 Sagittal section from the same fetus as in Fig. 60. In this section cut more medially, the developing deciduous canine and first molar are shown in the lower jaw, and in the upper jaw the developing deciduous lateral incisor, canine, and both molars. The lower first deciduous molar illustrates very well the mapping out of crown form produced by the internal enamel epithelium. From a study of both figures early dentine formation may be seen in most of the deciduous tooth germs. C, deciduous canine; DM, deciduous molar. ×6.

As the enamel organ enters the late cap stage the cells at the interior become separated from one another, although maintaining contact by protoplasmic processes. This is the first indication of the stellate reticulum. This very delicate, loosely formed tissue becomes much more evident and greater in volume as the enamel organ approaches the bell stage of development (Fig. 54). The points of contact of the processes of the stellate reticulum cells represent desmosomal attachments of the

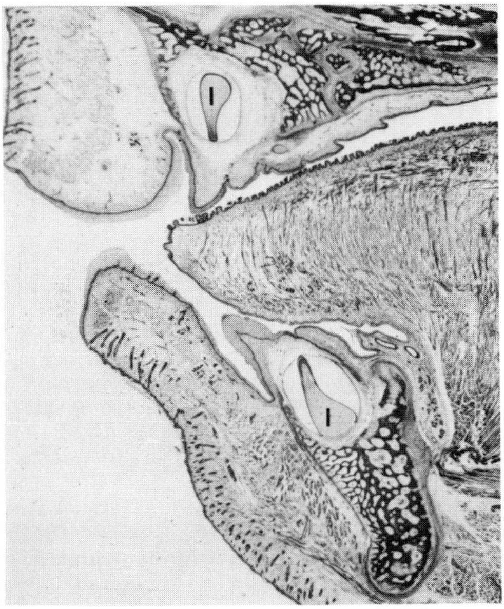

Fig. 62 Sagittal section of upper and lower jaws close to the median plane in human fetus of 156 mm C.R. length (Approx. 20 weeks). The different appearances of a tooth germ at the bell stage produced by sagittal, horizontal, and coronal sections may be appreciated by comparing the tooth germs for the deciduous central incisors as seen in this figure with those in Figs. 56 and 57. I. deciduous central incisor. × 7.

cells which elsewhere have been separated by the formation of extracellular material. For a time a heaped up mass of closely packed cells resting upon the internal enamel epithelium remains projecting into the stellate reticulum. This was described by Bolk as the enamel septum, dividing the stellate reticulum into buccal and lingual halves (Figs. 52, 54). It is not, however, at any time a complete septum, but a cone of epithelial cells everywhere surrounded by the stellate reticulum save at the base. As the late bell stage of the enamel organ is reached the enamel septum disappears. The enamel septum probably represents an area where active cellular proliferation persists for some time and so the cells remain close together.

At the late bell stage a further distinct layer of cells is seen in the

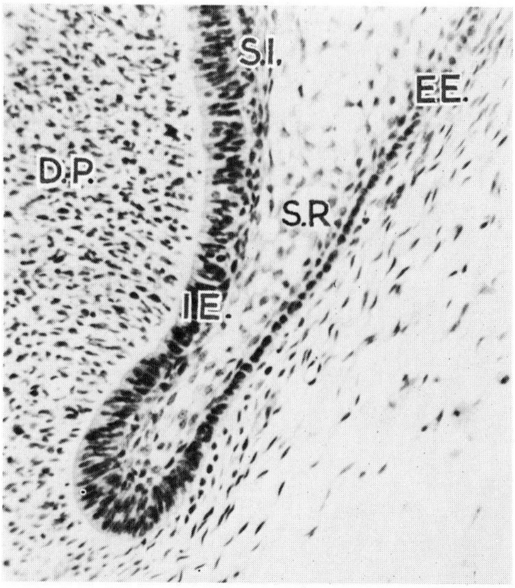

Fig. 63 The four layers of a fully formed enamel organ, at the rim of the enamel organ of a deciduous tooth germ. This region of the enamel organ is often called the cervical loop. (D.P.) dental papilla; (E.E.) external enamel epithelium; (I.E.) internal enamel epithelium; (S.I.) stratum intermedium; (S.R.) stellate reticulum. × 240

enamel organ. This is the stratum intermedium, two or three cells thick, and lying between the internal enamel epithelium and the stellate reticulum. When the enamel organs of the deciduous teeth are fully differentiated (fourth month of fetal life) they consist of (Fig. 63):

1. The external enamel (or dental) epithelium composed of cubical or low columnar cells.
2. The stellate reticulum forming the bulk of the enamel organ and composed of star-shaped (stellate) cells.
3. The stratum intermedium consisting of a layer of somewhat flattened cells, two or three cells thick.
4. The internal enamel (or dental) epithelium composed of columnar cells, which, as soon as enamel formation begins, are known as ameloblasts.

The formation of dentine and enamel begins very quickly after the enamel organ shows this differentiation.

It should be realised that growth of the enamel organ does not cease with its differentiation into these four layers. The enamel organ has at that point mapped out only a minute part of the future crown of the tooth. Growth of the deciduous enamel organs occurs throughout the rest of the fetal period, and so continues even after dentine and enamel formation has well started. The major growth site is then at the actively proliferating cervical loop of the enamel organ. Here additions are made to all four layers of the enamel organ until the full size of the crown has been produced (Fig. 63).

Differentiation of dental papilla. During the differentiation of the enamel organ changes, though much less striking, also occur in the dental papilla. At first the dental papilla is composed of closely packed mesodermal cells (Fig. 53) but by the time the bell stage of the enamel organ is reached delicate fibres have appeared amongst them. Capillaries also become evident (Figs. 59, 64). These are needed not only for

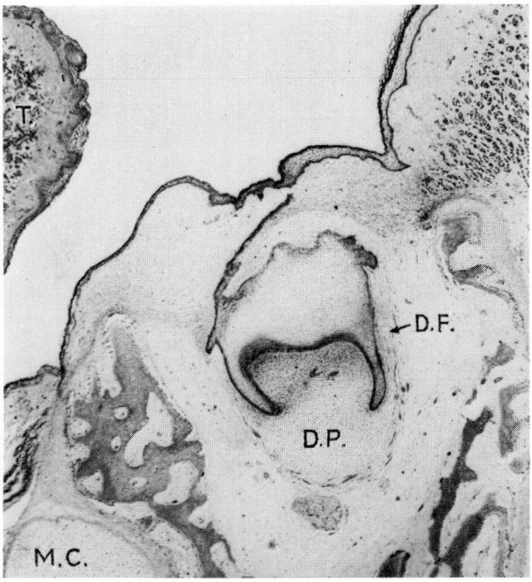

Fig. 64 Developing tooth germ. Enamel organ at the bell stage. Coronal section of deciduous lower first molar from human fetus of 95 mm C.R. length (approx. 16 weeks). (D.F.) dental follicle; (D.P.) dental papilla; (M.C.) Meckel's cartilage; (T.) tongue. × 28.

the nutrition of the tissue of the dental papilla, but are associated with the approaching activity of dentine formation.

At the bell stage of the enamel organ nerve fibres enter the papilla before odontoblasts have differentiated, but this innervation remains very simple until birth. At birth and soon after a sudden and conspicuous increase in innervation occurs in the deciduous teeth. There does not seem to be any connection between this innervation and cell differentiation or with tooth function.

Dental follicle. With growth of the tooth germ, more and more of the dental papilla is surrounded by the growing enamel organ. From a very early stage, however, a mesodermal cellular condensation appears in contact with the outer surface of the external enamel epithelium; this is continuous with the dental papilla around the rim of the enamel organ (Fig. 53). This is the primordium of the dental follicle or sac which, when fully developed, forms a fibrovascular capsule around the developing tooth (Fig. 64). At the bell stage of the tooth germ a plexus of nerve fibres appears in the follicle close to the surface of the enamel organ. The dental follicle is responsible for the nutrition of the enamel organ, maintains its proper relationship with the oral mucosa during growth, and controls the form and size of the bony cavity in which the developing tooth germ lies. The follicle finally becomes

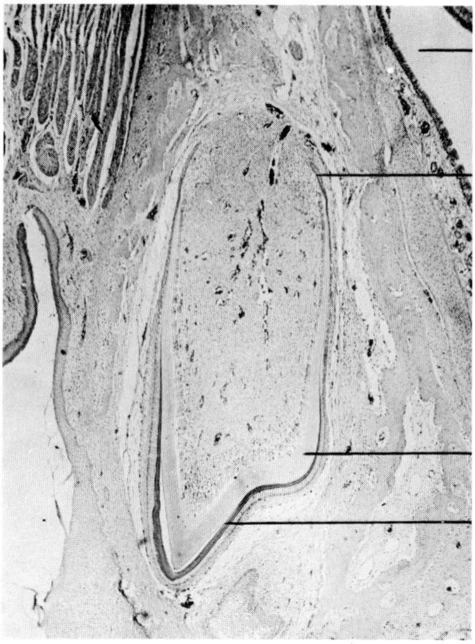

Fig. 65 Developing tooth germ showing the epithelial sheath of Hertwig. Section of the upper jaw of a full-term kitten. × 25.

the periodontal membrane whereby the fully formed tooth is attached to its socket after eruption.

Sheath of Hertwig. After the enamel organ has mapped out the full size and form of the crown of the developing tooth, further growth at the region of the cervical loop is related to development of the root area of the tooth. Henceforward the external and internal enamel epithelia are not separated by stratum intermedium and stellate reticulum, but grow as a two-layered epithelial wall, the sheath of Hertwig. This maps out the shape of the root area of the tooth in the same way as the enamel organ does for the crown of the tooth (Fig. 65). In the case of a tooth with a single root, the sheath of Hertwig is a simple tubular structure, but in multi-rooted teeth it must obviously be more complex, for though starting as a single tube for the undivided part of the root area, it is continued later as either two or three separate tubes, depending on the number of roots (Fig. 66). This is achieved by the inward growth of horizontally directed processes of epithelium from Hertwig's

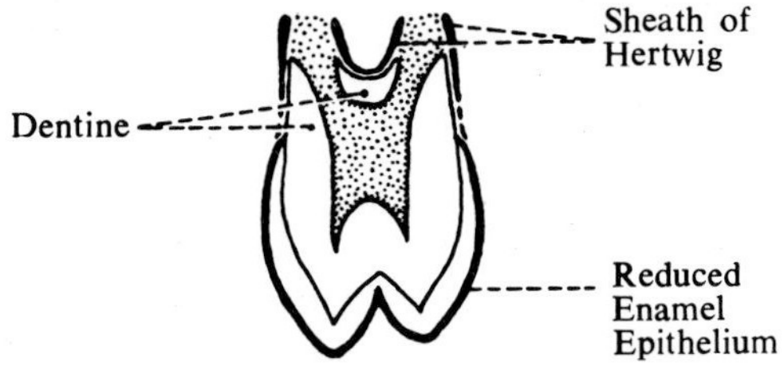

Fig. 66 Diagram of a vertical section through a two-rooted upper premolar showing the mapping out of the roots by the sheath of Hertwig.

sheath at the region where the separate roots are given off (Fig. 67A). These processes, corresponding in number to the number of roots, meet and fuse so as to produce separate epithelial surrounded openings instead of the original single opening (Fig. 67B). From this point the individual roots are mapped out each by its own tubular extension of the sheath of Hertwig.

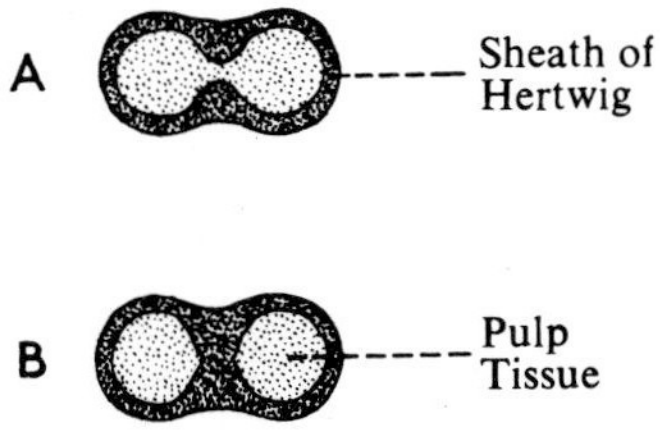

Fig. 67 Diagrammatic illustration of horizontal sections through the growing end of the sheath of Hertwig related to a two-rooted tooth. (A) The appearance of the processes which subdivide the area bounded by Hertwig's sheath. (B) Fusion of the processes and consequent delineation of the two roots.

THE DIFFERENTIATION AND FUNCTION OF THE TOOTH GERM

Recent experimental work on tooth development in Amphibians and in the mouse have led most authorities to regard the mesodermal component as of fundamental importance in the early stages. It is thought that areas of presumptive mesoderm in the jaws are responsible for the initiation of the dental lamina and that the papillary condensations are equally essential for the production of the early bud stages of the tooth germs. This view is contrary to the older one in which the ectodermal component in the form of dental lamina and the bud stage of the enamel organ was thought to appear first in development and to induce a mesodermal reaction. However, at later stages when a fully differentiated layer of internal enamel epithelium has developed the inductive effect is exerted by ectoderm on mesoderm, especially in the formation of a layer of odontoblasts on the surface of the dental papilla.

Apart from the question of primacy of the ectodermal and mesodermal components in dental development the source of origin of the mesoderm has attracted attention. It has been shown in amphibians that streaming of neural crest cells to the areas of dental development takes place and that the odontoblasts are derived from these cells. On these grounds the mesodermal element in amphibian tooth development has been described as ectomesenchyme. A similar origin has been postulated for the mesodermal element in the case of mammalian tooth development, for streams of cells reach the mandibular and maxillary processes beneath the surface ectoderm before the latter has shown the typical changes associated with tooth development.

The fully differentiated enamel organ of a tooth germ consists of (1) the external enamel epithelium, (2) the stellate reticulum, (3) the stratum intermedium, and (4) the internal enamel epithelium. At the growing rim of the enamel organ the external and internal enamel epithelial layers are continuous with one another. The basal lamina, separating the epithelial tissue of the enamel organ from the adjacent mesoderm, covers the surface of the external enamel epithelium, separating it from the vascular tissue of the follicle, continues around the rim of the enamel organ, and within the cup of the enamel organ separates the internal enamel epithelium from the dental papilla.

All the calcified tissues of the teeth, enamel, dentine, and cement develop between the internal enamel epithelium and its rootward continuation as the inner layer of Hertwig's sheath on the one side, and the surface of the dental papilla on the other. The basal lamina, separating the dental papilla and the internal enamel epithelium, represents the enamel-dentine (amelo-dentinal) junction separating the ectodermal derivative, enamel, from the mesodermal derivative, dentine. Enamel is laid down in the area between the epithelial surface of the basal lamina and the outward retreating ameloblasts; the thickness of the enamel in any part of the crown depends on the distance the ameloblasts migrate from the basal lamina. Dentine is laid down in the area mapped out between the mesodermal surface of the basal lamina and the inward retreating dentine-forming cells (odontoblasts) of the dental papilla. The thickness of the dentine in any part of the tooth depends on the distance the odontoblasts have migrated from the basal lamina (Fig. 68). The continual formation of dentine leads to progressive reduction in the size of the pulp cavities and root canals of the tooth.

Cement is laid down on the surface of the dentine which is not covered by enamel and after Hertwig's sheath commences to break up. In some animals a form of cement is also deposited on the surface of the enamel.

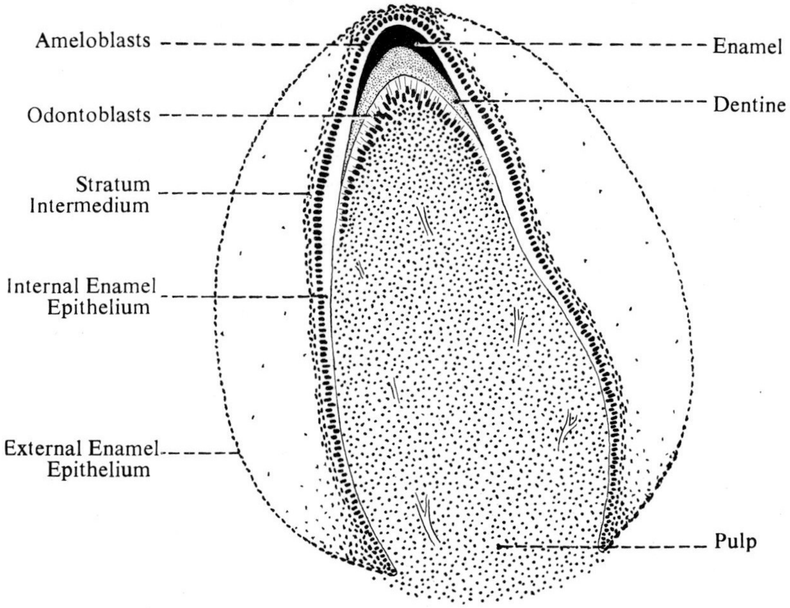

Fig. 68 Diagrammatic illustration of a developing human tooth after the commencement of dentine and enamel formation. Note the lengthening of the cells of the internal enamel epithelium during their differentiation before odontoblast formation begins. Note also the subsequent shortening of these cells in becoming ameloblasts and starting the formation of enamel.

The internal enamel epithelium and the inner layer of Hertwig's sheath have the following functions:

1. They determine the form and size of the crown and root portions of the tooth. In the early stages of development the form-determining function of the internal enamel epithelium is not dependent on the co-ordinated activity of various parts of the epithelium but is the function of the epithelium as a whole. If developing tooth germs are cut in half, each half does not form only one half of a tooth but has the power of forming *in vitro* a complete tooth germ with the normal number of cusps. At a later stage in differentiation this generalised form-determining property is lost and development depends on the normal growth of various regions of the internal enamel epithelium.

2. By their 'evocative' effect on the surface cells of the dental papilla they initiate the differentiation of the dentine-forming cells. It has been shown that in tooth germs grown *in vitro* the presence of the internal enamel epithelium is essential for the differentiation of odontoblasts.

3. Where the internal enamel epithelium becomes the fully differentiated ameloblast layer, enamel is laid down on the surface of the dentine. Dentine is always the first of the calcified dental tissues to appear. In some animals (*e.g.*, edentates) no enamel is formed and the crown

portion of the tooth consists of dentine without an enamel covering; in other animals (*e.g.*, rodents) enamel is not formed over certain parts of the crowns. In these cases where enamel is absent the cells of the internal enamel epithelium do not differentiate into ameloblasts; the function of the enamel organ is limited to (1) and (2) above.

4. The reduced enamel epithelium (that part of the enamel organ remaining on the enamel-covered surfaces after enamel formation is complete) and Hertwig's sheath may possibly protect the enamel and dentine from the erosive action of the adjacent vascular tissues before eruption of the crown into the mouth cavity and before cement is deposited on the surface of the developing root of a tooth. During eruption the reduced enamel epithelium is important in establishing the relation and attachment between tooth and gingival epithelium.

Over the crown portion of the developing tooth a rich capillary plexus is formed in the substance of the follicle and in contact with the external enamel epithelium and its covering basal lamina. In the early stages of enamel organ differentiation and prior to the commencement of calcification of the dentine, the capillaries do not enter the enamel organ. After calcification commences in the separate cusps of the cheek teeth or along the incisive edge of the anterior teeth, capillary loops invaginate the external enamel epithelium and the basal lamina and dip into the enamel organ as far as the stratum intermedium. Before calcification commences in the dentine, both the differentiating odontoblasts and ameloblasts can draw their nutrition from the blood vessels of the dental papilla. During this period the stellate reticulum reaches its phase of maximum development and apparently draws most of its fluid content from the follicular capillary plexus through the external epithelial layer of the enamel organ. Once dentine commences to calcify, the ameloblasts which rest upon each isolated centre of calcification are partly cut off from the capillary plexus of the pulp by an increasing crust of calcifying dentine. They can, however, draw upon the store of tissue fluid which has been built up in the stellate reticulum. Further demands for nutrition are met by the penetration of the follicular capillaries into the substance of the enamel organ (Fig. 69).

Over those places in a developing tooth germ where calcification has commenced, the amount of stellate reticulum is greatly reduced and in what remains of the reticulum the cells become more closely packed together. Calcification commences in the separate cusps of the molars and premolars and along the incisive edges of the anterior teeth before the growth of the internal enamel epithelium has fully mapped out the definitive form and size of the crown surface of the teeth (Fig. 70). Each little isolated centre of calcification is, for a while, moving away from the others. The surrounding stellate reticulum forms a delicate, cushioning, semi-fluid medium through which each centre of calcification can move as it rests upon the underlying more turgid tissue of the expanding dental papilla without the danger of fracture or deformity of its formative cells. Once the crown surface has approached to adult dimensions, calcification spreads over the surface of the crown until all the centres are united. When the cusps first form they are pointed and elongated as in Insectivores. They become more rounded later in development.

It has been suggested that the internal enamel epithelium should be thought of as a layer surrounded on each side by a pressure-exerting tissue. On one side is the water-imbibing stellate reticulum, and on the

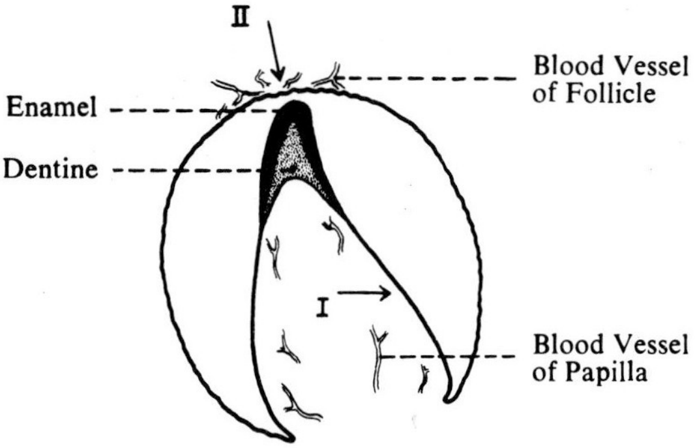

Fig. 69 Diagram showing the difference in the source of the nutritional supply to the ameloblasts (I) before and (II) after dentine and enamel formation has begun.

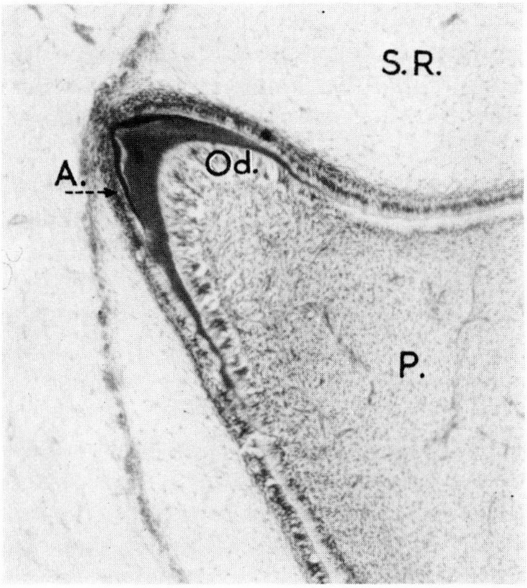

Fig. 70 Commencement of dentine and enamel formation at cuspal region of a deciduous molar. Note the disappearance of the stellate reticulum over this area. (A.) ameloblasts; (Od.) odontoblasts; (P.) pulp; (S.R.) stellate reticulum. Human fetus of 135 mm C.R. length. × 70.

other the growing dental papilla. The power of water absorption of the stellate reticulum probably resides in its rich mucopolysaccharide content; this appears to be a chondroitin sulphate which is water absorbent. The pressures on either side of the internal enamel epithelium cancel each other, so that any changes of shape in this layer are due to inherent growth activities. Cusp formation on this basis can be accounted for by the folding of the internal enamel epithelium; the tip of a cusp being a region of precocious cell maturity where deposition of dentine and enamel occurs early, the depressions between the cusps being areas where proliferation of the epithelial cells of the internal enamel epithelium continues longer.

Teeth should be considered not only as individual units but as part of a system. As one passes along a dentition from the first incisor to the last molar there is a series of form gradations which appears to indicate the presence of morphogenetic fields which influence the developing tooth germs in different parts of the jaws to develop in divergent ways. These fields can often be classified as corresponding to the incisor, canine, and premolar-molar regions of the dentition and each of these regions appears to have some degree of evolutionary independence. The process of 'incisivation' usually reaches its maximum in the central incisors, that of 'caninisation' in the canine teeth and of 'molarisation' in the middle of the premolar-molar series. There is often, however, some overlapping so that the process of 'caninisation' may involve the most lateral incisor and one or more of the premolars, and 'molarisation' may extend forward to involve the premolars. Furthermore, in some dentitions the morphogenetic field responsible for the canines is absent or deficient, so that the canines may not develop at all as in the typical rodent dentition, or may take on the morphology of an incisor as in sheep and oxen. In their early development all tooth germs are somewhat similar in form, specialisations such as cusp formation, ridge formation, etc., take place later in their development. The morphogenetic process appears to be inherent in the cells of the internal enamel epithelium or perhaps at an earlier stage along the dental lamina.

In development teeth go through an early phase when most of the component cells show active division. Later the tooth adds to its stock of functioning cells by growth at certain well-defined regions until the completion of the root.

Clinical considerations. Throughout the whole period of development of the tooth germs of both dentitions, from the first appearance of the enamel organs to the subsequent mapping out of the form of the crown by the enamel organ and that of the root by the sheath of Hertwig, a great variety of divergencies from the normal may occur. These abnormalities may involve the number, form, or size of the teeth. There is little direct knowledge of the mode of origin of these abnormalities, but it can be theoretically decided, in most instances, at which developmental stage the abnormality is likely to have been produced.

Variations from the usual number of teeth may be found as either less or more than the normal total. In both instances the permanent dentition is much more commonly affected than the deciduous dentition. Where less than the normal number of teeth are found the condition is produced by the failure of the correct number of enamel organs to appear; it may involve one or more teeth, or occasionally all the teeth (anodontia). Teeth which are found in excess of the normal number are known as supernumerary teeth. They are very uncommon in the deciduous dentition. It is possible that those which appear with the permanent dentition are:

1. Extra late-erupting deciduous or permanent teeth derived from the dental lamina in series with the deciduous enamel organs.
2. The result of a splitting (dichotomy) of a deciduous or permanent enamel organ, or
3. Members of a post-permanent dentition derived from the budding-off of a lamina from a permanent enamel organ.

Supernumerary paramolar teeth developing alongside (on the buccal side of) the permanent molars may be a 'predeciduous' dentition or separate derivatives of the dental lamina.

Variations in the form of a tooth may range from the details of tooth form to gross deformities. Additional cusps or roots may be found, or the normal number may fail to appear, roots may be fused, or the tooth may be so greatly distorted as to show a loss of its typical appearance, *e.g.*, extreme forms of dilated composite odontome. This type of abnormality arises during the period when the form of the tooth is being determined by the enamel organ or the sheath of Hertwig. It has been shown that there is a higher frequency of abnormal teeth in individuals suffering from mental retardation.

Variations in the size of a tooth are produced during the same period and may involve the whole tooth or only crown or root. Variations in size are, of course, only to be considered as abnormal when the teeth are unusually large or small.

Abnormal proliferations of the odontogenic epithelium may occur which do not produce teeth. The proliferations may remain cellular (ameloblastomata) or may lead to the production of single or multiple masses of the calcified dental tissues arranged in irregular and haphazard fashion. These are known as complex composite and compound composite odontomes respectively.

Just as cysts can arise from epithelial remnants left isolated in the tissues during the formation of the face and mouth region, so various cystic conditions may occur later in life which originate from remnants of some part of the formative dental epithelium. These are cysts of eruption, dental cysts, and dentigerous cysts.

BIBLIOGRAPHY

Bernick, S. & Levy, B. M. (1968). Studies on the biology of the periodontium of marmosets: I. Development of bifurcation in multirooted teeth in marmosets (*Callithrix jacchus*). *J. dent. Res.* **47**, 21.

Butler, P. M. (1956). The ontogeny of molar pattern. *Biol. Rev.* **31**, 30.

Diab, M. A. & Stallard, R. E. (1965). A study of the relationship between epithelial root sheath and root development. *Periodont.* **3**, 10.

Gaunt, W. A. (1959). The vascular supply to the dental lamina during early development. *Acta Anat.* **37**, 232.

Glasstone, S. (1954). The development of tooth germs on the chick chorioallantois. *J. Anat., Lond.* **88**, 392.

Kollar, E. & Baird, G. (1970). Tissue interactions in embryonic mouse tooth germs. *J. Embryol. exp. Morph.* **24**, 159, & **24**, 173.

Kraus, B. S., Clark, G. N. & Oka, S. W. (1968). Mental retardation and abnormalities of the dentition. *Amer. J. Ment. Def.* **72**, 903.

Ooë, T. (1959). On the development of position of the tooth germs in the human deciduous molar teeth. *Okajimas Fol. anat. Jap.* **32**, 97.

Pannese, E. (1960–62). Observations on the ultrastructure of the enamel organ. *J. Ultrastruct. Res.* **4**, 372; **5**, 328; **6**, 186.

Ruch, J. V., Karcher-Djuricic, V. & Gerber, R. (1973). Les déterminismes de la morphogenèse et des cytodifferénciations des ébauches dentaires de souris. *J. Biol. buccale.* **1**, 45.

Takagi, M. (1967). Studies on the dental innervation of tooth germs in the developmental stage. *J. Osaka dent. Univ.* **1**, 50.

Tonge, C. H. (1976). Morphogenesis and development of teeth. In *Scientific Foundations of Dentistry*. Eds. Cohen, B. & Kramer, I. R. H. London: Heinemann.

Turner, E. P. (1963). Crown development in human deciduous molar teeth. *Arch. oral Biol.* **8**, 523.

4. The Development of the Jaws

During the period of the early development of the deciduous teeth the jaws also begin to form. About the time the dental lamina appears in the maxillary and mandibular processes the first indication of bone formation for the jaws is seen; and by the time that the deciduous tooth germs are beginning the formation of dentine and enamel, these tooth germs have come into close relationship with the jaws, since they lie in cavities, the alveoli, formed by the bone of the mandible and the maxilla. It is therefore necessary to reconsider the development of the mandibular and maxillary processes from the embryonic stage in order to follow the parallel development of the bony jaws.

DEVELOPMENT OF THE MANDIBLE

Meckel's cartilage. The mandible is formed in the lower or deeper part of the first visceral (mandibular) arch. It is preceded there by Meckel's cartilage, which represents the primitive vertebrate mandible. In the human embryo Meckel's cartilage attains its full form by the 15 mm C.R. stage (six weeks) and then stretches downward and forward as an unbroken rod of cartilage from the cartilaginous otic capsule to the middle line; there its ventral end turns upward in contact with the cartilage of the opposite side, to which it is joined by mesenchyme. It is surrounded in its whole length by a thick investment of fibrocellular tissue. The dorsal end of the cartilage gives rise to the malleus of the middle ear; the remaining part of the cartilage is largely associated with the development of the mandible, the membrane bone which forms the replacing skeletal structure (Fig. 45).

The mandibular nerve. Meckel's cartilage at this stage of development has a close relationship to the mandibular nerve, the nerve of the first visceral arch, and its branches, acting as their skeletal support. The main nerve issues from the skull medial and ventral to the dorsal end of the cartilage and comes into direct relationship with it about the junction of its dorsal and middle thirds (Fig. 71). Here, after giving off its other branches, it divides into the lingual and inferior alveolar (dental) nerves. The lingual nerve passes forward on the medial side of the cartilage, whereas the inferior alveolar (dental) nerve lies lateral to its upper margin, and running forward parallel to it terminates by dividing into mental and incisive branches; the incisive branch continues its course parallel to the cartilage.

The body of the mandible. The further history of Meckel's cartilage is bound up with the development of the bony mandible in which, however, it takes very little direct part. The mandible first appears as a band of dense fibrocellular tissue which lies on the lateral side of the inferior dental and incisive nerves. Ossification occurs in this tissue at the 17–18 mm C.R. stage (seventh week) in the angle formed by the incisive

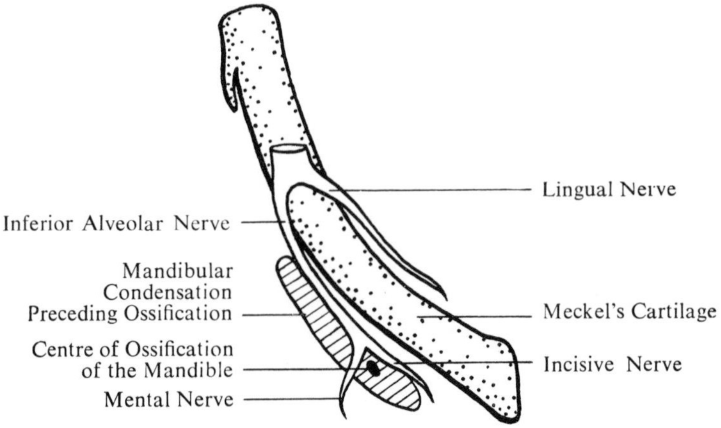

Fig. 71 Diagram to illustrate the early development of the mandible.

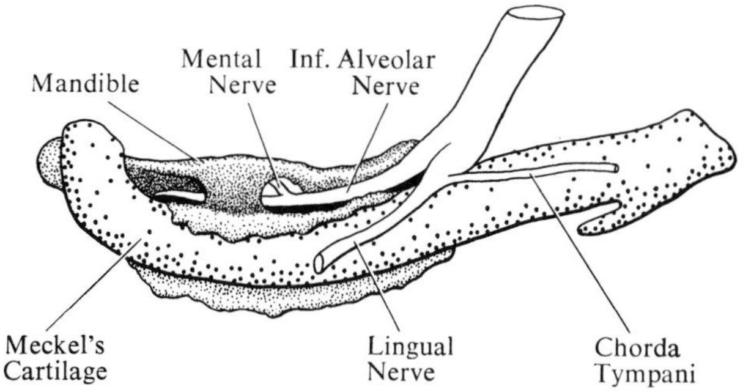

Fig. 72 Diagrammatic illustration of the development of the mandible after the bridging over of the mental and incisive nerves has commenced; and seen from the lingual aspect.

and mental nerves (Fig. 71); that is, in the region of the future mental foramen, and from this centre the formation of bone spreads rapidly backward below the mental nerve, which then lies in a notch in the bone, and on the lateral side of the inferior alveolar (dental) nerve. The bone in front of the region of the notch for the mental nerve grows medially below the incisive nerve and soon afterwards spreads upwards between this nerve and Meckel's cartilage; in this way the incisive nerve is contained in a trough of bone formed by lateral and medial plates which are united beneath the nerves (Figs. 72, 83). At the same stage

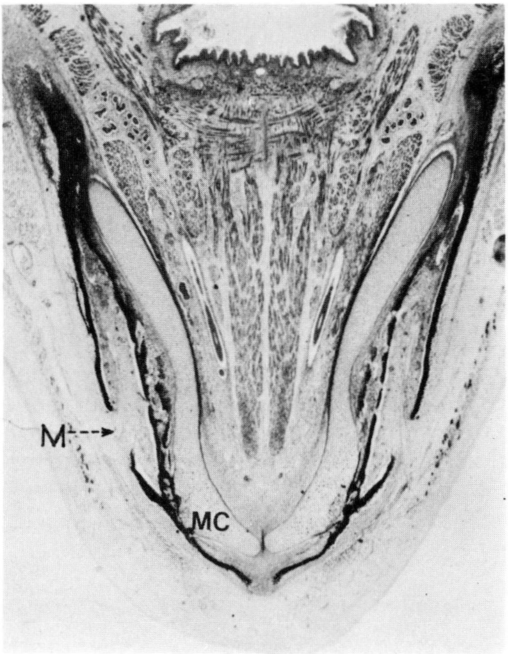

Fig. 73 Horizontal section of the developing lower jaw. Resorption of Meckel's cartilage has begun towards its ventral (anterior) end in the region where the bone is directly applied to the cartilage. Behind this region both lateral and medial plates of bone appear. (M) mental foramen and nerve. Human fetus of 43 mm C.R. length (approx. 10 weeks). (MC) Meckel's cartilage. × 14.

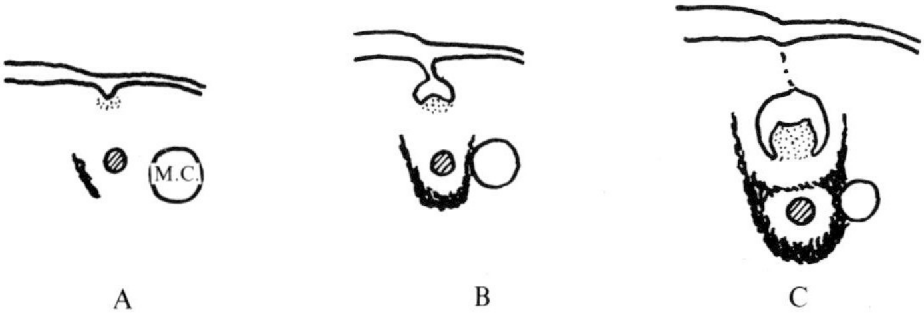

Fig. 74 Diagram illustrating the development of the body of the mandible in relationship to the inferior alveolar nerve, Meckel's cartilage and the developing teeth. Bone is shown in solid black, the nerve trunk is cross-hatched. (A) A plate of bone has formed lateral to the nerve trunk and Meckel's cartilage, MC (B) The nerve trunk is contained in a trough of bone; the tooth germ is at the cap stage of the enamel organ. (C) Upward growth of the lateral and medial plates has extended the trough of bone to contain the tooth germ which has reached the bell stage of the enamel organ.

the notch containing the mental nerve is converted into the mental foramen by the extension of bone over the nerve from the anterior to the posterior edge of the notch (Fig. 72). The bony trough grows rapidly forward towards the middle line where it comes into close relationship with the similar bone formation of the opposite side but from which it is separated by connective tissue (Fig. 73). Union between the two halves of the bony mandible takes place before the end of the first year. By the growth of bone over the incisive nerve from the lateral and medial plates the trough of bone is converted into the incisive canal.

A similar spread of ossification in the backward direction produces first a plate of bone in relation to the whole of the lateral aspect of the inferior alveolar (dental) nerve, then a bony trough in which the nerve lies, and very much later the canal for it. Thus by these processes of growth the original primary centre of ossification produces the body proper of the mandible as far back as the mandibular foramen and as far forward as the symphysis; that is the part of the mandible which surrounds the inferior alveolar (dental) and incisive nerves—the neural element. At this stage the developing tooth germs lie some little distance superficial to the mandible and are not contained by it (Figs. 74, 75).

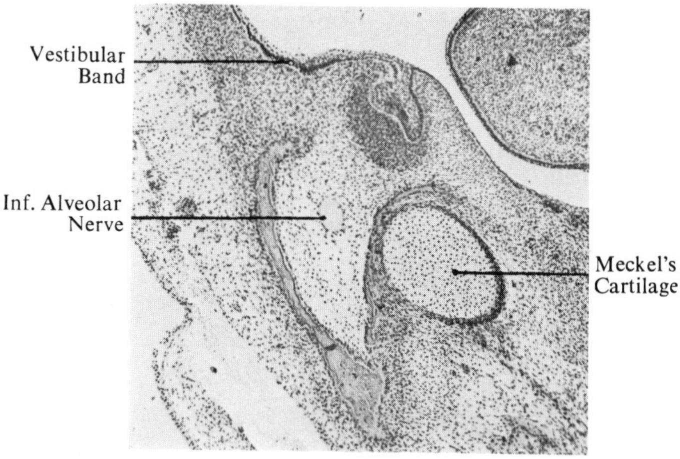

Fig. 75 Coronal section of the developing lower jaw at the level of the tooth germ for the deciduous first molar. The mandibular bone forms a well-defined trough containing the inferior alveolar (dental) nerve. Note in this part of the mouth the shallow vestibular band and its relative remoteness from the dental lamina. Human fetus of 27 mm C.R. length (approx. 8 weeks). ×45.

The alveolar bone. As the enamel organs of the deciduous tooth germs reach the early bell stage the bone of the mandible begins to come into close relationship to them. This is brought about by the upward growth, on each side of the tooth germs, of the lateral and medial plates of the mandibular bone above the level where the roof of the canal for the incisive and inferior alveolar (dental) nerves is formed (Fig. 74). By this growth the developing teeth come to lie in a trough of bone. This trough is later divided into separate small basins or alveoli for the teeth by the formation of septa between its two walls (Fig. 76).

The fate of Meckel's cartilage. With the exception of the very terminal part of Meckel's cartilage at the middle line, the anterior part of the mandible, from in front of the mental foramen, includes the cartilage in its substance. This part of the cartilage is first surrounded by an extension of bone from the medial plate and then is gradually resorbed and replaced by an extension of ossification from the membrane bone around it. During the later fetal period and at least until the time of birth one or two nodules of cartilage are seen in the fibrous tissue of the symphysis; these nodules are remnants of the ventral end of Meckel's cartilage. The rest of Meckel's cartilage disappears completely except for a part of its fibrous covering which persists as the spheno-mandibular and spheno-malleolar ligaments. The most dorsal part of the cartilage ossifies to form the incus and the malleus, and the latter is attached to the spine of the sphenoid by the spheno-malleolar ligament.

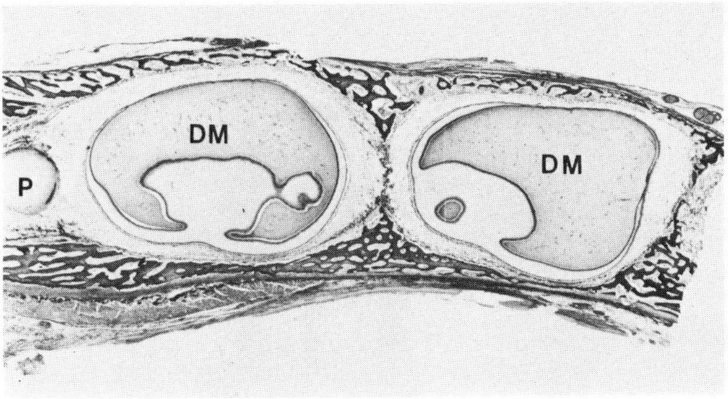

Fig. 76 Horizontal section through a human fetal mandible of six months showing the deciduous molars in their alveoli. Immediately behind the deciduous molars is the tooth germ for the first permanent molar. DM, deciduous molar; P, permanent molar. ×7.

The ramus. The backward extension of the mandible to form the ramus is produced by a spread of ossification from the body, behind and above the mandibular foramen. From this region the mandible diverges laterally from the line of Meckel's cartilage. Just as earlier the body of the mandible is first indicated by a fibrocellular condensation in which ossification occurs, here too the ramus and its processes are first mapped out by an extension of this condensation. The formation of bone in this tissue occurs rapidly so that the coronoid and condylar processes are to a large extent ossified by the 40 mm C.R. stage (tenth

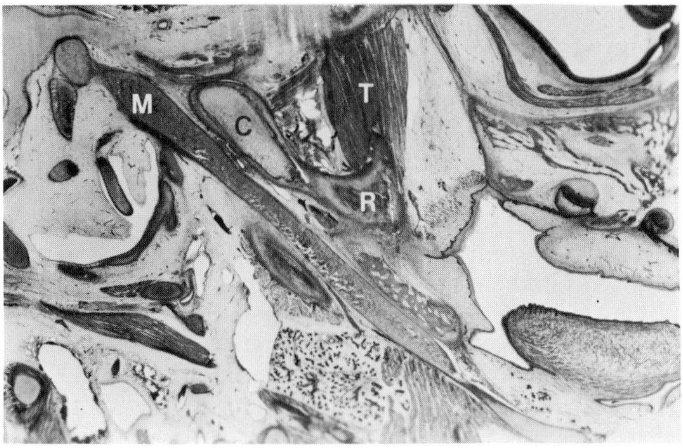

Fig. 77 Sagittal section of the head of a human fetus of 65 mm C.R. length. Meckel's cartilage may be traced from its posterior end in the middle ear to its anterior end in the lower jaw. Above and in front of Meckel's cartilage and running into the ramus of the mandible is the condylar cartilage. C, condylar cartilage; M, Meckel's cartilage; R, ramus of mandible; T, temporalis muscle. × 8. (*By courtesy of Prof H. J. J. Blackwood.*)

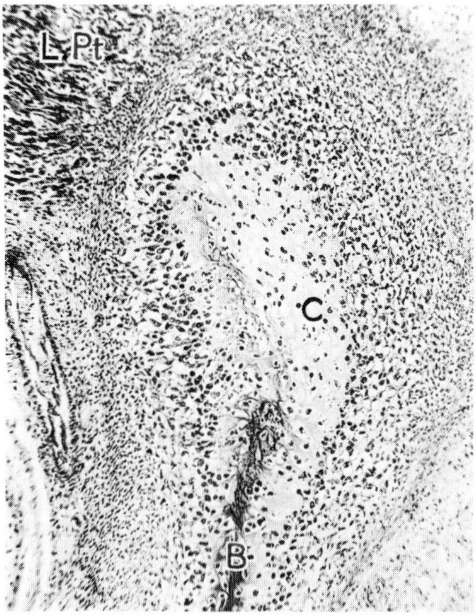

Fig. 78 First appearance of the secondary cartilage in the condyle of the mandible. (**B**) bone; (**C**) secondary cartilage; (**L Pt**) lateral pterygoid muscle. Coronal section of human fetus of 48 mm C.R. length. × 77.

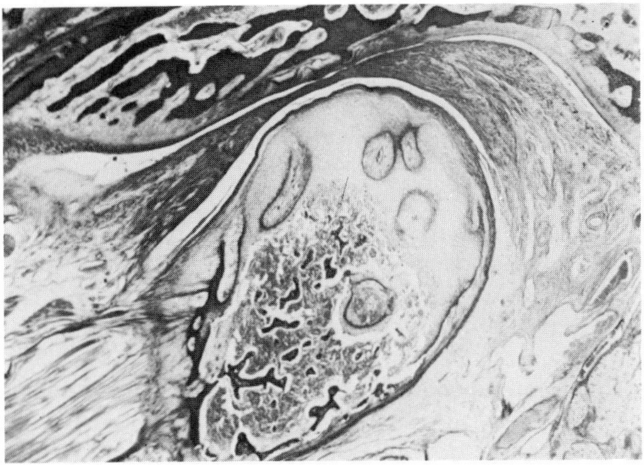

Fig. 79 Sagittal section through the mandibular joint of human fetus of 210 mm C.R. length (seventh month). The condylar cartilage is reduced to a zone beneath the articular surface. A number of vascular canals are present in the cartilage. Note the already dense fibrous structure of the articular disc apart from its most posterior part. × 12.

week). The further growth of these processes is modified by the appearance of secondary cartilages.

The secondary cartilages. These cartilages, which occur at various sites in the region of membrane bone formation, are described as secondary or accessory, since they are not part of and have no connection with the primary cartilaginous skeleton (to which Meckel's cartilage belongs). They also differ in their behaviour and histological appearance from the typical hyaline cartilage of which the primary cartilaginous skeleton is composed. The secondary cartilages increase in size by the proliferation and transformation of the cells of the thick layer of fibrocellular tissue which covers them. These cartilages have less intercellular matrix than hyaline cartilage.

The condylar cartilage. In the mandible there are three main sites of secondary cartilage formation. The largest and first of these to appear

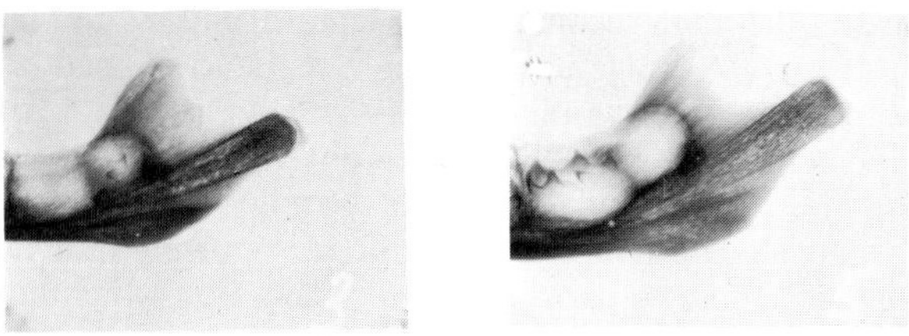

A B

Fig. 80 Radiographs of the mandible. (A) Five months fetal life. (B) At birth. In both jaws the bone which has replaced the condylar cartilage is seen as a cone-shaped area in the ramus. (*By courtesy of Dental Record.*)

is the condylar cartilage, and it is of great importance in the growth of the mandible. It first appears at about the 50 mm C.R. stage (twelfth week). At this stage it is seen as a fringe of cartilage on the superior and lateral aspects of the bone in the condylar process, which merges on one side into this bone and on the other into the fibrocellular layer which delimits the condylar region (Fig. 78). Through additions from the cells of this covering layer of fibrocellular tissue, the cartilage soon forms a cone-shaped mass which not only occupies the whole of the condylar process but reaches forward and downward into the ramus as far as the level of the mandibular foramen. The cartilage in the anterior older part of the tissue begins to show endochondral ossification. This continues until, by the fifth month of fetal life, the only area of cartilage left unresorbed is a zone immediately beneath the proliferating tissue of the condylar articular surface (Fig. 79). Thus in the fifth month of fetal life the original cone of cartilage is largely replaced by bony trabeculae, which run through the ramus and contrast strongly with the membrane bone of the ramus (Fig. 80).

The zone of cartilage left beneath the articular surface of the condyle persists throughout not only the whole fetal period but until at least the end of the second decade (Fig. 81). During this period the thickness of the zone of cartilage gradually diminishes as the proliferative activity of the cells of its covering fibrocellular layer grows less, until eventually the cartilage disappears and the replacing bone forms the whole of the condyle. Since the cartilage remains during the whole of the normal growth period it increases the length of the mandible throughout that time. By the fifth month of fetal life large vascular canals have appeared in the condylar cartilage; these are still present at birth. They are probably related to the nutritive requirements of the rapidly growing cartilage (Fig. 79).

Other secondary cartilages. The coronoid cartilage forms a strip along the anterior border and summit of the coronoid process. It first appears about the 80 mm C.R. stage. The cartilage is covered superficially by a thick fibrocellular layer and rests on the membrane bone below. All trace of the cartilage has disappeared long before birth.

The third of the main secondary cartilages of the mandible appears after the 100 mm C.R. stage at the symphyseal end of each half of the bony mandible. The two symphyseal cartilages are separated from each other by the connective tissue of the symphysis, the cells of which add to the cartilages. These cartilages enable the mandible to grow in width while they persist. The symphyseal cartilage is entirely independent of Meckel's cartilage and its perichondrium. The union which takes place at the symphysis between the two halves of the mandible shortly after birth obliterates them so that they take no further part in the growth of the mandible.

At birth the mandible, though perfectly recognisable as such, differs in several respects from the adult bone. The chief differences are the

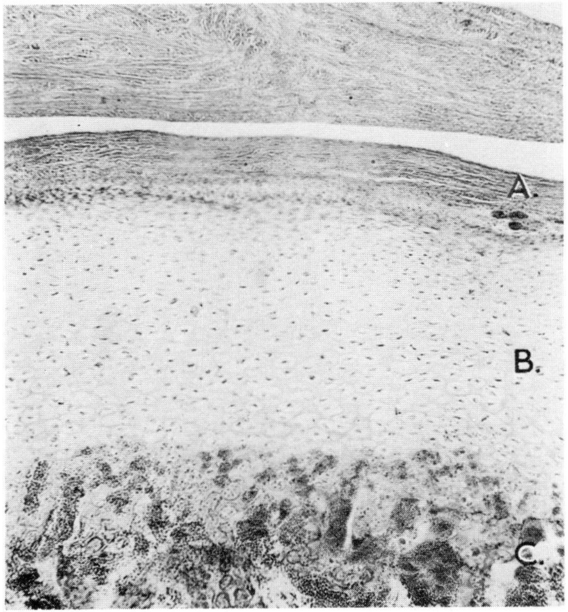

Fig. 81 Mandibular condyle and articular disc at birth. (A.) Layer of fibrocellular perichondrial tissue forming the articular surface of the condyle. (B) Zone of secondary cartilage. (C) Area of resorption of the cartilage and replacement by bone. × 80.

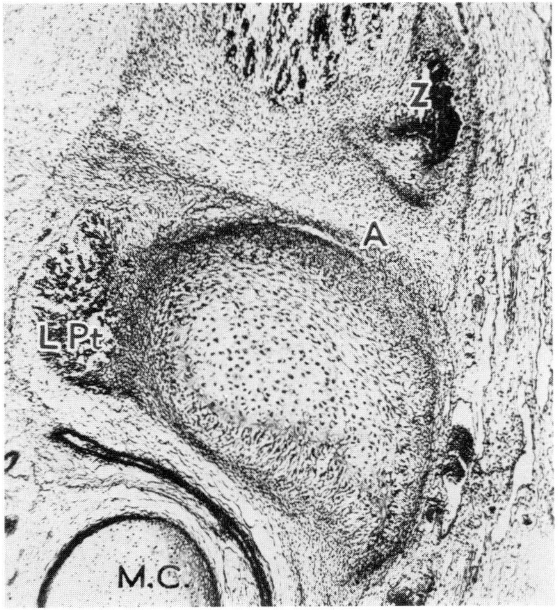

Fig. 82 Developing mandibular joint. The lower joint cavity has just started to appear. (A) articular disk; (L Pt) lateral pterygoid muscle; (M.C.) Meckel's cartilage; (Z) zygomatic arch. Coronal section. Human fetus of 57 mm C.R. length (approx. 12 weeks). × 60.

wide mandibular angle, and the small size of the ramus compared with the body (Fig. 132). The chin is usually poorly developed at birth. Much of its growth takes place after puberty. Its function appears to be that of a strengthening of the weakest part of the arch of the mandible, replacing in human evolution the simian shelf (see p. 394).

DEVELOPMENT OF THE TEMPORO-MANDIBULAR JOINT

The temporo-mandibular joint is first indicated by the growth of the tissue condensation of the developing mandible, which everywhere precedes ossification, towards a corresponding condensation in the temporal region. The mandibular condensation maps out the shape of the condyle. At this stage the mandibular and temporal elements of the joint are still separated by a wide interval. The closer approximation of the mandible to the temporal region is brought about by the development of the secondary cartilage in the condylar process. By the rapid growth of the cartilage the previously wide interarticular interval is largely obliterated. The only intervening tissue left is a strip of dense tissue immediately above the upper surface of the condyle. This tissue appears at the same time as the condensation for the condyle and it is connected to the lateral pterygoid muscle from its first appearance. The strip of tissue becomes the articular disc (Fig. 82). The formation of the joint cavities above and below this strip of tissue occurs as the condyle becomes approximated to the temporal element of the joint. Joint cavity development is virtually complete between the 65 and 70 mm C.R. stages. The cavities continue to increase in size with the growth of the condyle and of the articular fossa. The articular eminence is hardly apparent at birth and only begins to attain its typical form after the establishment of the deciduous dentition. Small areas of secondary cartilage appear in the temporal region. They appear later than the condylar cartilage and disappear before birth.

DEVELOPMENT OF THE MAXILLA

The maxilla proper (excluding the premaxilla) is developed in the maxillary process of the mandibular arch. Like the mandible its first appearance is as a membranous ossification, but unlike the mandible its further development and growth are little affected by the appearance of secondary cartilage. Ossification in the maxilla commences slightly later than in the mandible, about the 18 mm C.R. stage. The centre of ossification first appears in a band of fibrocellular tissue which lies to the outer side of the cartilage of the nasal capsule, and immediately lateral to and slightly below the infraorbital nerve where it gives off its anterior superior alveolar (dental) branch. The ossification centre lies above that part of the lamina from which develops the enamel organ of the canine tooth germ. From this centre ossification spreads backward towards the developing zygomatic bone below the orbit, and forward in front of the anterior superior alveolar nerve below the terminal part of the infraorbital nerve towards the developing premaxilla. At this stage the forming bone takes the shape of a curved strip, arranged vertically with the convex side directed medially (Fig. 83). From the anterior extension there develops the upward directed frontal process which, with a corresponding process of the premaxilla, forms the frontal process of the adult bone. The developing facial and frontal processes of the premaxilla and maxilla rapidly unite with one another so that from an early stage no suture appears between them on the face.

Early in development the developing maxilla forms a bony trough for the infraorbital nerve and, by downward growth, an outer alveolar plate in relation to the canine and deciduous molar tooth germs. The maxilla continues to grow mainly upward, downward, and backward and with the development of a palatal process also spreads towards the midline

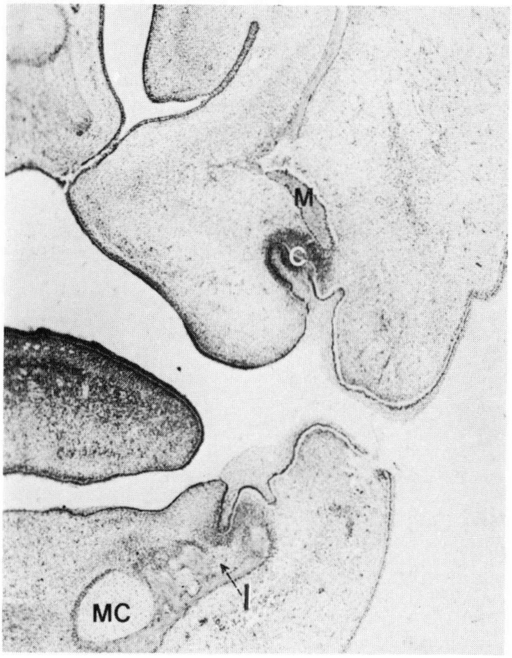

Fig. 83 Coronal section through developing mandible and maxilla at the level of the upper deciduous canine tooth germ. In the lower jaw the bone forms a shallow trough for the incisive nerve and medially has spread around part of Meckel's cartilage. In the upper jaw the palatal process is just coming into contact with the nasal septum. (I) incisive nerve. Human fetus of 27 mm. C.R. length (approx. 8 weeks). (C) deciduous canine; (M) developing maxilla; (MC) Meckel's cartilage. × 30.

in the substance of the anterior part of the united palatal folds. About the 27 mm C.R. stage a mass of secondary cartilage appears in the zygomatic process, and by its proliferation for a time adds considerably to the bulk of this part of the maxilla. This area of cartilage is still present at 40 mm (Fig. 84). During this period the palatal process extends backward; at the union of palatal process and the main part of the developing maxilla a large mass of bone is produced. From this region, on the inner side of the dental lamina and tooth germs, the medial alveolar plate develops somewhat later than the lateral alveolar plate (Fig. 85). The trough of bone thus formed is still later divided by septa into alveoli, as happens in the mandible. Small areas of secondary cartilage may develop along the growing margins of the alveolar plates as in the mandible, and in the middle line of the developing hard palate between the two palatal processes.

The fate of the nasal capsule. The nasal capsule is the primary skeleton of the upper face (Fig. 45) and therefore analogous to Meckel's cartilage in the lower part of the face. In the upper portion of the lateral wall of the cartilage the facial part of the ethmoid bone develops, and in the upper and back parts of the septal cartilage the perpendicular part of the ethmoid develops. The two portions of the ethmoid are united after birth by the ossification of the cribriform plate in the roof of the capsule. In the lower portions of the lateral walls of the capsule the

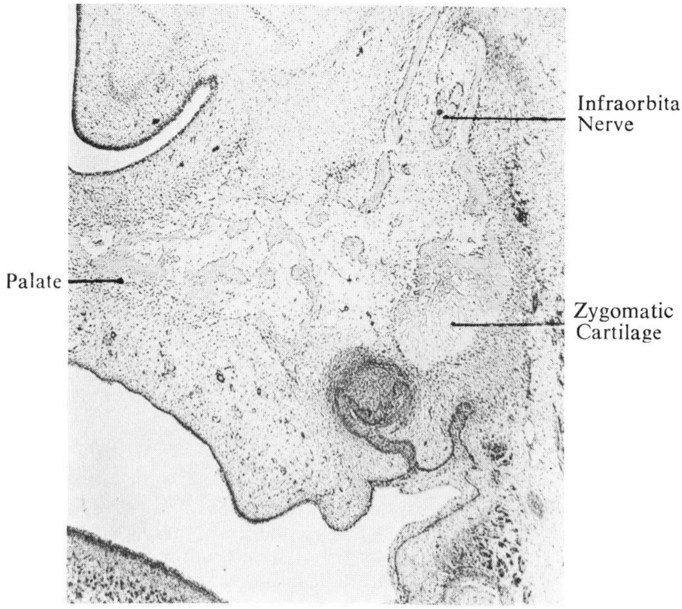

Fig. 84 Developing maxilla. Coronal section of human fetus of 40 mm C.R. length at the level of the upper first deciduous molar tooth germ. ×40.

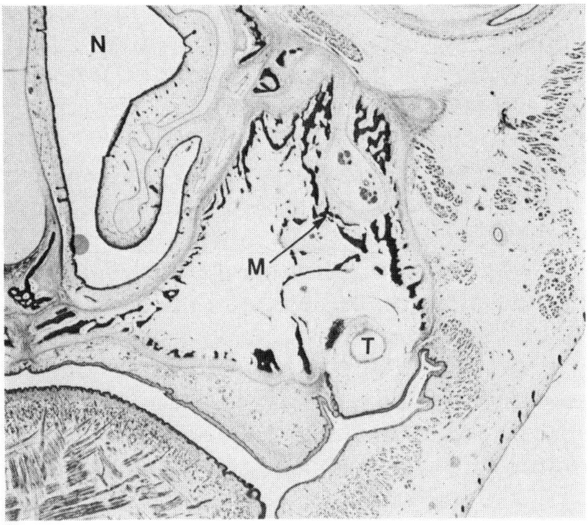

Fig. 85 Coronal section of human fetus of 100 mm C.R. length showing developing maxilla. M, developing maxilla; N, nasal cavity, T, enamel organ of developing tooth.

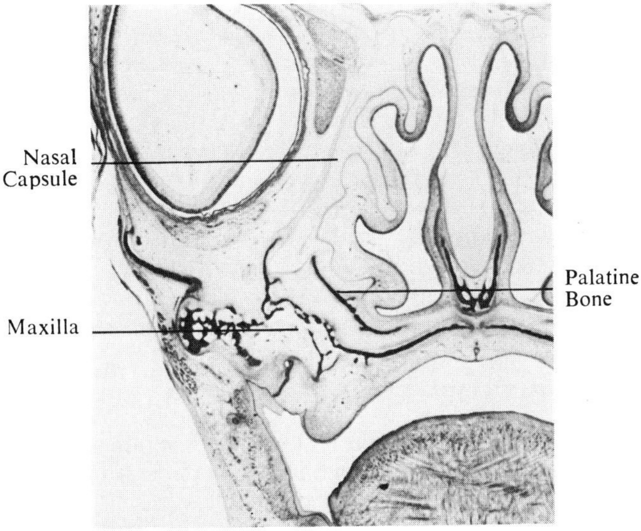

Fig. 86 Coronal section of the head of a human fetus of 70 mm C.R. length (approx. 13 weeks) showing the relationship of the developing palatine bone to the nasal capsule and the maxilla. × 10.

inferior turbinate bones (conchae) develop. The intermediate region of the capsule between the facial ethmoid and inferior turbinate atrophies, and it is in this region that the maxillary sinus extends outwards from the nasal cavity to invade the maxillary bone. The front of the nasal septum remains cartilaginous throughout life.

The maxillary sinus. The maxillary sinus first appears about the fourth month of fetal life as a small out-pocketing of the mucosa from the lateral wall of the nasal cavity. It is at first separated from the developing maxilla by the cartilage of the nasal capsule and only comes into direct relationship with the bone after the cartilage has atrophied. In its gradual extension the sinus comes into relation with the maxilla above the level of the palatal process and hollows out the interior of the bone, so separating its upper or orbital surface from its lower dental region. At birth, however, these parts are still close together, and it is only very gradually that the maxilla increases in height with an associated increase in the size of the sinus. The final height of the maxilla is not reached until near the time of the completed eruption of the permanent teeth. The sinus may increase in size, however, during adult life by extension into the alveolar process.

COMPARISON OF MANDIBULAR AND MAXILLARY DEVELOPMENT

Both bones commence as centres of ossification in close relation to a nerve at a place of bifurcation; and in close relation to elements of the cartilaginous facial skeleton. Both bones have neural and alveolar elements; both develop secondary cartilages in their backward extensions. Whereas the condylar cartilage, however, remains active as a growth centre for a long period in relation to the mandibular joint, the zygomatic cartilage of the maxilla is restricted in its appearance and activity to a limited period of fetal life and is related to the suture between it and the zygomatic bone. The maxilla has no muscular processes and the mandible no palatal process. In its growth the maxilla depends upon surface deposition and growth at the sutures at which it articulates with adjacent bones; the mandible depends for its growth on surface deposition and the replacement of cartilage by bone.

DEVELOPMENT OF THE PREMAXILLA

The premaxilla is formed in the region of the junction of the maxillary and fronto-nasal processes, though it is impossible to decide to what extent each of these processes contribute to the region in which the premaxilla develops since they have fused and so lost their identity before bone formation commences.

At seven weeks of age a separate centre of ossification has appeared for the premaxilla. This, however, retains its separate identity for only a very short period for during the eighth week union takes place with the maxillary ossification. In this way a single mass of bone, which may be described as the maxillary corpus, is early produced on each side. Slightly later two distinct frontal processes arise from this corpus, one from the premaxillary element and the other from the original maxillary part. For some time a hiatus remains between these two processes, but by 15 weeks the gap has disappeared on the facial aspect. A heavy trabecularised network of bone appears on the labial aspect of the canine alveolus which spreads and fuses with the underlying frontal processes. From the premaxillary part of the corpus arise the alveolar processes which surround the developing incisor tooth germs.

This complex and rapidly altering pattern of development explains much of the great diversity of views that have been expressed on the ossification of the premaxilla in man.

Though on the facial aspect all trace of union between the maxilla and premaxilla has disappeared before birth, on the palatal aspect the suture between the premaxilla and maxilla can still be seen until after birth extending from the region of the incisive foramen forward to the alveolar process between the canine and lateral incisor.

DEVELOPMENT OF THE PALATINE BONE

The palatine bone develops in a fibrocellular condensation (membranous ossification) on the medial (inner) side of the cartilaginous nasal capsule. Ossification commences in the seventh to eighth week of fetal life in the region of the tuberosity in close relation to the descending palatine nerves. Ossification extends upwards as the vertical plate and horizontally as the palatal process. By the end of the second month (30 mm C.R. length) all the processes of the bone are visible. At first the vertical plate of the palatine bone is separated from the maxilla by the back part of the lateral wall of the nasal capsule (Fig. 86). With atrophy of this part of the cartilage the vertical plate of the growing palatine bone comes to overlap the inner side of the nasal surface of the maxillary bone and helps to form the medial wall of the maxillary sinus.

Clinical considerations. In cases of facial clefts the later developing bones fail to unite or meet one another so long as the clefts persist. If teeth do not develop the alveolar processes are not formed. Bilateral failure of growth of the condylar cartilages leads to gross underdevelopment of the lower jaw. Unilateral growth failure produces a marked asymmetry of the lower part of the face. Underdevelopment or even absence of the maxillary air sinuses does not appear to affect the size of the maxillae.

BIBLIOGRAPHY

Baume, L. J. (1962). Ontogenesis of the human temporo-mandibular joint. I. Development of the condules. *J. dent. Res.* **41**, 1327.

Blackwood, H. J. J. (1965). Vascularization of the condylar cartilage of the human mandible. *J. Anat. Lond.* **99**, 55.

Coleman, R. D. (1965). Development of the rat palate. *Anat. Rec.* **151**, 107.

Kraus, B. S. & Decker, J. D. (1960). The prenatal inter-relationships of the maxilla and premaxilla in the facial development of man. *Acta Anat.* **40**, 278.

Moffett, B. C. (1957). The prenatal development of the human temporomandibular joint. *Contr. Embryol. Carneg. Instn.* **36**, 19.

Noback, C. R. & Moss, M. L. (1953). The topology of the human premaxillary bones. *Amer. J. phys. Anthrop.* **6** (N.S.), 181.

Sperber, G. H. (1976) *Cranio-facial Embryology*. 2nd ed. Bristol: Wright.

Symons, N. B. B. (1952). The development of the human mandibular joint. *J. Anat. Lond.* **86**, 326.

Wood, N. K., Wragg, L. E., Stuteville, O. H. & Oglesby, R. J. (1969). Osteogenesis of the human upper jaw: Proof of the non-existence of a separate pre-maxillary centre. *Archs. oral Biol.* **14**, 1331.

Yuodelis, R. A. (1966). The morphogenesis of the human temporomandibular joint and its associated structures. *J. dent. Res.* **45**, 182.

5. The Later Development of the Teeth

In this chapter a general account is given of the development of the tooth in relation to the surrounding tissues from the beginning of dentine and enamel formation until the crown and root are completed and the tooth has erupted to the occlusal plane. A detailed description of the development of the individual dental and parodontal tissues is given in Chapters 11–16.

The dental follicle. This first appears, early in tooth development, as a cellular condensation of mesodermal origin continuous with the basal part of the dental papilla and surrounding the enamel organ of the tooth germ (Fig. 53). It becomes related to a similar condensation beneath the epithelium of the developing gums which eventually forms the connective tissue layer, the lamina propria, of the oral mucosa. Many of the cells of the dental follicle become fibroblasts and produce a fibrous tissue sac which, when fully formed, encloses the whole tooth germ, both enamel organ and dental papilla. The developing tooth is thus suspended within the fibrous compartment which is attached to a localised region of the oral mucous membrane (Fig. 87). In this way each tooth germ in each of the dental arches is maintained in constant relationship to the oral mucosa throughout the period of growth of the mouth cavity and jaws, and, furthermore, each developing tooth is kept in relation to the region of the mouth cavity into which it later erupts (Fig. 88).

The collagen fibres of the follicular sac at first run in a circumferential manner around the tooth term and there is very little attachment to the adjacent alveolar bone. When root formation commences the fibres in this region become reorientated to form the periodontal membrane and become firmly embedded in the alveolar bone and in the cement covering the developing root of the tooth (Fig. 227).

The base of the follicle, which is related to, and supports, the dental papilla, is pierced by the vessels and nerves entering and leaving the developing pulp. Other vessels run in the substance of the follicle and form an inner capillary plexus in relation to the external enamel epithelium, and an outer plexus, which develops between the surface of the follicle and the adjacent alveolar bone.

There is some difference of opinion as to whether the dental follicle is represented solely by the investing layer of tissue which is applied to the outer surface of the enamel organ and dental papilla or by the whole of the tissue intervening between the developing tooth-germ and

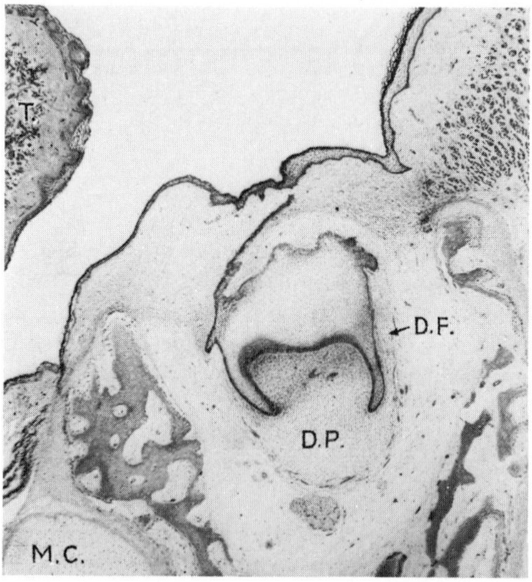

Fig. 87 Developing tooth germ. Enamel organ at the bell stage. Coronal section of deciduous lower first molar from human fetus of 95 mm C.R. length (approx. 16 weeks). (D.F.) dental follicle; (D.P.) dental papilla; (M.C.) Meckel's cartilage; (T.) tongue. ×28.

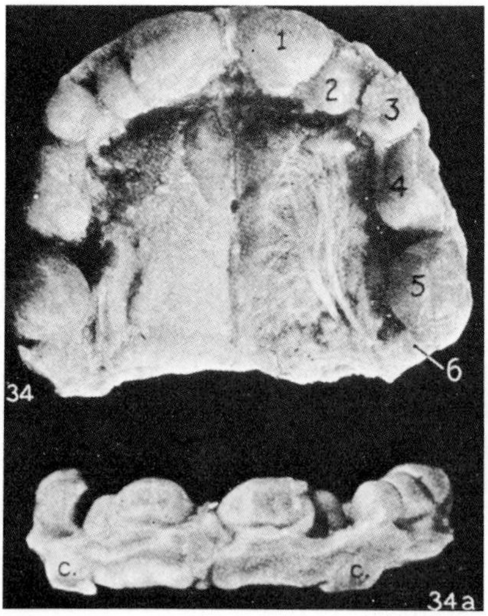

Fig. 88 Upper surface of palate of fetus of 26½ weeks, 231 mm C.R. length, showing arrangement of dental follicles displayed by removal of all the hard parts. (1) Central incisor dental follicle, (2) lateral incisor, (3) canine, (4) first molar, (5) second molar, (6) first permanent molar. (34a) shows the same specimen from the front. (West, 1925. *Contrib. Embryol.*, Washington, Carnegie Inst. *By courtesy of Dental Board of United Kingdom.*)

the surrounding alveolar bone (Fig. 87). Although a well defined investing layer can be distinguished at the early stages of tooth development, by the later part of fetal life this distinction becomes difficult to make. The fibrous sac which constitutes the dental follicle then would appear to comprise the whole of the tissue between developing tooth and the alveolar bone.

Alveoli. At first each deciduous tooth germ developing within its follicle is quite independent of the growing bone of the jaw and has no firm attachment to it. With further development the bone becomes built up on the outer and inner surfaces of the follicles of the deciduous teeth so that these come to occupy a trough of bone. Later, transverse partitions of bone subdivide the trough into a series of small compartments or alveoli, one for each developing tooth (Figs. 76, 132). Superficially each of these alveoli is covered over by the oral mucous membrane, to which the follicles are attached.

Meanwhile the dental follicle has developed its inner and outer vascular plexus. The inner plexus lies between the follicle and the external enamel epithelium and is concerned with the nutrition of the enamel organ and with enamel formation. The outer plexus lies on the surface of the follicle and is concerned with resorption of the bony alveolus, which is necessary to enlarge the bony cavity so as to make room for the growing tooth germ.

Formation of dentine and enamel begins in the deciduous tooth germs at four to six months of fetal life and continues relatively uninterrupted until all the enamel and the coronal part of the dentine have

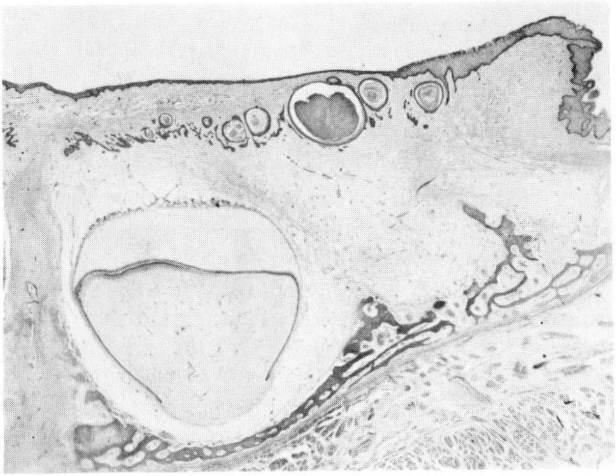

Fig. 89 Coronal section of lower jaw through developing deciduous central incisor. Between the developing tooth and the oral epithelium is the disintegrating dental lamina which shows a number of cyst-like masses. Human fetus of 210 mm C.R. length. × 12.

been laid down. This stage is not reached until some time after birth and varies with the particular tooth (see Table 1, p. 122). The crowns of the deciduous teeth having reached their full dimensions, a short period of quiescence occurs during which no further tooth substance is formed until eruption begins. The comparable phase in the development of the permanent dentition is more prolonged.

After dentine and enamel formation has started in the deciduous tooth germs, the dental lamina begins to disintegrate so that only remnants of it are left in the tissue between the crowns of the deciduous teeth and the oral epithelium. Some of these remnants are capable of proliferating and produce small epithelial masses, the so-called glands of Serres. Most of the epithelial masses degenerate and form globular structures composed of concentric layers of cornified looking material. These have variously been called epithelial pearls or cell nests (Fig. 89). Some of these structures may proceed to cyst formation.

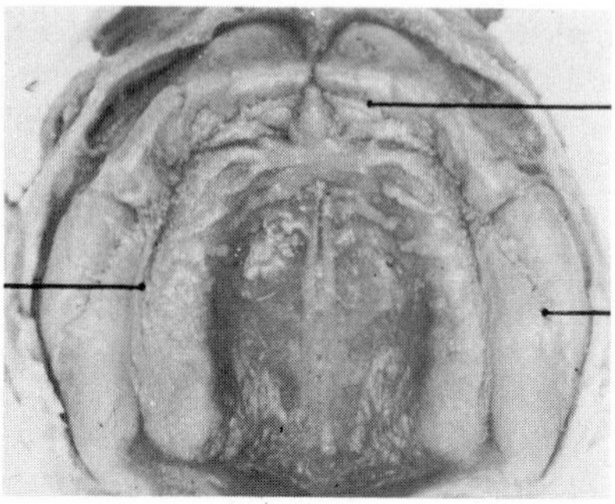

Fig. 90 Upper jaw and palate of human fetus of 225 mm C.R. length (middle of seventh month). The gum pads have fundamentally the same arrangement as at birth. Twice the natural size.

When the tooth germs for the permanent successional teeth first appear in fetal life they are lodged in the same follicles as their deciduous predecessors. This arrangement is maintained until the deciduous teeth begin to erupt when the permanent teeth form follicles of their own which later lie in bony cavities known as crypts (Figs. 91, 92).

Gum pads. During fetal development the oral mucous membrane of the gums becomes greatly thickened so as to produce pads of gum in both upper and lower jaws (Fig. 90). The gum pads cover the alveoli containing the unerupted deciduous teeth and are marked out into segments by transversely running grooves, each segment corresponding to an underlying deciduous tooth and its follicle. This arrangement is present at birth and persists until the deciduous teeth begin to appear in the mouth cavity. The gum pads are bounded lingually by a linear depression, the dental groove (Fig. 90). This corresponds to the place of origin of the epithelial ingrowth, which gives rise to the enamel organs

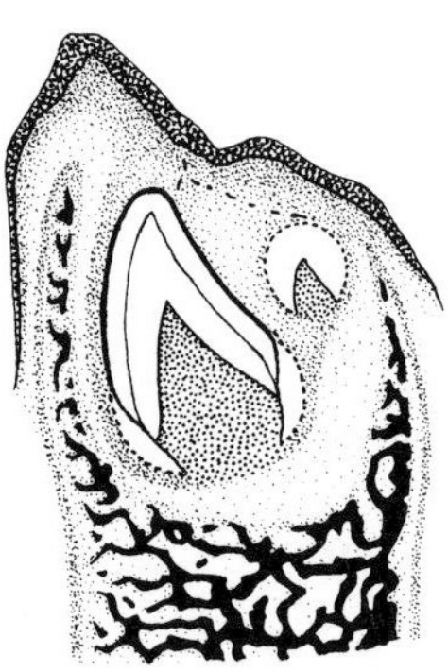

Fig. 91.

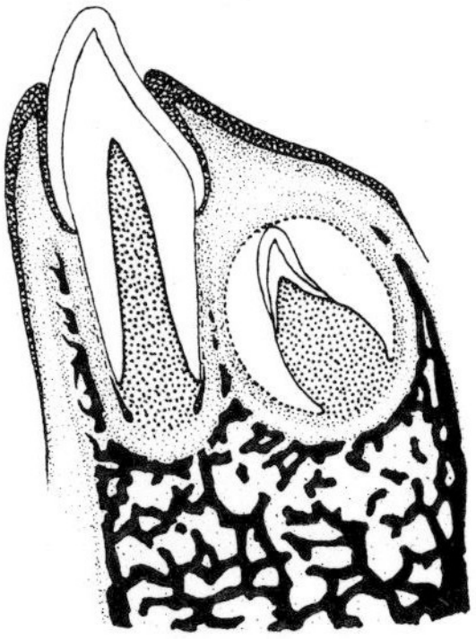

Fig. 92

Fig. 91 Diagrammatic illustration of a sagittal section through the lower jaw of a child at birth showing the relationship between a deciduous incisor and the tooth germ for its permanent successor. At this stage both share the same alveolus and follicle. The crown of the deciduous tooth is largely completed; dentine and enamel formation has not begun in the permanent tooth.

Fig. 92 Diagrammatic illustration of a sagittal section through the lower jaw of a child of about seven months showing the relationship between an erupting deciduous incisor and its developing permanent successor. As the deciduous tooth erupts a separate follicle and crypt begin to form for the permanent tooth, in which dentine and enamel formation has commenced. The root of the deciduous incisor is only partly formed and Hertwig's sheath is still active.

of the teeth (Fig. 62). In the upper jaw there is an additional groove, lingual to the dental groove; this is the gingival groove which marks off the gingiva from the palate proper (Figs. 90, 113).

When the jaws of the newly born child are closed there is usually contact between the gum pads of the two jaws in the molar region and a space left between them at the front of the mouth through which the tongue may protrude.

Gubernacular cords and crypts. As the deciduous teeth begin to erupt, the successional permanent teeth, which until that time are lodged in the same dental follicles as their predecessors, gradually acquire separate follicles (Figs. 93, 95).These gain a separate attachment to the oral mucous membrane through strands or cords of fibrous tissue known as the gubernacular cords. The permanent molars developing at the back of the mouth also have their follicles related to the oral mucous membrane by gubernacular cords. Hence each tooth of both the deciduous and permanent series develops within its own fibrous sac or follicle and is maintained, by this follicle, in its proper relationship to the other units of the dentition and to the mouth cavity.

At the same time as the successional permanent teeth develop dental follicles distinct from those of their predecessors they become lodged in separate bony cavities (Fig. 135).The bone of the jaw grows around each follicle to produce a bony cavity, the crypt. The crypt is, however, not complete as there is an opening in its roof through which the follicle of the tooth germ communicates with, and is attached to, the oral mucous membrane by the gubernacular cord (Figs. 93, 95). After the deciduous teeth have erupted into the mouth cavity the gubernacular cords lie in bony canals which pass from the crypts of the permanent teeth to the surface of the alveolar bone on the lingual aspect of the

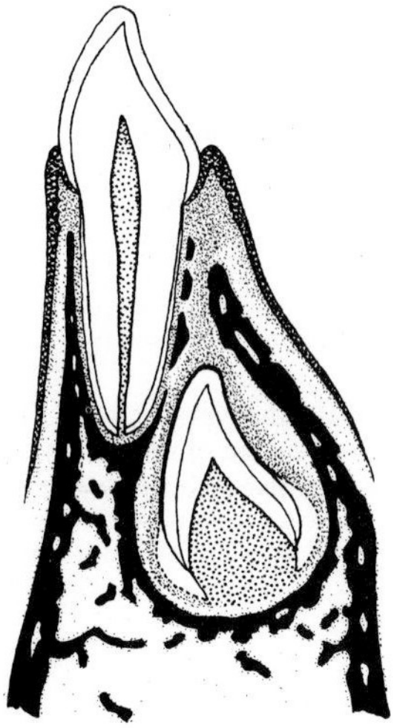

Fig. 93

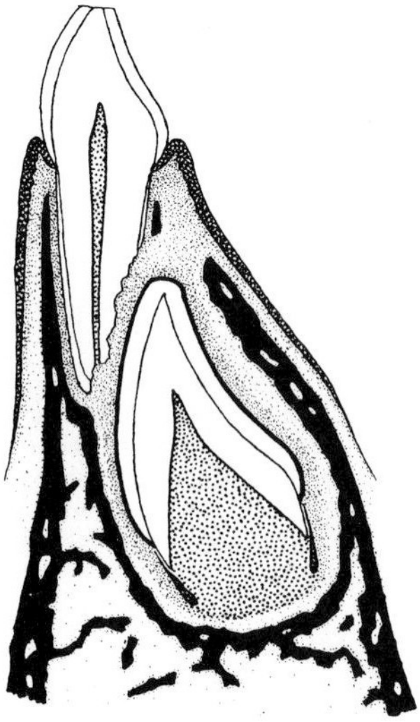

Fig. 94

Fig. 93 Diagrammatic illustration of a sagittal section through the lower jaw of a child of two and a half years showing the relationship between a fully erupted deciduous incosor and its permanent successor. At this stage the deciduous tooth is contained in a bony socket. The crown of the permanent incisor is largely formed and is contained in a fully formed crypt.

Fig. 94 Diagrammatic illustration of a sagittal section through the lower jaw of a child of about seven years showing the relationship between a deciduous incisor and the replacing permanent incisor. With the beginning of the eruption of the permanent tooth the bone forming the roof of its crypt and part of the root of the deciduous tooth have been removed by resorption.

deciduous teeth (Figs. 93, 95, 109); in the case of the premolars, however, the openings of their gubernacular canals are frequently found within the socket of the corresponding deciduous molar. Each permanent molar tooth as it develops in turn is also lodged in a crypt situated in the back part of the upper and the lower alveolar processes (Figs. 133, 135, 138). During tooth eruption the gubernacular cords decrease in length but increase in thickness, producing a widening of their canals (Figs. 93, 94). In addition the gubernacular tissue becomes less dense.

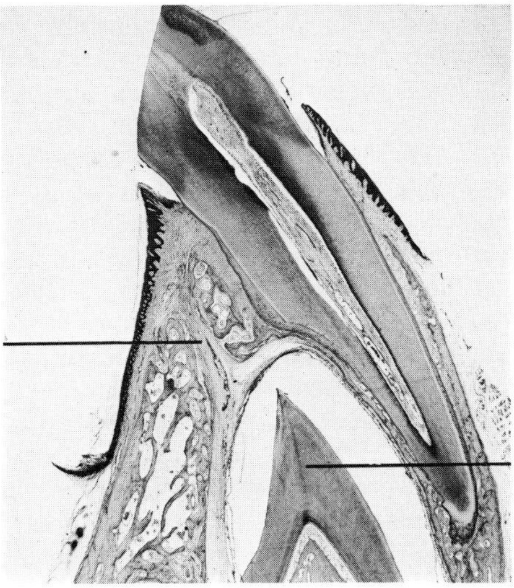

Fig. 95 Section through a functioning deciduous tooth and its underlying permanent successor in a Rhesus monkey. Lingual to the deciduous tooth the gubernacular canal passes from the roof of the crypt for the permanent tooth towards the surface of the alveolar bone. Epithelial remnants of the dental lamina are present in the substance of the gubernacular cord. ×7. (*By courtesy of Dr R. Sprinz.*)

TOOTH ERUPTION

It should be clearly understood that the process of eruption involves not only the actual emergence of a tooth into the mouth cavity but the total movements whereby the tooth is carried from its position in alveolus or crypt towards the mouth, and after appearing in the mouth cavity is brought into and maintained in occlusion with the opposing teeth.

The mechanism of tooth eruption involves a number of correlated processes including pulpal growth, root formation, periodontal membrane formation, bone deposition and resorption—and much discussion has turned on the relative importance of these factors.

Theories of eruption. There have been a number of theories put forward to account for the eruption of the teeth, the main ones being:

1. Root growth. The crown of the tooth is elevated into the mouth cavity through the thrust provided by the development of the root.
2. Bone growth. Bone deposition beneath the developing tooth at fundus of the socket pushes the tooth towards the mouth.
3. Pulpal proliferation. Cellular division and growth particularly in the basal region of the pulp creates pressure which raises the crown away from the underlying follicle.
4. Tissue fluid or blood pressure. An increase in tissue fluid or blood

pressure within the enclosed system formed by alveolar bone, follicular tissue and the calcified crown provides the motive force in eruption.

5. Periodontal membrane. Traction from some component of the periodontal membrane pulls the tooth towards the mouth cavity. The traction may be produced by a shortening of the oblique principal fibres as newly formed collagen matures with cross-linking and aggregation. Alternatively the motive force may reside in the movement of the fibroblasts of the periodontal membrane.

The first four theories have in common that they have been held for a long time and postulate a force which pushes the tooth, whereas the fifth is dependent on the pulling force of the periodontal membrane. Many observations have been brought forward to support each of the first four theories, and indeed to casts doubts on each of them. The observations have arisen from (a) clinical practice, e.g. on root length relative to the pre-eruptive position of the tooth or on the amount of root formation in cases of accelerated tooth eruption, from (b) histological studies, e.g. on the number of mitoses in the pulp tissue of erupting teeth or on the amount of fundic bone formation beneath such teeth, and from (c) experimental work. Most of the experimental investigations have been carried out on the continuously growing and erupting incisor of the rat.

In the more recent experiments with the rat incisor the tooth to be operated on is first cut out of occlusion with the opposing incisors and is constantly kept out of occlusion during the experiment. In this way an unimpeded eruption rate for the operated tooth is established which avoids the errors which may result from variations in the rate of attrition through leaving the incisor in occlusion during the conduct of an experiment. Destruction of the growing base of the rat incisor can be carried out to test the root growth and pulp proliferation theories. If the adjacent alveolar bone is also destroyed the closed system required by the tissue fluid or blood pressure theory is interfered with. In another variation of this experimental approach the rat incisor is divided into two and a gap established between the distal and proximal parts. Any movement of the distal part must then be independent of the tissues of the basal region of the tooth.

Drugs which alter the blood pressure or interfere with mitotic activity have been injected into rats with an unimpeded eruption rate of the incisor in order to test the blood pressure and the pulpal proliferation theories respectively.

A considerable body of experimental work provides support for the theory that some component of the periodontal membrane is responsible for tooth eruption. In the rat incisor with an unimpeded eruption rate in which the growing base of the tooth had been destroyed an eruption rate equivalent to that of control animals was found. In transected incisors the distal half showed a normal eruption rate. Without any continuity with a growing base it would seem that this segment could only erupt by virtue of the attached periodontal membrane. There is however residual doubt in that earlier experimental work of a similar kind produced conflicting findings in the eruption rates of the operated teeth.

Apart from the theoretical arguments related to the changes in dimension of maturing collagen fibrils the concept of the periodontal fibres acting as the traction force in tooth eruption appeared to be supported by the findings in the initial work on animals with experimentally induced lathyrism. Collagen formation is disorganised in this disease and consequently it could be anticipated that the eruption rate would be slowed or stopped. In some experiments a slowing in eruption rates was observed but later work has shown no change.

Although the inconclusive results from the experiments on lathyritic animals throw doubts on the concept of the periodontal fibres as the primary factor in producing tooth eruption this does not exclude the possibility that the periodontal fibroblasts may act in such a role. A number of observations on the structure and activity of the mature fibroblasts of the periodontal membrane support this hypothesis. The fibroblasts in the part of the periodontal membrane close to the tooth show numerous microfilaments in organised systems in the peripheral parts of the cells. This is a feature which is common to all motile cells. Moreover these fibroblasts move occlusally at a rate equal to that of the eruption of the tooth, unlike the fibroblasts related to the alveolar bone of the socket which are relatively static. If the periodontal fibroblasts exert a traction effect on the tooth it may be mediated through the periodontal fibres.

It is possible that tooth eruption is brought about by a number of factors possibly acting at different stages in the process. The elimination of one factor in an experimental situation without any consequent effect on the eruption of the tooth does not necessarily mean that this factor is unimportant in the normal situation, for there may be a compensation produced by other factors.

Histological aspects of eruption. Prior to the commencement of dentine and enamel formation the tooth germ grows in all dimensions within its follicle and its expanding bony cavity (alveolus or crypt). When the crown of the tooth is completed the pulp is contained between the calcified crown and the base of the follicle (Fig. 91). As the calcified crown moves away from the base of the follicle on the commencement of eruption the sheath of Hertwig, which previously lay inactive beneath the crown of the tooth, begins to proliferate and initiates root formation (Figs. 92, 96A). During the whole process of active tooth eruption, root formation continues.

As root formation proceeds the more crownward part of Hertwig's sheath disintegrates allowing contact between the follicle and the dentine of the root (Fig. 96A). Development of cementoblasts takes place from undifferentiated follicular cells and these lay down a layer of cement on the surface of the dentine by which follicular collagen fibres

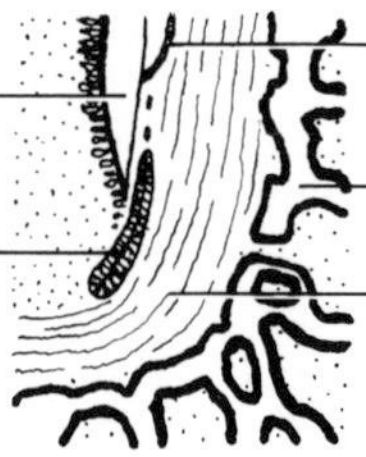

Fig. 96A Diagrammatic illustration of a vertical section of a developing tooth showing early root formation and the beginning of the disintegration of Hertwig's sheath.

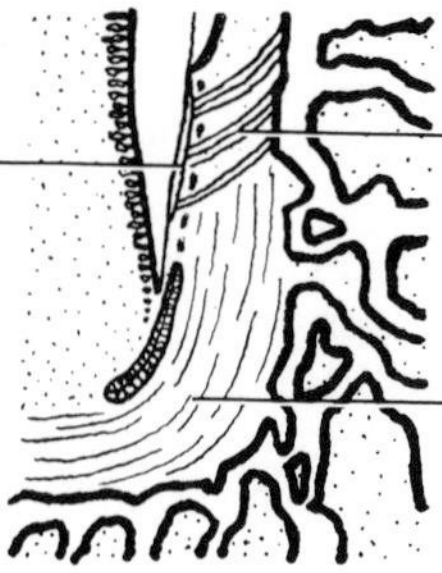

Fig. 96B Diagrammatic illustration of a vertical section of a developing tooth showing somewhat more advanced root formation than in Fig. 96A. A layer of cement has been deposited and the formation of a periodontal attachment has replaced part of the dental follicle.

are attached to the root and so take part in the formation of the periodontal membrane (Fig. 96B). Follicular collagen fibres are also attached to the surrounding alveolar bone by the deposition of new bone. Remnants of the sheath of Hertwig persist in the periodontal membrane and are known as the epithelial debris or rests of Malassez.

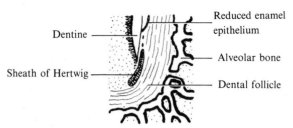

In the case of the deciduous teeth the erupting crown moves through the more superficial part of the follicle and the overlying gum tissue. This process is facilitated by a loosening of the overlying connective tissue produced by an increase in its vascularity and by the presence of the epithelial cell remnants, and little cysts which are derived from the disintegrated dental lamina (Fig. 89). Sometimes a cyst which is larger than normal is produced. This appears between the erupting tooth and the superficial surface of the gum and is called a cyst of eruption. Such cysts usually disappear when the tooth penetrates the gum. In some cases, however, such a cyst becomes abnormally large, and if the crown of the erupting tooth becomes enveloped by the cyst, a dentigerous (tooth containing) cyst is produced. In the case of permanent teeth the roof of the crypt is resorbed as the tooth moves towards the mouth cavity, and the gubernacular canal becomes greatly enlarged as the tooth erupts along the line of the gubernacular cord, which becomes vascular and looser in texture (Figs. 93, 94).

The crown of the erupting tooth is covered by the reduced enamel epithelium derived from the epithelium of the enamel organ. During eruption this approaches and then comes into contact with the overlying epithelium of the gum. Union of the epithelial layers produces an area of epithelial tissue through which the crown of the tooth enters the mouth cavity (Figs. 100, 101).

During tooth eruption the alveolar bone plays only a secondary part in the process. As the tooth moves towards and into the mouth cavity and root formation proceeds (Fig. 97), that part of the follicle between the growing root and the alveolar bone becomes converted into the periodontal membrane (see p. 271). The basal part of the follicle, however, remains and passes beneath the base of the erupting and growing tooth. At the time of emergence of an erupting tooth into the mouth cavity the root is about three-quarters formed. Pulp expansion continues between the calcified crown and root of the tooth and the basal part of the follicle until active eruption ceases and growth of the root is complete. With the conversion of the follicle into the periodontal membrane the alveolus or crypt becomes a tooth socket and the alveolar bone is more closely adapted to the form of the root or roots of the tooth.

If the tooth follicles should, at any time during growth of the teeth and of the jaws, become detached from the gum the tooth germs may lose their developmental connection with the oral mucosa, become buried deeply in the jaws, or erupt in some abnormal position as into the nasal cavity, pterygo-palatine fossa, or beneath the chin. This is much more likely to occur in permanent teeth, due to rupture of the gubernacular cord following fracture of the jaw or as the result of scar tissue formation around the follicle following some infective process.

The process of active eruption should be distinguished from that by which the functional teeth are carried with the growing alveolar bone upwards and forwards in the lower jaw, and downwards and forwards in the upper jaw; the latter process continues for some years after the teeth are brought into occlusion by active eruption.

A form of active eruption may occur even after the teeth have become functional. Where attrition produces a progressive wearing down of the occlusal surfaces the teeth erupt to the extent of the loss of tooth substance.

The reduced enamel epithelium. When the enamel is completely formed it is covered by the shrunken remains of the enamel organ, which henceforth is commonly referred to as the reduced enamel epithelium. It is made up, at this stage, of two layers; an inner, composed of the ameloblasts, and an outer, representing the rest of the enamel organ (Fig. 98). The ameloblasts become considerably reduced in length and in some cases may be cuboidal (Fig. 99). The outer layer is only a few

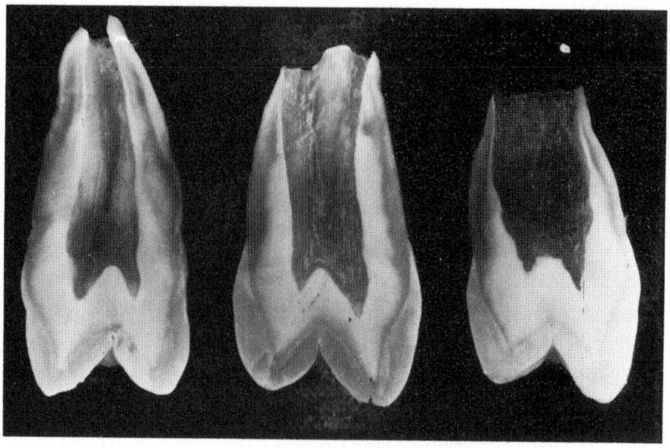

Fig. 97 Recently erupted premolars sectioned vertically to show increasing amounts of root formation.

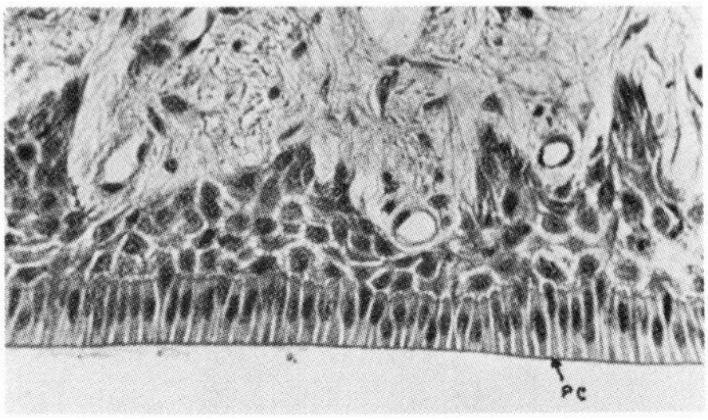

Fig. 98 The enamel epithelium of a permanent molar of a monkey after enamel formation. There are two layers—the reduced ameloblasts and an 'outer layer' composed of squamous type cells. In light microscope pictures such as this there appears to be a cuticle (PC) between the ameloblasts and the enamel. Such a cuticle is not found in electron micrographs. ×205. (*By courtesy of Prof W. D. McHugh and the 'Dental Practitioner'.*)

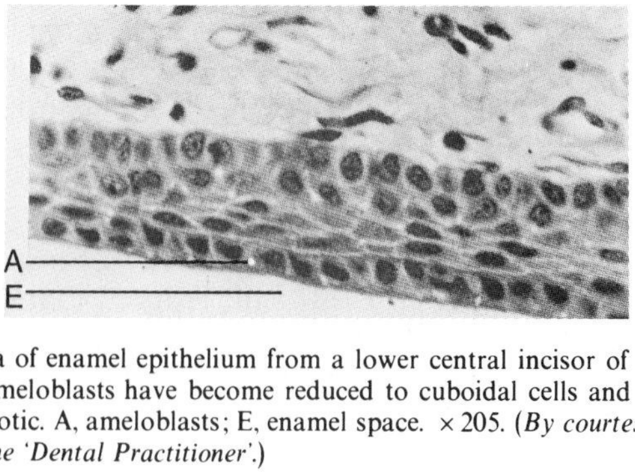

Fig. 99 An area of enamel epithelium from a lower central incisor of a 26-month-old monkey. The ameloblasts have become reduced to cuboidal cells and their nuclei are becoming pyknotic. A, ameloblasts; E, enamel space. ×205. (*By courtesy of Prof W. D. McHugh and the 'Dental Practitioner'.*)

cells thick and since these are polygonal and are interconnected by intercellular bridges they resemble the cells of the stratum spinosum of the oral epithelium.

The reduced enamel epithelium normally covers the whole of the enamel and at the cervical margin is continuous with the epithelial sheath of Hertwig (Fig. 100). During the period when the crown of the tooth lies in its follicle before eruption commences, this epithelial covering prevents the tissues of the follicle from coming into direct contact with the enamel so that normally no cement is deposited on the crown of the tooth.

After eruption of the tooth begins, and as the crown moves towards the oral epithelium, the ameloblasts also assume a polygonal shape and become morphologically indistinguishable from the outer cells of the reduced enamel epithelium.

As the tooth nears the oral epithelium mitotic figures appear in the

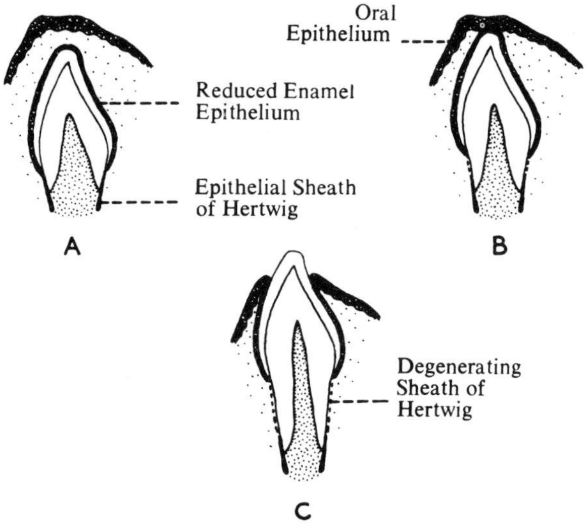

Fig. 100 Diagram to illustrate the eruption of a tooth and the formation of the epithelial attachment. (A) Tooth just before the commencement of eruption. (B) Fusion of the reduced enamel epithelium with the oral epithelium as the tooth nears the mouth cavity. (C) The emergence of the tip of the tooth into the mouth cavity.

outer cells of the reduced enamel epithelium and cellular processes from it reach out towards the oral epithelium.

Epithelial attachment and gingival crevice. When, during the process of eruption, the crown of the tooth reaches the oral mucous membrane, the reduced enamel epithelium fuses with the epithelial layer of the mucous membrane (Figs. 100B, 101). As a result of this fusion the epithelial cells immediately above the tip of the crown of the tooth are cut off from their nutritional supply. Through this area the crown of the tooth emerges into the mouth cavity; and without any bleeding since its pathway is epithelial lined.

Once a part of the tooth has emerged in the mouth cavity the reduced enamel epithelium is known as the epithelial attachment or junctional

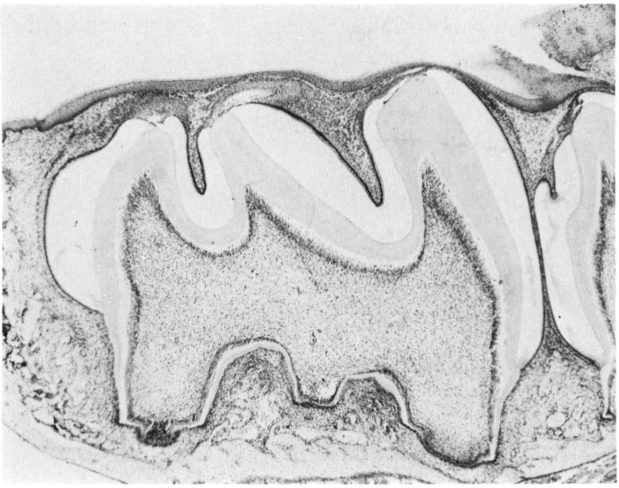

Fig. 101 Sagittal section through the lower jaw of a 17-day-old rat. The crown of the first molar is virtually fully formed and it is about to erupt into the mouth cavity. Over the cusps union of oral and reduced enamel epithelial has already taken place; adjacent to these areas an irregular proliferation of the reduced enamel epithelium has occurred. × 24.

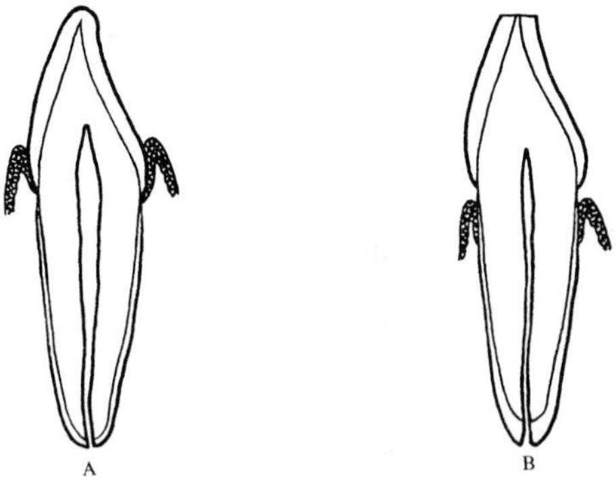

Fig. 102 Diagram to illustrate the altering position of the epithelial attachment at different stages. (A) At the time when the tooth has recently become functional in the mouth cavity. (B) After the tooth has been functional for many years and a loss of tooth substance has taken place due to attrition. The compensating increase in thickness of the cement is also indicated.

epithelium, since it is through it that the surrounding gingival tissues are directly related to the crown of the tooth. Immediately adjacent to the epithelial attachment is a shallow trough, the gingival sulcus or crevice, bounded on one side by the surface of the tooth and on the other by the gingival margin (Fig. 100C). With the continued eruption of the tooth the gingival margin and gingival crevice retreat further rootward on the tooth, leaving progressively more of it uncovered by epithelium.

The gingival migration proceeds at a fairly rapid rate until the tooth reaches the plane of the occlusion and comes into contact with the opposing tooth or teeth. At this stage the gingival margin has reached a level so that about two-thirds to three-quarters of the enamel surface is exposed in the mouth cavity, whereas the remaining one-quarter to one-third is still covered by the epithelial attachment (Fig. 102A).

Even after the tooth has reached the occlusal plane the gingival margin and crevice tend to shift gradually further rootward on the enamel so that eventually they reach the cement-enamel junction. A considerable time before this stage is reached the epithelial attachment commences to proliferate on to the cement so that part of the epithelial attachment is on the enamel and part on the cement. Finally, with the

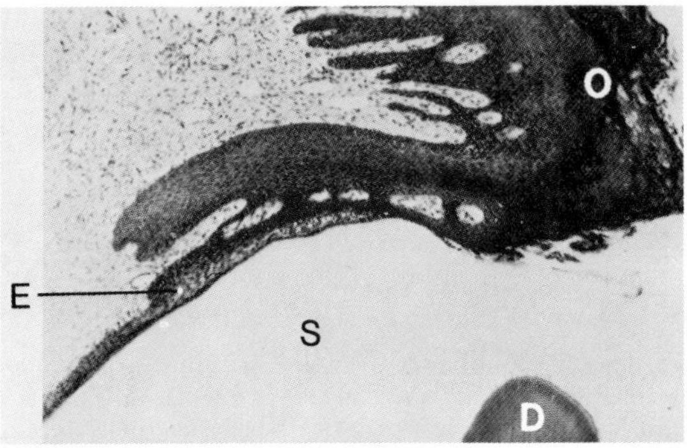

Fig. 103 The tissues over the erupting cusp of a lower first molar of a two-year-old monkey. A large process of oral epithelium can be seen growing down in the connective tissue a little distance from the proliferating outer layers of the enamel epithelium. These fuse to form a gingival cuff. D, dentine; E, enamel epithelium; O, oral epithelium; S, enamel space. × 50. (*By courtesy of Prof W. D. McHugh and the 'Dental Practitioner'.*)

continued rootward shift of the gingival margin and crevice, accompanied by the proliferation of the epithelial attachment on the cement, the stage is reached where not only the whole extent of the epithelial attachment is on the cement but the gingival margin and crevice are also related to the cement, and an area of the root is exposed in the mouth (Fig. 102B).

The process of actual bodily movement of the tooth relative to the tissues of the jaw is referred to as active eruption, whereas in distinction the process whereby the tooth is progressively uncovered by the rootward shift of the epithelial attachment is usually known as passive eruption; a better name would be coronal exposure.

It has been shown that as the tooth emerges into the mouth cells derived from the region of fusion of the oral epithelium and the enamel epithelium grow down around the crown and fuse with the outer cells of the enamel epithelium. The latter cells also show a proliferative activity. The cuff of epithelium so formed spreads gradually in a cervical direction and may replace the epithelial layer which was previously formed by the enamel epithelium alone (Fig. 103).

At the site of junction between the cells of the oral epithelial downgrowth and the cells derived from the outer layer of the reduced enamel epithelium there is a change in the orientation of the cells (Fig. 104). The superficial cell layers of the oral epithelium are arranged parallel to the gingival surface whereas those derived from the reduced enamel epithelium are parallel to the enamel surface and have a 'but-on' arrangement to the gingival surface. This produces a plane of reorientation between the cells of these two epithelial layers. It seems likely that exudation of gingival fluid takes place along this pathway.

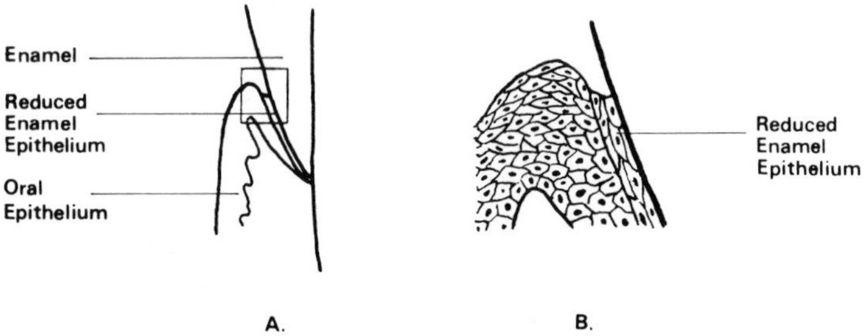

Fig. 104 A. Diagrammatic representation of the region of fusion of oral epithelium and reduced enamel epithelium around a recently erupted tooth. B. Diagram of the boxed area in A as seen in higher magnification, showing the cellular arrangement at the junction between the reduced enamel epithelium and the downgrowth of the oral epithelium.

There has been a great deal of controversy regarding the nature of the relationship of the gingival epithelium to the surface of the tooth. According to some workers there was a true continuity of tissue between the epithelium and the organic matrix of the enamel, whereas in the opinion of others there was merely a physical contact between the epithelium and the enamel surface. The first view entailed the concept of an epithelial attachment between gingiva and crown so that the normal gingival crevice is restricted to a shallow sulcus superficial to the epithelial attachment. In the other case a potential gingival crevice, at least, would extend to the enamel-cement junction.

The original simple concept of an epithelial attachment which has its origin in a developmental union between the reduced enamel epithelium and the organic matrix of the enamel became untenable when it was seen that the reduced enamel epithelium becomes replaced, at least in part, by a downgrowth of squamous cells from the oral epithelium once the tooth has appeared in the mouth cavity. Further evidence of change in this region has been provided by autoradiographic techniques which indicate that cells of the epithelial attachment can migrate rapidly along the tooth surface and that the whole epithelium of the attachment has a rapid turnover rate. Yet the demonstration of hemidesmosomes and a basal lamina on the cells of the epithelium adjacent to the enamel surface clearly points to some form of attachment between epithelium and crown (see p. 192 and Fig. 153).

Anatomical and clinical crowns. Due to the alteration in position of the gingival tissues relative to the tooth, the area of tooth surface exposed in the mouth cavity varies considerably at different stages. In order to avoid confusion the terms anatomical crown and clinical crown are used. The anatomical crown refers to the enamel covered area of the tooth: the clinical crown is that part of the tooth which is exposed in the mouth cavity and which may be greater or less in extent than the anatomical crown according to the stage reached in passive eruption. Two main divisions in the process may be distinguished:

1. Where the bottom of the gingival crevice is on the enamel surface and the epithelial attachment or cuff is either wholly or partly on the enamel surface; the clinical crown is less than the anatomical crown (Fig. 102A).
2. Where the bottom of the gingival crevice is on the cement and the epithelial attachment or cuff is wholly on the cement; the clinical crown is greater than the anatomical crown (Fig. 102B).

Between these two stages there is a short period where the bottom of the gingival crevice is exactly at the enamel-cement junction; the clinical and anatomical crowns are then exactly equal.

The proliferation of epithelium on to the cement is impossible while the gingival, transeptal, and alveolar crest fibres remain intact. There is a difference of opinion as to whether these fibres degenerate as a result of the proliferation of the epithelium or whether the epithelial cells can only proliferate after the collagen fibres have commenced to break down.

Clinical considerations. Where passive eruption (coronal exposure) accompanies active eruption it must be considered as a physiological process whereby the area of the epithelial attachment is kept relatively constant, so that in spite of the active eruption the gingival tissues are kept properly related to the tooth. Thus in cases of early attrition of the teeth, as occurs in primitive races, there is a definite correlation of the two processes. In civilised races a marked passive eruption is often found which is not associated with any attrition once the teeth have reached the occlusal plane. This recession of the gums produces abnormally long clinical crowns, since there is little if any attrition to wear down the occlusal surfaces or incisive edges. It must be considered as abnormal and indeed is accelerated by inflammatory conditions of the gingival tissues.

BIBLIOGRAPHY

Beertsen, W. (1975). Migration of fibroblasts in the periodontal ligament of the mouse incisor as revealed by autoradiography. *Archs. oral Biol.* **20,** 659.

Berkovitz, B. K. B. (1975). Mechanisms of tooth eruption. In *Applied Physiology of the Mouth*, ed. C. L. B. Lavelle. Bristol: Wright.

Berkovitz, B. K. B. & Bass, T. P. (1976). Eruption rates of human upper third molars. *J. dent. Res.* **55,** 460.

Berkovitz, B. K. B., Migdalski, A. & Solomon, M. (1972). The effect of the lathyritic agent amino-acetonitrile on the unimpeded eruption rate in normal and root-resected rat lower incisors. *Archs. oral Biol.* **17,** 1755.

Berkovitz, B. K. B. & Thomas, N. R. (1969). Unimpeded eruption in the root-resected lower incisor of the rat with a preliminary note on root transection. *Archs. oral Biol.* **14,** 771.

Bodegom, J. C. (1969). *Experiments on Tooth Eruption in Miniature Pigs.* Nijmegen: Janssen.

Cahill, D. R. (1969). Eruption pathway formation in the presence of experimental tooth impaction in puppies. *Anat. Rec.* **164,** 67.

Diab, M. A., Stallard, R. E. & Zander, H. A. (1966). The life cycle of the epithelial elements of the developing molar. *Oral Surg.* **22,** 241.

Listgarten, M. A. (1966). Phase-contrast and electron microscopic study of the junction between reduced enamel epithelium and enamel in unerupted human teeth. *Arch. oral Biol.* **11,** 999.

McHugh, W. D. (1961). The development of the gingival epithelium in the monkey. *Dent. Practit.* **11,** 314.

Main, J. H. P. & Adams, D. (1966). Experiments on the rat incisor into the cellular proliferation and blood-pressure theories of tooth eruption. *Arch. oral Biol.* **11,** 163.

Manson, J. D. (1963). A study of bone changes associated with tooth eruption. *Proc. R. Soc. Med.* **56,** 515.

Ness, A. R. (1964). Movement and forces in tooth eruption. In *Advances in Oral Biology*, ed. P. H. Staple. London: Academic Press.

Ness, A. R. (1967). Eruption—A review. In *The Mechanisms of Tooth Support.* Bristol: Wright.

Orban, B., Bhatia, H., Kollar, J. A. & Wentz, F. M. (1956). The epithelial attachment (The attached epithelial cuff). *J. Periodont.* **27,** 167.

Pitaru, S., Michaeli, Y., Zagicek, G. & Weinreb, M. M. (1976). Role of attrition and occlusal contact in the physiology of the rat incisor: IX The part played by the periodontal ligament in the eruptive process. *J. dent. Res.* **55,** 819.

Schroeder, H. E. & Listgarten, M. A. (1971). *Fine structure of the developing epithelial attachment of human teeth.* Vol. 2. Monographs in Developmental Biology. London: Karger.

Scott, J. H. (1948). The development and function of the dental follicle. *Brit. dent. J.* **85,** 193.

Stallard, R. E., Diab, M. A. & Zander, H. A. (1965). The attaching substance between enamel and epithelium—a product of the epithelial cells. *J. Periodont.* **36,** 40.

West, C. M. (1925). The development of the gums and their relationship to the deciduous teeth in the human fetus. *Contr. Embryol. Carneg. Instn.* No. 79, **16,** 25.

6. The Establishment of the Deciduous and Permanent Dentitions

In the preceding chapters a description has been given of the formation of the teeth and their eruption to a functional position in the mouth. This involves for each tooth a period of early development in a cellular state, followed by a period of formation of the hard tissues of the crown, and then by a period of root formation which generally coincides with the eruption of the tooth. In this chapter a consideration is made of the way in which these processes in the individual teeth are timed so as to permit the proper arrangement of the dentition both before and after eruption.

Although the small jaws of the child must accommodate the members of both dentition from fetal life until about seven years this is possible because of the following factors.

1. While the crowns of the deciduous teeth are forming in the jaws the permanent teeth are at the tooth germ stage (Fig. 91).

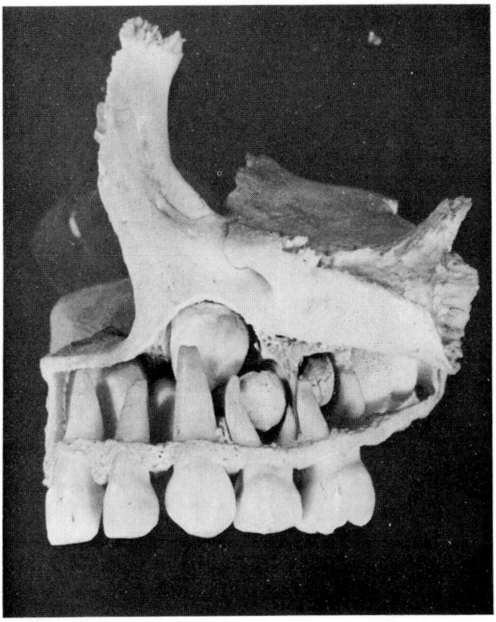

Fig. 105 Left half of upper jaw showing the relationship of the developing permanent teeth to the roots of the functioning deciduous dentition. (*By courtesy of Dr R. Sprinz.*)

Table 1 Chronology of tooth development

Tooth		Tooth germ fully formed	Dentine formation begins	Formation of crown complete	Appearance in mouth cavity	Root complete
Deciduous	Incisors	3–4 months fetal life	4th–6th month fetal life	2–3 months	6–9 months	$1–1\frac{1}{2}$ years after appearance in mouth cavity
	Canines			9 months	16–18 months	
	1st Molars			6 months	12–14 months	
	2nd Molars			12 months	20–30 months	
Permanent	Incisors	30th week fetal life	3–4 months (Upper lateral incisor 10–12 months)	4–5 years	Lower 6–8 years Upper 7–9 years	2–3 years after appearance in mouth cavity
	Canines	30th week fetal life	4–5 months	6–7 years	Lower 9–10 years Upper 11–12 years	
	Premolars	30th week fetal life	$1\frac{1}{2}–2\frac{1}{2}$ years	5–7 years	10–12 years	
	1st Molars	24th week fetal life	Before birth	$2\frac{1}{2}–3$ years	6–7 years	
	2nd Molars	6th month	$2\frac{1}{2}–3$ years	7–8 years	11–13 years	
	3rd Molars	6th year	7–10 years	12–16 years	17–21 years	

Modified from Schour, I. and Massler, M. (1940) and Kraus, B. S. (1959).

2. By the time the crowns of the permanent teeth are forming the deciduous teeth are erupted or erupting (Figs. 92, 93).

3. Since there is a period of about six years between the appearance of each of the permanent molars this allows sufficient time for jaw growth to accommodate the lengthening of the dental arches.

Table 2 Table illustrating the relation in time of the deciduous and permanent dentitions

		Year	
		Birth	
			Appearance of Deciduous Incisors
		1	↓
		2	↓
			Deciduous dentition established
		.	
		.	
		.	
		6	Appearance of 1st Permanent Molar
Period of lengthening of dental arch by the Permanent Molars	Period of replacement of Deciduous dentition by Permanent dentition	7	↓
		.	
		.	
		.	
		.	
		12	
		13	
		.	
		.	
		.	
		17	↓
			Appearance of 3rd Permanent Molar
		18	Permanent dentition established

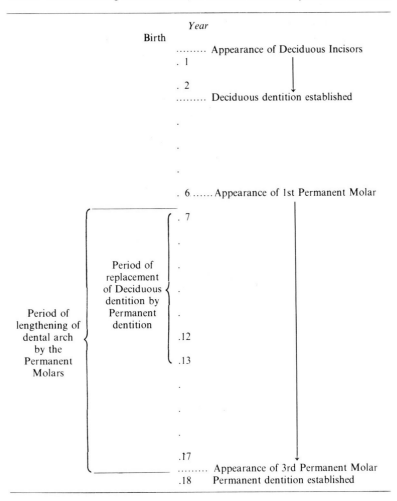

Deciduous teeth. The teeth of the deciduous dentition begin to appear in the mouth cavity from about six months, usually commencing with the lower central incisors. They appear at intervals, the second molar being the last of the dentition to appear, and the whole dentition is

established and functional by two or two and a half years. The order of eruption of the deciduous teeth can be expressed by the formula.

$$I_1 \, I_2 \, DM_1 \, C \, DM_2.$$

The eruption of the first deciduous molar before the canine may be related to its role in stabilising the occlusion between the upper and lower dental arches. Root formation in a deciduous tooth is complete about one to one and a half years after the tooth appears in the mouth cavity. The formation of a deciduous tooth takes between 2 and 4 years from the appearance of its tooth germ to the completion of its root. The deciduous teeth form the whole of the functioning dentition for some four years (Fig. 105). During this time the cusps of the teeth become worn; if this attrition is heavy the mandible may move forward relative to the upper jaw, establishing an edge-to-edge bite of the incisors.

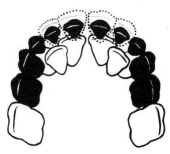

Fig. 106 Diagram illustrating the relative positions of the anterior teeth of the deciduous and permanent dentitions before and after eruption of the permanent teeth. Deciduous teeth shown in solid black; permanent teeth unshaded. The permanent incisors after eruption are indicated with broken outline; before eruption with continuous line. (*By courtesy of Prof S Friel.*)

The teeth in the deciduous arches may either be spaced or in contact mesially and distally with their neighbours. This spacing usually appears at the time of the eruption of the deciduous teeth.

Permanent teeth. During the period of the eruption of the deciduous teeth and their establishment as the functioning dentition the crowns of the successional permanent teeth, lying in their crypts, are forming (Fig. 134). The first permanent molar starts to calcify earlier, about the time of birth, before the beginning of the eruptive movements of the deciduous teeth. The second permanent molar begins to calcify towards the end of the third year and the third molar at around nine years. As an approximation it may be taken that the process of formation of a permanent tooth occupies a period of about twelve years; the first molar, the lower incisors, and the upper central incisor, however, take about ten years, whereas the upper canine takes longer. After the crowns of the permanent teeth are formed there is an interval of quiescence, until with the commencement of eruption tooth formation again becomes active. For, as in the case of the deciduous teeth, root formation does not properly begin until the teeth start their movement towards the mouth cavity. The roots of the permanent teeth are completed two to three years after the tooth first appears in the mouth.

While the crowns of the permanent incisors and canines lie unerupted in the jaws they are situated lingual to the roots of their deciduous predecessors (Fig. 105). The crowns of the canines, and particularly of the upper canine, are placed at a deeper level than those of the incisors (Figs. 105, 135). Moreover, the crowns of the lateral incisors are generally in a more lingual position than the other anterior teeth. This facilitates the packing of the crowns of the permanent teeth into the jaws beneath the much smaller deciduous incisors and canines (Fig. 106). The developing premolar crowns are at first to be found between the roots of their respective deciduous predecessors, the deciduous molars (Figs. 106, 134), but by six years of age they lie at a deeper level in the jaws relative to the deciduous molars, and beneath the apices of the molar roots (Fig. 135).

Change of dentition. The first of the permanent teeth to erupt are usually the first molars; these teeth appear in the mouth cavity at or soon after six years of age. In many children, however, the lower central incisors appear before the first permanent lower molars. With the appearance of the first permanent molars there is initiated the process of the elongation of the dental arch by the eruption of the permanent molars. The replacement of the deciduous teeth by their permanent successors commences generally a little later with the eruption of the incisor teeth; usually the lower incisors are ahead of the upper. The lower central incisors appear around seven years, followed soon afterwards by the upper incisors. The establishment of the first permanent molars and of the central incisors, therefore, takes place much about the same time followed not long afterwards by the lateral incisors. There then follows a period of rest extending over a year or longer before the next group of permanent teeth erupts. This consists of the canines and premolars, which replace the deciduous canines and deciduous molars respectively. The appearance in the mouth cavity of the second permanent molars is close in time to that of the canine-premolar group and these molar teeth further extend the length of the dental arch. After a second and longer rest period the final elongation of the arch is produced by the appearance of the third molars (seventeen to twenty-one years). With these teeth the permanent dentition is complete. The order of eruption of the permanent teeth can be expressed by the formula,

$$(M_1\,I_1)I_2(CP_1\,P_2\,M_2)M_3.$$

Variability of eruption time is lowest for the first permanent molars and highest for the canines, second premolars and third molars.

The first permanent molars develop in their crypts in line with and immediately behind the second deciduous molars. As these teeth erupt they are guided into position in the mouth cavity by the distal surface of the second deciduous molars (Fig. 107). If both upper and lower deciduous molars are in correct occlusal relationship to each other it then follows that the first permanent molars, upper and lower, must erupt in correct position and establish the occlusal relationship proper for them. The first permanent molars act as the keystones of the permanent dentition, establishing and maintaining its correct position during the

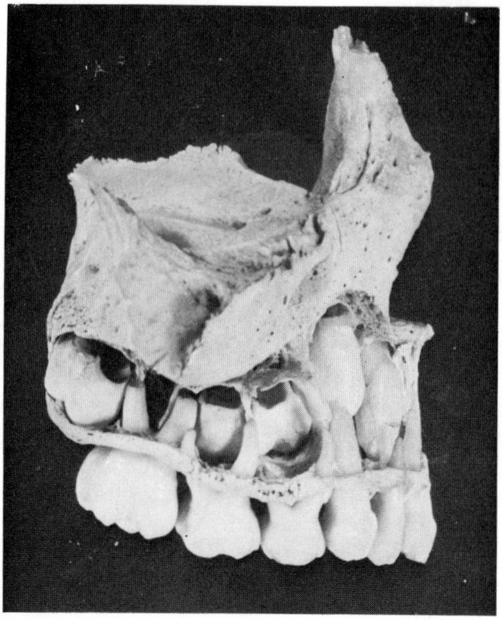

Fig. 107 Right half of upper jaw. At this stage the functioning dentition is made up of the deciduous teeth and the first permanent molar. (*By courtesy of Dr R. Sprinz.*)

period that the deciduous dentition is replaced by the more anterior permanent teeth.

The replacement of the deciduous by the permanent dentition involves important growth changes, such as the shedding of the deciduous teeth, the eruption of the permanent teeth, and the reformation of the alveolar bone to form new sockets for the replacing permanent teeth. As the relationship in size varies between individual deciduous teeth and their successors, regional adjustments must be made to make use of the available space.

In the incisive region, where the permanent teeth are considerably larger than their predecessors, the extra space required is made available largely by increased growth in width at the front of the alveolar arches, which may show itself in a spacing between the roots and sometimes between the crowns of the deciduous teeth towards the end of their

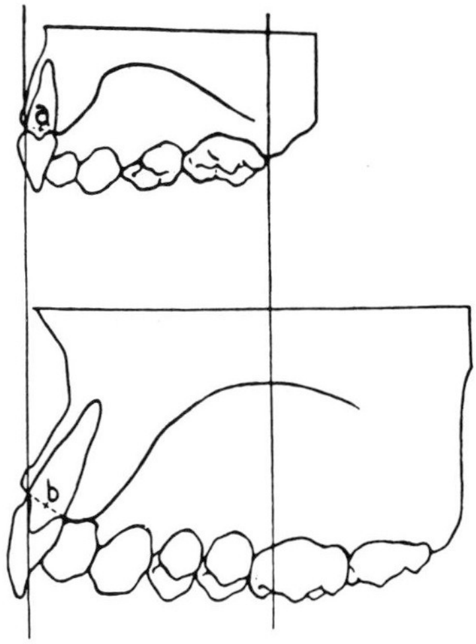

Fig. 108 The deciduous incisors (*a*) are arranged more vertically than the permanent incisors (*b*); the premolars usually occupy less space mesio-distally than the deciduous molars and the permanent first molar moves forward to close the surplus space. (*By courtesy of Prof S. Friel.*)

period of use. In those deciduous dentitions in which spacing has always existed the establishment of the larger permanent teeth is greatly facilitated. Furthermore, in the case of the upper teeth, the direction of eruption is usually forward as well as downward, so that their incisive edges come to occupy a more forward and larger arch than that of the deciduous incisors (Fig. 108). The fully erupted permanent incisors are therefore less vertical in their sockets than their predecessors.

The mesio-distal length of the premolars is less than that of the deciduous molars which they replace, and this difference is more marked in the lower than in the upper jaw. As a result space is made available for the larger permanent canines at the front of this region and for a forward movement of the first permanent molars, more especially the lower ones, at the back of this region (Fig. 108). The average combined mesio-distal lengths of the incisor and canine teeth of the deciduous and permanent dentitions are as follows (from G. V. Black):

Deciduous Teeth		*Permanent Teeth*	
Lower jaw	Upper jaw	Lower jaw	Upper jaw
26·6 mm	37·2 mm	36·4 mm	46·0 mm

The average combined mesio-distal lengths, on one side, of the deciduous molars and of the premolars are:

Deciduous Molars		*Premolars*	
Lower jaw	Upper jaw	Lower jaw	Upper jaw
17·6 mm	15·5 mm	14·0 mm	14·0 mm

In most deciduous dentitions the distal surfaces of the upper and lower second deciduous molars are in the same vertical plane so that the first permanent molars are not immediately guided into the definitive occlusal relationship as they erupt. This relationship may, however, be established later. It may be produced by a forward movement of the lower deciduous molars in those dentitions were a space between the deciduous lower canines and the molars exist. Alternatively the correct occlusal relationship of the first permanent molars may finally be established by the rather greater mesial movement that the lower tooth makes compared with the upper on the replacement of the deciduous molars by the premolars. The mesio-buccal cusp of the upper first permanent molar then occludes outside but opposite the buccal groove of the lower first permanent molar (Fig. 28).

With the eruption of the first permanent molars and the other permanent cheek teeth, the interlock between the cusps of the upper and lower dental arch is restored. In adult life these cuspal relationships are altered by attrition, and if this is heavy, may even be abolished.

A comparable loss of tooth substance may take place through attrition of the approximal surfaces of the teeth. As a result the teeth move bodily and remain in contact. This movement is usually referred to as physiological mesial drift. The transeptal fibres of the periodontal membrane are important in producing it. Histologically there is evidence of resorption of the mesial surfaces of the sockets of the teeth and of bone deposition on the distal surfaces. Also associated with this movement of the teeth are various compensating changes in the parodontal tissues.

Sex differences in dental development. In girls calcification begins earlier than in boys and the teeth appear earlier in the mouth cavity. These differences are shown before the tenth year and cannot be ascribed directly to the timing of sex hormone secretions. Moreover, in precocious puberty there is no evidence of any advance in tooth development or eruption. The time of eruption of the second permanent molar may, however, be correlated with the onset of puberty in certain individuals.

THE SHEDDING OF THE DECIDUOUS TEETH

Each member of the deciduous dentition is in turn replaced by a permanent tooth. The process by which the deciduous teeth are removed to allow the succeeding permanent teeth to take their functional positions in the mouth is known as the shedding of the deciduous teeth. This loss of the deciduous teeth is mainly due to the resorption of their roots, which is associated with the eruption of the permanent teeth. The shedding of the deciduous teeth is a normal physiological process. It usually commences earlier in girls than in boys.

The permanent teeth, when they commence to erupt, are lodged in bony crypts. In the crypts they are surrounded by the vascular connective tissue of the follicle. Thus each permanent tooth is separated from its deciduous predecessor by the bone forming the roof of its crypt and by the follicular tissue. It is, however, connected to the oral mucous membrane through the fibrous gubernacular cord, which occupies a canal in the alveolar bone. The openings of these canals on the alveolar bone are just lingual to the crowns of the deciduous teeth (Figs. 24, 93, 109).

The pressure exerted by the erupting permanent teeth on the overlying tissues first leads to a resorption of the bone separating them from

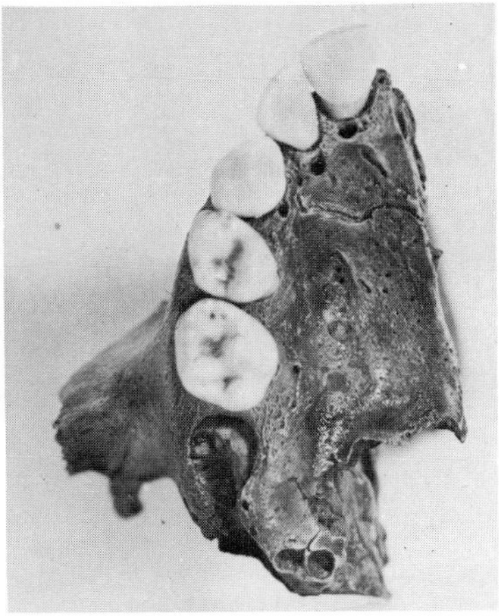

Fig. 109 Palatal aspect of maxilla of young child. Note the openings of the gubernacular canals lingual to the deciduous incisors and canine. The openings of the gubernacular canals associated with the developing premolars are not visible in this specimen; frequently they open into the sockets of the deciduous molars. The calcified crown of the first permanent molar may be seen in its crypt immediately behind the deciduous teeth.

the deciduous teeth. The actual resorption is effected by large multinucleated cells, osteoclasts, which appear in the outer part of the follicle. After the bone separating the permanent and deciduous teeth has been removed, the tissues of the follicle come into contact with the roots of the deciduous teeth and a resorption of these roots then begins (Figs. 94, 110). This resorption, like that of the bone, is carried out by large multi-nucleated cells. These cells lie in concavities, known as Howship's lacunae, on the roots of the deciduous teeth. The resorption affects first the cement and then both the cement and the dentine of the deciduous teeth and proceeds crownwards as the underlying permanent teeth continue to erupt (Fig. 112). The enamel is not usually affected. During eruption the enamel of the permanent teeth is separated from the follicular tissues by the reduced enamel epithelium, which acts as a protective capsule.

At the commencement of eruption the permanent incisors and canines lie apically and lingual to the roots of their deciduous predecessors (Figs. 95, 107). As a result the resorption produced during their eruption first affects the lingual aspect of the apical region of the deciduous roots (Fig. 94). As eruption continues they come to lie more directly beneath their deciduous predecessors, so that the resorption affects the whole cross-section of the deciduous root. At the commencement of eruption each premolar lies directly deep to the deciduous tooth

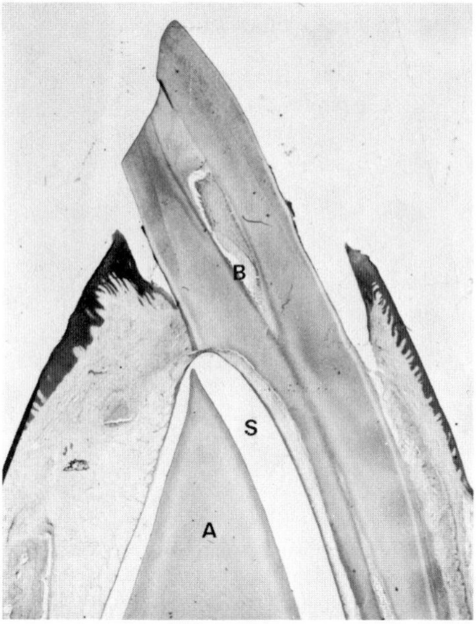

Fig. 110 Resorption of deciduous tooth. A, permanent tooth; B, deciduous tooth; S, space occupied by enamel before decalcification in the histological preparation of the section. Labio-lingual section from jaw of New World monkey. × 12.

which it replaces; thus resorption first affects the apical region of the roots of the deciduous molars. In some cases the roots may show very unequal rates of resorption.

At an earlier stage in development the premolars lie between the roots of the deciduous molars and resorption may take place on the distal surface of the mesial root and on the mesial surface of the distal root in lower molars, also on the buccal surface of the palatal root in upper molars (Fig. 134). This early resorption, however, is brought about by the growth of the developing premolar crowns and is not concerned with their eruption. Subsequently with growth in height of the alveolar bone the deciduous molars move vertically away from the premolar crowns, so that the premolars no longer lie between their roots but are placed apically to them (Fig. 135). The small resorptions caused earlier are repaired by deposition of cement.

Resorption of the roots of the deciduous teeth continues until the whole or the greater part of the roots are removed and the teeth are finally shed, the replacing permanent teeth then being able to occupy their positions. The pulp tissue in the crowns of the deciduous teeth remains apparently unaffected during this process. Occasionally even after the whole root area of a deciduous tooth has been resorbed the

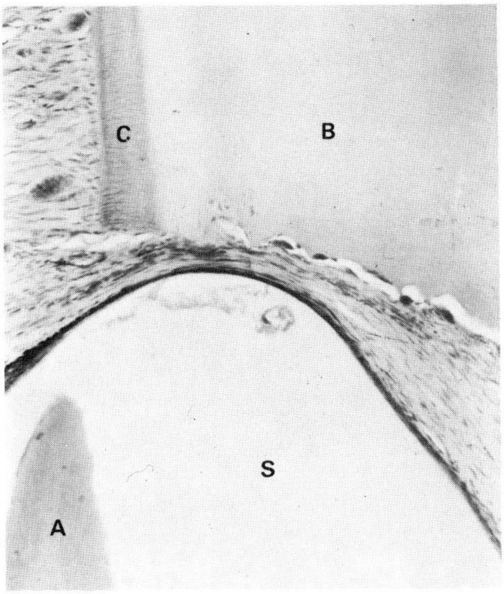

Fig. 111 Higher magnification of the resorption of the deciduous tooth shown in Fig. 110. A, permanent tooth; B, deciduous tooth; C, cement of deciduous tooth; S, space previously occupied by enamel of permanent tooth. Note the osteoclasts which lie in lacunae on the resorbed surface of the deciduous tooth, and the layer of reduced enamel epithelium which delimits the enamel space. × 100.

crown remains in position in the jaw for some time, still remaining attached by the gingivae and by the connection of its vital pulp to the underlying tissues. Resorption of the roots of the deciduous teeth does not progress smoothly but takes place intermittently, there being bursts of activity and intervening rest periods. During the phases of quiescence a certain degree of repair of the resorbed areas often takes place by a deposition of cement. Sometimes as the result of an over-active repair process anchylosis of a deciduous tooth occurs, due to localised union of the repairing cement and the adjacent bone. When this takes place the eruption of the replacing permanent tooth is prevented or takes place in an abnormal direction.

Though the shedding of the deciduous teeth is mainly brought about by the resorption of their roots with the consequent loss of attachment to the alveolar bone, it is accelerated by a second factor. This is the increasing strain which is thrown on the teeth through the more powerful development of the masticatory muscles during growth. The small root area of the deciduous teeth is inadequate to carry the increased load, and so abnormal stresses are thrown on their attachments. This leads to increased resorption of their roots, and this in turn makes them

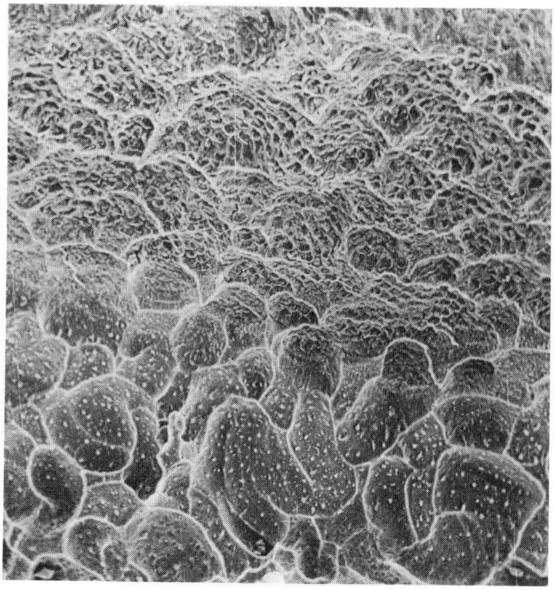

Fig. 112 Resorbing surface of human deciduous molar showing Howship's lacunae in both dentine and enamel. Dentine shown in the lower part of field. The peritubular zones in the dentine and the enamel prisms are both standing slightly above the resorbing surface. Original magnification × 500. (*Courtesy of Dr A. Boyde.*)

less able to bear the force of mastication. Thus a vicious circle is set up.

Sometimes fragments of the roots of deciduous teeth become isolated from the crown during the shedding of these teeth. These fragments may remain in the tissues between the roots of the erupted permanent teeth (Fig. 138). They occur most frequently in the case of the second deciduous molars as the span of the widely divergent roots of these teeth is considerably greater than that of the crowns of the replacing premolars. Thus parts of the roots of these teeth are not involved in the resorption processes and may be left buried in the jaw.

In certain cases deciduous teeth remain in position in the mouth long after the time at which they are normally shed. This may be due to:

1. The non-formation of a replacing permanent tooth. The tooth

most frequently congenitally absent from the permanent dentition is the lower second premolar followed in frequency by the upper lateral incisor.

2. The failure of a replacing tooth to erupt. This is most commonly the upper canine.

3. Anchylosis of a deciduous tooth to the alveolar bone.

In the first two classes the retained deciduous teeth often remain functionally useful for many years. However, they are usually lost through an eventual resorption of their roots. This resorption is probably caused by the heavy masticatory stresses of adult life which fall on these teeth; as their roots are small compared with those of the permanent teeth the area of attachment for the periodontal fibres is insufficient.

Where a deciduous tooth becomes anchylosed it fails to rise in the jaw with the increase in height of the alveolar bone, and so gradually appears at a lower level in the jaw compared with the adjacent teeth. The 'submergence' of such a tooth may continue to the extent that it becomes buried in the alveolar bone.

BIBLIOGRAPHY

Alexander, S. A. & Swerdloff, M. (1979). Mucopolysaccharidase activity during human deciduous root resorption. *Arch. oral Biol.*, **24**, 735.

Brothwell, D. R. (1963). *Dental Anthropology*. Oxford: Pergamon Press.

Butler, P. M. (1967). The prenatal development of the human first upper permanent molar. *Arch. oral Biol.* **12**, 551.

Butler, P. M. (1968). Growth of the human second lower deciduous molar. *Archs. oral Biol.* **13**, 671.

Christensen, G. J. & Kraus, B. S. (1965). Initial calcification of the human permanent first molar. *J. dent. Res.* **44**, 1338.

Fanning, E. (1961). A longitudinal study of tooth formation and root resorption. *N.Z. dent. J.* **57**, 202.

Friel, S. (1954). The development of ideal occlusion of the gum pads and the teeth. *Amer. J. Orthodont.* **40**, 196.

Furseth, R. (1968). The resorption process of human deciduous teeth studied by light microscopy, microradiography and electron microscopy. *Archs. oral Biol.* **13**, 417.

Garn, S. M., Lewis, A. B., Koshi, K. & Polacheck, D. L. (1958). The sex differences in tooth calcification. *J. dent. Res.* **37**, 561.

Johnson, H. W. (1961). Epithelial activity in the exfoliation of the deciduous tooth and emerging permanent teeth. *J. dent. Res.* **40**, 1231.

Kraus, B. S. (1959). Calcification of the human deciduous teeth. *J. Amer. dent. Ass.* **59**, 1128.

Picton, D. C. A. (1962). Tilting movements of teeth during biting. *Arch. oral Biol.*, **7**, 151.

Schour, I. & Massler, M. (1940). Studies in tooth development: The growth pattern of human teeth. *J. Amer. dent. Ass.* **27**, 1918.

Smith, R. G. (1980). A clinical study into the rate of eruption of some human permanent teeth. *Arch. oral Biol.*, **25**, 675.

Yilmaz, R. S., Darling, A. I. & Levers, B. G. H. (1980). Mesial drift of human teeth assessed from ankylosed deciduous molars. *Arch. oral Biol.*, **25**, 127.

7. Tooth Movement and Associated Tissue Changes

It is customary to consider the movements of the teeth as falling into three phases in their relationship to the eruption of the teeth. The three phases are as follows:

1. Pre-eruptive, the period during which the erupted teeth lie deep in the jaws in their alveoli or crypts and before the movement produced by active eruption takes place.

2. Eruptive, the period during which the teeth move vertically towards the mouth cavity, pierce the oral mucous membrane to enter the mouth cavity and then move on to reach the occlusal plane. These movements have been described (pp. 111–119).

3. Post-eruptive or functional, the period after the teeth have reached the occlusal plane.

Apart from the active eruption of the teeth during the second phase the other movements of the teeth are associated either with growth of the teeth themselves and of the jaws, or with tooth loss and wear of the teeth. Movements of the teeth associated with growth may occur at any time during the first two decades of life but particularly occur during the first or pre-eruptive phase. Movements of the teeth associated with wear of the teeth occur during the third or functional phase.

Movements of the teeth associated with growth may be considered in two phases: (a) Those occurring before eruption begins and (b) those occurring either during eruption or after the teeth have become functional.

Unerupted teeth. When they first appear as thickenings along the free edge of the dental lamina the deciduous tooth germs are separated from one another by a relatively considerable interval. With growth of the tooth germs within their follicles the space between the germs becomes reduced and the developing teeth, especially in the canine-incisor region, become crowded together (Fig. 56). By this time each tooth lies in its alveolar compartment, but by its attachment through the dental follicle to the oral mucous membrane it remains in a relatively superficial position (Fig. 113).

During this phase ot ıncrease in the size of each tooth germ, that is before dentine formation stabilises the size of each tooth crown, room is provided by movements of the tooth germs within the alveolar bone. The second deciduous molar migrates backward and the teeth in front of the first deciduous molar migrate forward. In the mandibular arch each half is lengthened by growth in front at the symphysis and behind

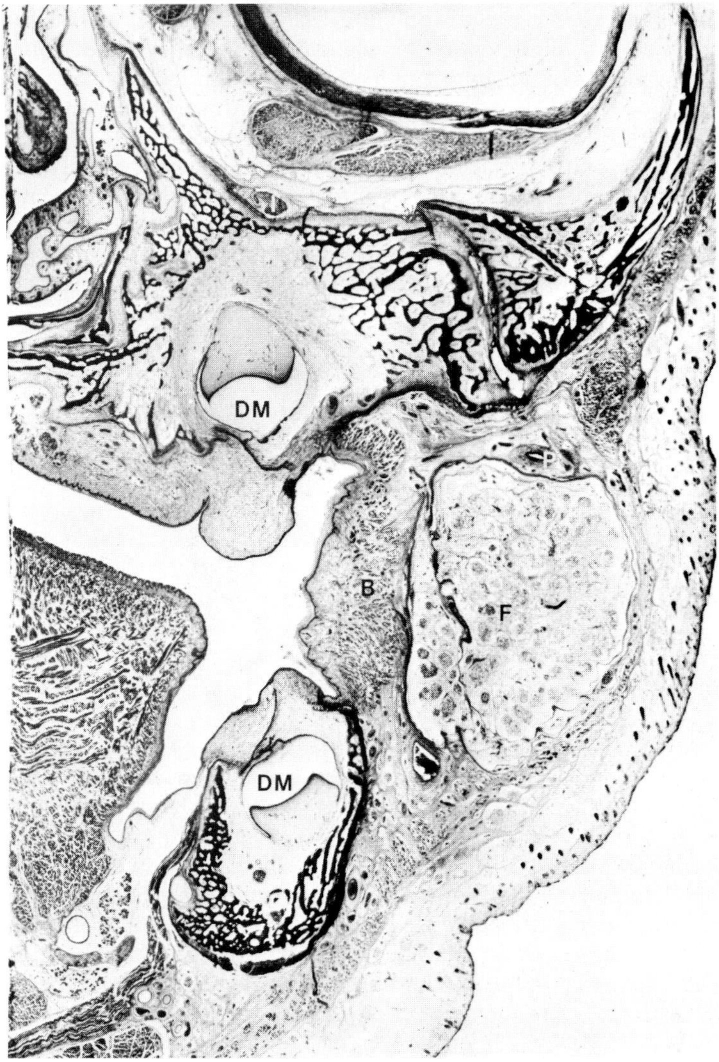

Fig. 113 Coronal section through the head of a human fetus of 120 mm C.R. length. Note the tooth germs of the second deciduous molars, the structure of the fetal bone, the buccal pad of fat, the parotid duct, the buccinator muscle, and the infraorbital nerve. B, buccinator muscle; DM, deciduous molar; F, buccal pad of fat; I, infraorbital nerve; P, parotid duct. × 10.

at the condyle and posterior border of the ramus (Fig. 114). In the upper jaw each maxillary element extends both in front and behind by surface deposition and by growth at the anterior aspect of the mid palatal suture. To a large extent the growing tooth germs expand eccentrically in an outward or facial direction, though it is possible that there is some bodily outward movement of the whole dentition. They are accommodated by a progressive shifting of the labial or buccal wall of the alveoli.

The processes of growth of the tooth germs, tooth eruption, and tooth migration are all the result of growth changes involving the tooth germs, tooth pulps, and alveolar bone, and although they can be analysed as separate phases they overlap one another to a considerable extent. In all phases of tooth development, however, the alveolar bone is continually adapted by a process of bony reconstruction to the growing, erupting, and migrating teeth. The adaptation of the bone, whether as

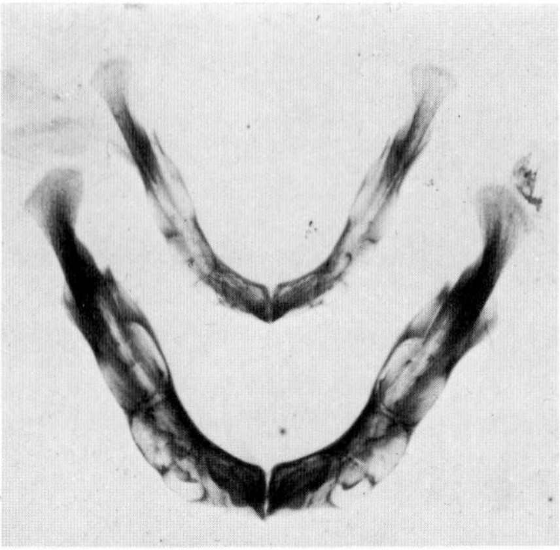

Fig. 114 Radiograph of five month fetal and full term human mandibles. (90 per cent actual size.)

alveolus, crypt, or socket, is the result of the activity of the vascular tissue of the dental follicle or periodontal membrane. In areas where bone resorption is active, osteoclasts are seen on the bony surfaces (Figs. 115, 116); where bone deposition is proceeding osteoblasts form an epithelial-like lining on the surface of the bone (Figs. 115, 116). The permanent teeth within their crypts undergo a corresponding process of growth associated with expansion of the crypts and of migration through the growing jaws. The teeth are maintained in correct relationship to the overlying gum through the attachments of their gubernacular cords.

Functional teeth. After the teeth have erupted they continue to migrate forward and outward with the growing jaws throughout childhood. This appears to occur particularly in the upper jaw (Fig. 125). The chief tissue changes in the periodontal membrane, tooth sockets, and alveolar bone are as follows:

1. Bone resorption on the buccal and mesial walls of the sockets and bone deposition on the lingual and distal walls.

2. Bone deposition on the outer (facial) surface of the alveolar bone, which maintains the proper thickness of the buccal alveolar plate, and also at the alveolar margins.

3. Bone resorption on the inner (lingual) surface of the alveolar bone so as to retain the proper thickness of the lingual alveolar plate.

4. Replacement and reattachment of the periodontal membrane as the tooth moves and its socket is reformed.

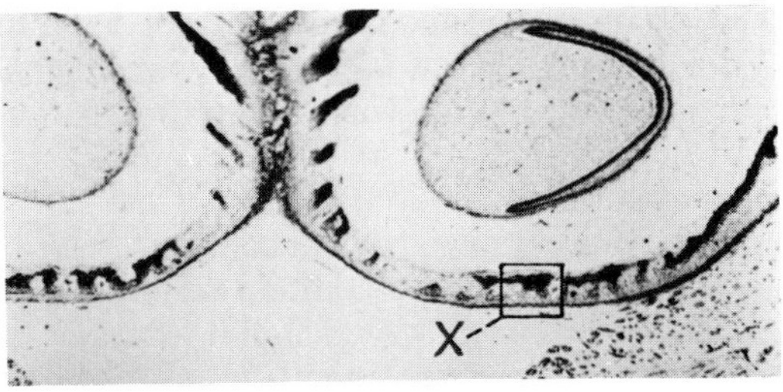

Fig. 115 Transverse section through fetal upper jaw showing the deciduous central incisors and the mesio-buccal aspects of their alveoli. × 14.

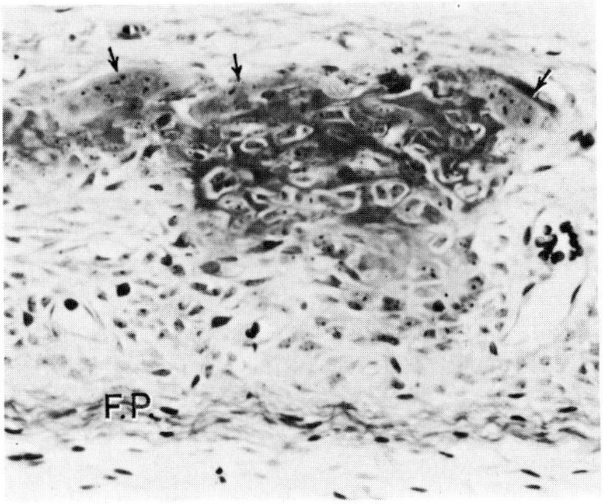

Fig. 116 High magnification of area (X) from Fig. 115 showing bone resorption on the inner aspect of the buccal alveolar wall. Osteoclasts are indicated by arrows. On the outer aspect of the bone numerous osteoblasts are engaged in bone formation. (F.P.) fibrous layer of the periosteum. × 225.

During the period of facial growth the functional teeth also move vertically as the depth of the jaws is increased by alveolar bone growth. This is well shown during the functional life of the deciduous dentition by a comparison of the jaws at three years of age and at six years (Figs. 134 and 135). In the earlier stage each premolar crown is embraced by the roots of a deciduous molar, whereas at the later stage the deciduous molars have been lifted away from the premolars by alveolar growth. The vertical movement of the teeth is also observed in noting the increasing distance between the apices of the lower deciduous teeth and the lower border of the mandible.

It should be remembered that during these growth movements the erupted teeth are in constant use and that tension is put upon all parts of the periodontal membrane by the forces of mastication and occlusion. This is of special importance in understanding the complex changes which take place on the buccal and mesial surfaces of the sockets. Here both pressure due to tooth migration and tension due to tooth function act together, so that both resorption and restoration of the walls of the sockets take place; the structure of the lamina dura is maintained and also the attachment of the periodontal membrane.

During tooth migration there is then a continual reformation of the socket around the moving tooth, a constant restoration and reattachment of the periodontal membrane, and a constant readjustment of the occlusal relations of the opposing teeth of the upper and lower arches. Meanwhile the teeth continue to function and such tissues as cement, periodontal membrane, and alveolar bone are modified or reconstructed to meet the needs of dental function.

Tooth loss. When a tooth is lost from the arch the teeth on either side of the space tend to tilt towards each other. The opposing teeth generally tilt and move somewhat vertically beyond the other teeth in the arch.

Loss of tooth substance due to attrition may occur either at the incisive edges and occlusal surfaces of the teeth or it may take place approximally at the contact areas. In the first situation the loss of tooth substance brings about slow imperceptible movement of the teeth in both arches in a vertical or axial direction. In this way loss of facial height is avoided. The reduction in tooth length which would be otherwise produced by attrition at the incisive edges or occlusal surfaces is compensated, to some extent at least, by the continued deposition of cement at the apices of the roots.

Loss of tooth substance at the contact areas is associated with the phenomenon known as physiological mesial drift. By this means the teeth in each arch are maintained in contact at their approximal surfaces. Mesial drift of the teeth is accompanied by modelling changes in the alveolar bone forming the sockets of the teeth involved (see p. 128). It has been usual to attribute physiological mesial drift of the teeth to the masticatory forces which fall on the cheek teeth, many of which have an axial implantation with a mesial inclination. However it has recently been indicated that mesial drift is produced by the transeptal fibres which link the individual members of each arch together. Shortening of the collagen macromolecules, which constitute these fibres, during their maturation could produce the necessary traction to effect the movement.

Clinical considerations. In orthodontic treatment mechanical appliances are used in order to bring the teeth into their normal position in the arches. The ideal is to produce tooth movement under conditions as close as possible to those which take place during growth migration. As the forces used are applied to the crowns of the teeth there are often tilting movements of the teeth, which render the pattern of tissue changes in the sockets somewhat complex (Fig. 237). If excessive force is used resorption of cement and even of dentine may take place as well as the resorption of bone. As a result of a failure of the proper correlation between the process of detachment and attachment of the fibres of the periodontal membrane, the teeth may become loose in their sockets. Sometimes extensive resorption of the roots of the teeth takes place. Abnormal tooth movements leading to abnormal occlusion of the teeth may occur as the result of such habits as thumb and finger sucking or from sucking the lower lip between the upper and lower incisors.

BIBLIOGRAPHY

Friel, S. (1945). Migrations of teeth following extractions. *Proc. R. Soc. Med.* **38**, 456.

Kenney, T. B. & Ramfjord, S. P. (1969). Patterns of root and alveolar-bone growth associated with development and eruption of teeth in rhesus monkeys. *J. dent. Res.* **48**, 251.

Orban, B. (1928). Growth and movement of tooth germs and teeth. *J. Amer. dent. Ass.* **15**, 1004.

Picton, D. C. A. & Moss, J. P. (1980). The effect on approximal drift of altering the horizontal component of biting force in adult monkeys (*Macaca irus*). *Arch. oral Biol.* **25**, 45.

Reitan, K. (1960). Tissue behaviour during orthodontic tooth movement. *Amer. J. Orthodont.* **46**, 881.

8. Growth of the Face

Some knowledge of the processes involved in growth of the face is necessary to understand the development of the dentition. In this chapter a general outline of facial growth is given.

GENERAL CONSIDERATIONS

Phases in cranio-facial growth. In early fetal life the skeleton of the craniofacial region is made up of cartilage—the primary cartilaginous skeleton or chondrocranium. Its chief elements are the paracordal region, the auditory or otic capsules, the nasal capsule and Meckel's cartilage (Fig. 45). The growing brain rests upon the basal chondrocranium and is elsewhere surrounded by a membranous capsule. At this period growth is rapid and generalised, involving growth of the cartilage and of the brain capsule as a whole.

Within the cartilage (endochondral ossification) and within the brain capsule (membranous ossification) centres of ossification appear which are at first widely separated. With development the individual bones approach one another until they come into near contact at synchondroses or sutures, which remain for some time as sites of localised growth. At various periods throughout life, from the fetal stage to old age, bones tend to unite with one another at the synchondroses or sutures. Between early fetal life and postnatal life growth becomes less active and less generalised, changing from an overall process to a system of localised growth sites (*e.g.* sutures, synchondroses, bony surfaces). There has been much difference of opinion regarding the relative importance of these sites in the growth of the skull, for the amount of growth and the period during which it occurs have, in most cases, not yet been clearly defined.

At one time the sutures were held to be primary growth centres, that is it was believed that the osteogenic tissue of the sutures was responsible for the thrusting apart of the related bones. It is now generally accepted that growth at sutures is a secondary phenomenon by which the bony elements, which would be carried apart from each other by growth of brain, eyeball, tongue or some other organ, are maintained in relationship. It has also been suggested that the areas of cartilage which persist in the skull after birth, such as the synchondroses in the skull base or the cartilage of the nasal septum also act in this sense as primary growth centres, relative to the adjacent bones.

Such ideas have been brought together in the wider concept of functional cranial components. In this view the cranial components which are concerned with the various functions of the head and neck are composed of (1) all those 'soft' tissues such as muscles, glands, viscera or visceral spaces which are related to a specific function, and (2) the related skeletal tissues which support or protect these 'soft' tissues. A specific function may involve as its related skeletal supporting or protecting unit only a part of one bone or alternatively parts or more than one bone. As an example of the former, in the mandible one recognises

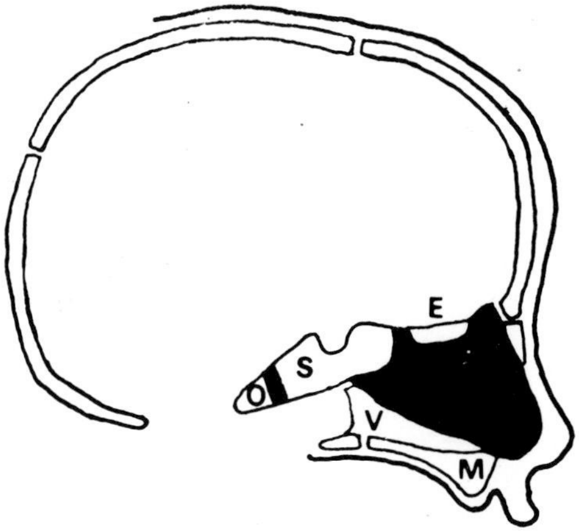

Fig. 117 Diagrammatic representation of a median sagittal section through the skull of a child a few months after birth. Cartilage is shown in black. O, occipital; S, sphenoid; E, ethmoid; V, vomer; M, maxilla.

distinct tooth-bearing and muscular parts. On the other hand the entire endocranial aspects of all the bones of the calvaria serve to protect the brain tissue.

The important aspect of the concept of functional cranial components is that all the parts of the head and neck are seen to be inter-related in function and in growth and that the bones of the skull are not considered, as they so often have been, as self-sufficient entities growing independently of the other tissues and organs.

Growth areas of the skull. The skull, for purposes of understanding its growth, can be divided into three regions:

1. *The cranial vault*, made up of membrane bones, the frontal, parietals, squamous part of the temporals, and part of the occipital and sphenoid bones (Fig. 117). In its growth the cranial vault is related to the growth of the brain, although the actual form of the skull is probably determined by independent factors.

2. *The cranial base*, made up mainly of cartilage replacing bones, the ex- and basi-occipitals, the body, lesser wings and part of the greater wings of the sphenoid, the petrous part of the temporal bones, and the

perpendicular plate of the ethmoid (Fig. 117). The growth of the cranial base is largely independent of brain growth.

3. *The face* consists of membrane bones which have been built up around the cartilage of the nasal capsule and Meckel's cartilage, and cartilage replacing bones, the labyrinths (lateral masses) of the ethmoid and inferior nasal concha, which have replaced parts of the nasal capsule (Fig. 118). Except for the nasal septum the cartilage is all removed

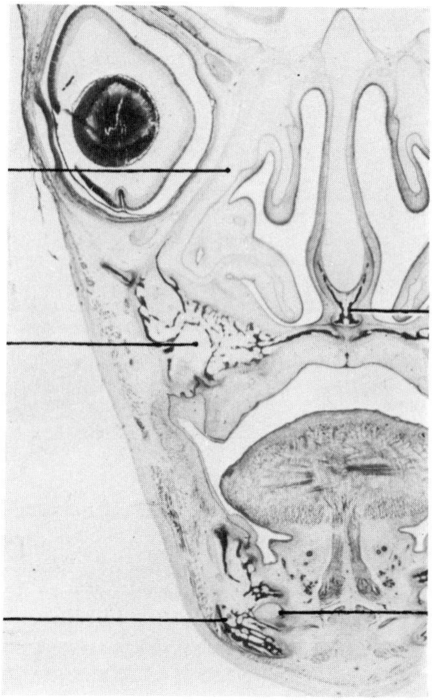

Fig. 118 Coronal section of the head of a human fetus of 70 mm C.R. length showing the cartilaginous skeleton of the face and the membrane bones built around it. × 10.

or replaced during late fetal life or shortly after birth. In the case of the mandible, however, certain secondary cartilages appear during fetal life and are important in growth. The facial skeleton consists of two parts, the mandible, which is movable at the mandibular joints, and the upper face, which is attached to the under surface of the front part of the cranial base. The facial skeleton is built around the organs of sight, respiration (nasal cavities), and mastication (tongue and teeth).

Methods of skull growth. Bone growth in the skull takes place by three methods:

1. The replacement of cartilage by bone (Fig. 119). This is very active

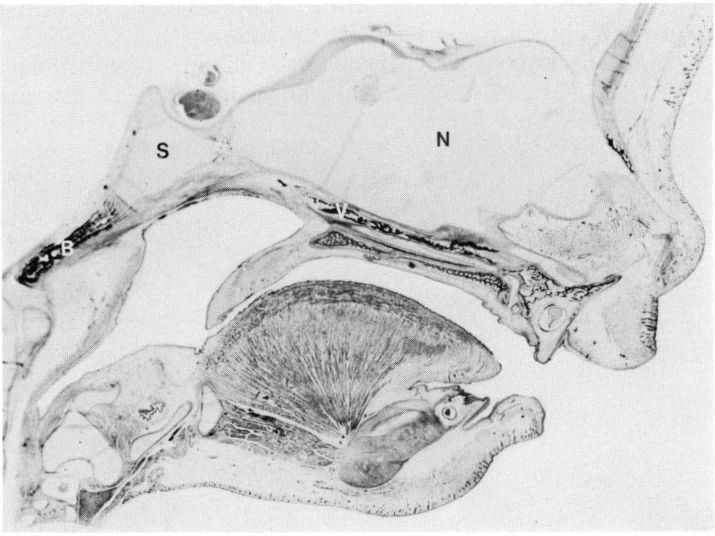

Fig. 119 Sagittal section through the head of a human fetus of $5\frac{1}{2}$ months showing the cartilage of the cranial base and nasal septum. Ossification of the basi-occipital is well advanced. B, basi-occipital; N, cartilage of the nasal septum; S, cartilage in the sphenoidal region; V, vomer.

in late fetal life especially at the base of the skull and is active after birth at three important sites:

a. The synchondrosis between the basi-occipital and basi-sphenoid bones (Fig. 117).

b. The cartilage of the mandibular condyles.

c. The nasal septum.

Growth at the synchondroses between sphenoid and ethmoid and between ethmoid and frontal is of more limited extent.

2. At the sutures. Suture growth is active in the cranial vault and upper face during late fetal life and for the first few years after birth. Suture growth probably continues to be of some importance up to about the end of the first decade. After this time it is of less significance.

At a growing suture the tissue between the bony edges can be divided into five layers (Figs. 120, 121). These are:

a. A layer of cellular tissue in which bone-forming cells are proliferating and depositing new bone at the growing suture edge of each bony unit. This later corresponds to and is continuous with the cellular osteogenic layer of the periosteum covering the other surfaces of the bone (cambial layer).

b. A layer of fibrous tissue corresponding to the fibrous layer of the periosteum (capsular layer). Part of this fibrous tissue extends from one bone to the other at each surface of the suture, uniting the bony elements. The two layers (a) and (b) are duplicated, being found in relation to each of the bony elements of the suture.

c. A middle layer of tissue between the fibrous layers containing blood vessels and transversely running fibres uniting the fibrous layers.

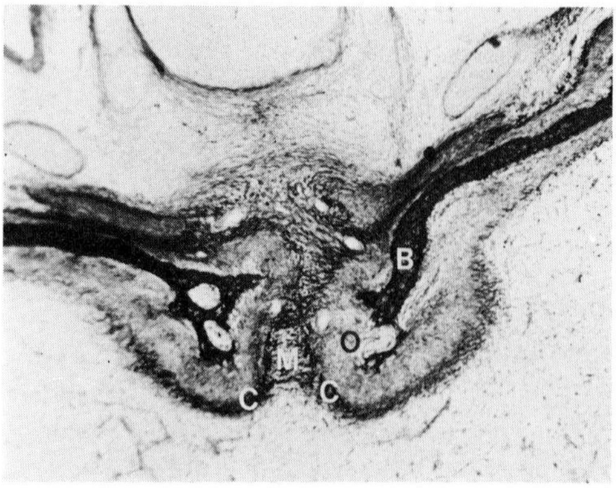

Fig. 120 Coronal section through the developing mid-palatal suture in a human fetus. Compare with Fig. 121. B, bone; C, capsular layer; M, middle layer, O, osteogenic cambial layer. × 50.

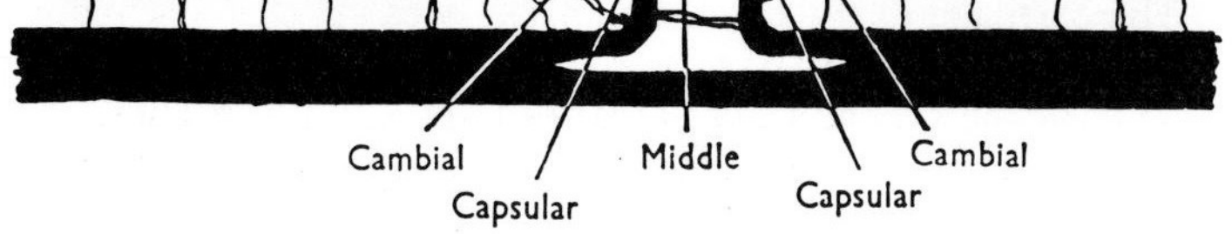

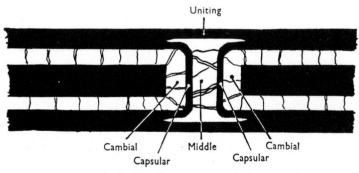

Fig. 121 Diagram of a suture showing the various layers in its construction. (*By courtesy of Prof J. J. Pritchard, Dr F. G. Girgis, and 'Journal of Anatomy'.*)

Therefore a growing suture has two sites of growth (osteogenic cellular layers), one for each of the bony elements. The amount of growth can vary in the two growth sites so that one bone can grow more than the other. The force which separates the bones at sutures is not, however, the soft tissue of the suture but some growing organ such as brain, eyeball, or tongue or the cartilages of the cranial base and nasal septum.

3. Surface deposition. This occurs over the external surfaces of the cranial and facial bones beneath the covering periosteum. It is more extensive in some areas than in others and is associated with resorption

of bone in regions such as the interior of the cranial cavity, the floor of the nasal cavity, the nasal air sinuses, and at the anterior border of the mandibular ramus. Bone deposition is the most important method of growth of the facial skeleton during late childhood and adolescence and may persist in certain regions into adult life.

REGIONAL GROWTH OF THE FACE

The upper face is closely related to the anterior segment of the cranium (frontal, ethmoid, and sphenoid bones); this segment of the cranium meets the occipital at the spheno-occipital synchondrosis at the base of the skull (Fig. 117), which is a site of growth until about puberty. Forward growth of the upper face is related in part to forward growth of the whole anterior cranial segment and takes place with it. The result of this growth is to increase the antero-posterior dimension of the naso-pharynx and to make room for the muscles of mastication by increasing the distance between the back of the face (pterygoid plates) and the vertebral column. During growth of the cranial base the glenoid fossae are usually carried somewhat backward and downward so that growth of the mandible in the forward direction must be greater in amount than the forward growth of the upper face in order to maintain normal occlusion between the upper and lower teeth.

The maxilla. During the first few years after birth there is a certain amount of growth at the sutures between the maxilla and other facial bones and also between these other bones (palatine, lacrimal, zygomatic and labyrinths of ethmoid) and the elements of the anterior cranial segment (Fig. 122). This growth takes place behind the maxilla in the pterygopalatine fossa and at the sutures of the orbital cavity. The maxilla is thrust downward and forward by the growing eyeballs and nasal septum, and this separation of the facial bones permits growth to take place at the sutures. Growth at the orbital surface of the maxilla takes place against the orbital contents, eyeball, muscles and the intervening

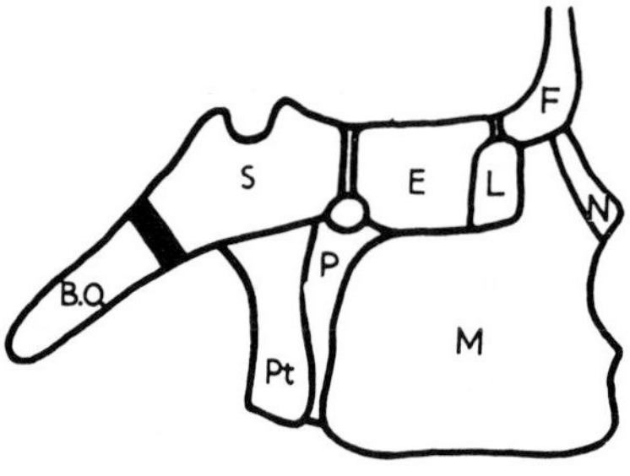

Fig. 122 The relation of the maxilla to the other bones of the face and the cranial base in man. (M) Maxilla. (N) Nasal bone. (F) Frontal bone. (L) Lacrimal bone. (E) Ethmoid. (P) Vertical plate of palatine bone. (S) Body of the sphenoid. (Pt) Pterygoid plate. (Bo) Basi-occipital.

fibro-fatty tissue, and at the posterior surface against the anterior border of the temporal muscle and the intervening fibro-fatty tissue. The result is a downward and forward displacement of the bone (Fig. 123). After the third year this circum-maxillary suture growth is less active, and

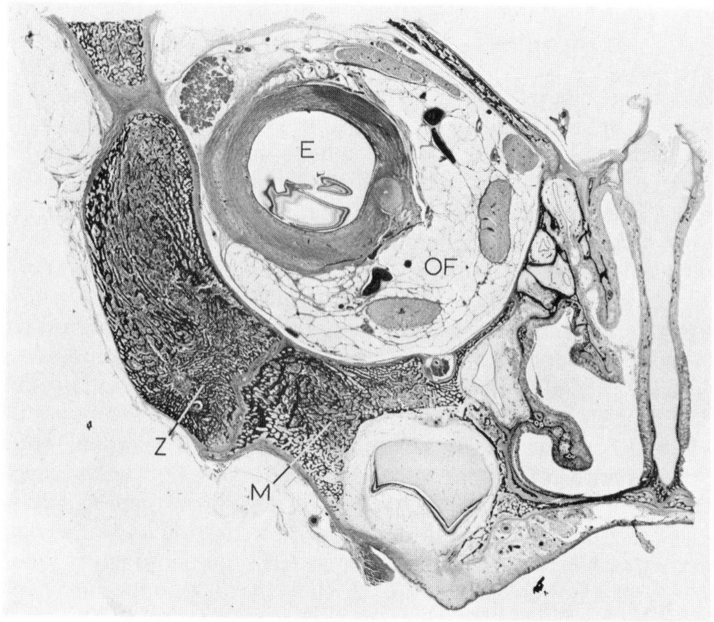

Fig. 123 Coronal section, new born infant, showing mass of orbital fat (OF) in contact with the superior surface of the maxilla (M). E, eyeball; Z, zygomatic bone. Original magnification ×6·5. (*By courtesy of Dr R. A. Latham and the Archs. oral Biol.*)

by the end of the first decade it is almost complete, although there may be a further spurt at the time of puberty.

Surface deposition and resorption. Apart from the areas of cartilage involved in the growth of the facial skeleton such as septal and condylar cartilages, the chief method of growth determining the final form of the facial skeleton is the balance between bone deposition and resorption in various regions of the skeleton. In this there is considerable variation between one individual and another, and in the same individual at different periods. Deposition is most active at the alveolar processes of both jaws, the under surface of the hard palate, the bridge of the nose, the back of the ramus, and the outer surfaces of the zygomatic arches (Fig.124). Bone resorption occurs in the interior of the maxillae, thereby increasing the size of the sinuses; the upper surface of the hard palate, thereby increasing the depth of the nasal cavities; to a variable extent on the inner surface of the mandible, the middle region of the facial surface of the maxillary bones, the facial aspect of the zygomatic buttress and the lateral wall of the orbital cavity. The overall effect is to increase the vertical component of facial growth and reduce the forward component, a characteristic feature of the modern human face as compared with that of anthropoid apes and early types of humanity.

During the juvenile period, when sutural growth is more active, the

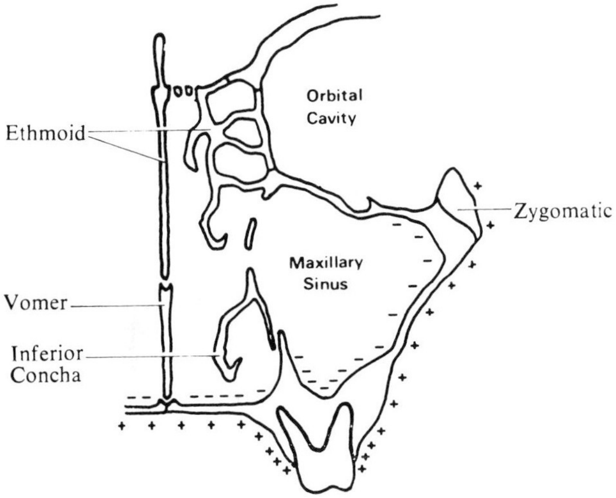

Fig. 124 Diagrammatic representation of a coronal section through the upper facial skeleton at the level of the first permanent molar showing the major sites of surface deposition and resorption. Deposition, +; resorption, −.

direction of facial growth is forward and downward in direction, becoming predominantly vertical during the second decade when the surface deposition-resorption mechanism is relatively more important (Figs. 125, 127).

Increase in the height of the mouth cavity is chiefly the result of continuous growth of the alveolar processes of both the upper and lower jaws. This is related to the downward component of mandibular growth and the elongation of the ramus, providing a space between the jaws to be 'filled in' by alveolar bone so that the teeth are maintained in occlusion.

Growth in width. During fetal life and at birth a complete sagittal suture system divides the cranio-facial skeleton into two halves. During fetal life and early infancy, growth at this suture system is largely responsible for the increase in width of the cranio-facial skeleton. Separation of the bones along the suture system is produced by growth of the brain, of the cartilage between the great wings and body of the sphenoid and of the roof of the nasal capsule.

During the first year after birth, however, the great wings unite with the body of the sphenoid, while the metopic suture and the mandibular

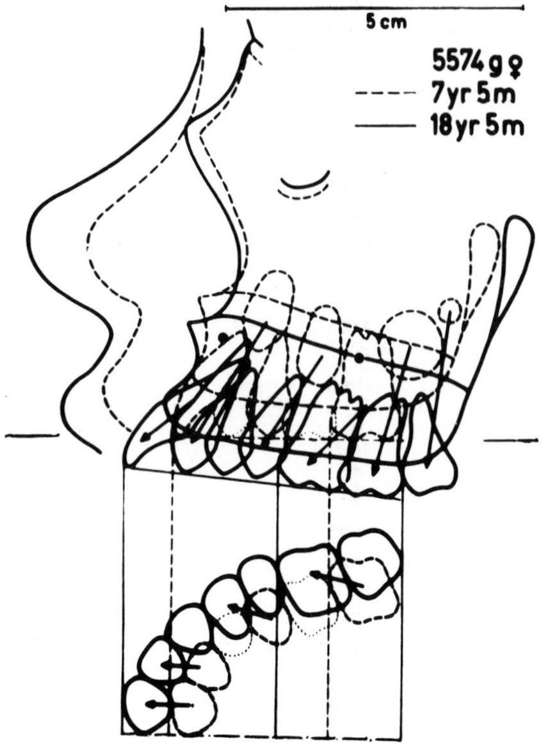

Fig. 125 Growth of the maxilla and dento-alveolar development, analysed by means of implants. (*By courtesy of Prof A. Björk and Trans. Europ. Orthodont. Soc.*)

symphysis are largely obliterated so that the frontal bone and the mandible become single bony elements. Ossification of the sphenoidal cartilage stabilises the middle region of the cranial base and the sphenoid becomes a single bone reaching from one temporal fossa to the other. Soon afterwards (by the third year) ossification of the cribriform plate region unites the bilateral facial elements of the ethmoid with the midline perpendicular plate, so that the ethmoid becomes a single bone extending from one orbital cavity to the other and stabilising the intraorbital and upper nasal regions of the facial skeleton. The maxilla can still move outwards relative to the ethmoid and growth can still take place at the zygomatico-maxillary and mid-palatal sutures, but with the attainment of adult dimensions of the orbital cavity at about seven years of age, growth at these sutures becomes considerably reduced and further growth during the later part of childhood is chiefly brought about by surface deposition of bone associated with internal resorption.

A factor in determining the growth in width of the dental arches is the outward as well as the vertical direction of growth of the alveolar processes.

Relation of teeth to facial growth. In the upper jaw, bone deposition is the chief factor producing the increase in length of the alveolar process necessary to make room for the permanent molars as they erupt at approximately six, twelve, and eighteen years. These teeth develop and their crowns are formed one after another in the alveolar bulbs at the back of the maxilla (Figs. 105, 107). From the alveolar bulbs they move forward into the space made available for them at the back of the alveolar process by the forward movement of the upper dentition through the alveolar bone as this increases in size as a result of bone deposition upon its outer, facial surface. During the first decade and to a limited extent during the second decade some space is made available by deposition of bone at the posterior surface of the maxilla. In the lower jaw a certain amount of space is made for the permanent molars by resorption of bone at the root of the anterior border of the ramus; by the greater difference in size between the deciduous molars and their successors the premolars; and, to a lesser extent than in the upper jaw, by a forward movement of the teeth through the alveolar bone. The lower teeth keep contact with the upper teeth during facial growth in part as the result of a forward movement with the alveolar bone, but in part also by a continuous forward growth of the whole mandible from behind which carries the lower teeth with it.

In animals such as the pig, and to a lesser extent in the non-human primates, where a great increase in alveolar length is required for the much larger permanent molar and canines, an important mechanism for growth in the upper jaw is at the suture between the maxilla and premaxilla. In the lower jaw the increase in alveolar length is brought about in part by a forward projection of the alveolar process over the body of the mandible in front. In man the suture between the maxilla and premaxilla closes before birth and the lower alveolar process remains at the same plane as or behind the body of the mandible, so producing the human chin.

Growth of the mandible. Before the middle of fetal life a typical bony mandible is produced, the condylar cartilage having been replaced by bone except at its growing articular surface. The continued proliferation of this cartilage until the end of the second or beginning of the third decade of life produces part of the increase in mandibular length as measured from condyle to symphysis, and at the same time increases the height of the ramus. Growth at the condyle usually occurs in a backward, upward, and outward direction, so that not only is the length of each half of the mandibular arch increased but also the distance between the condyles (Fig. 114). This keeps pace with the increasing width of the base of the skull and the consequent separation of the glenoid cavities of the temporal bones. Since the mandible is attached at the temporo-mandibular joints to the 'fixed' area of the skull base, the effect of the growth at the condyles is to help to carry the mandible progressively downward and forward (Fig. 126). The mandible is also carried forward and downward with the growing face through the

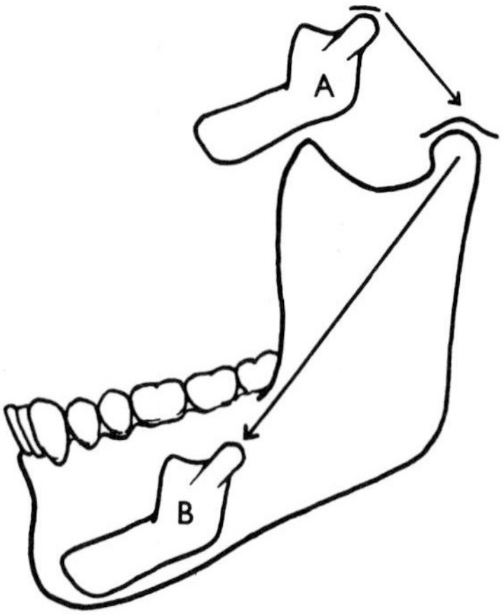

Fig. 126 Diagram to illustrate mandibular growth and change in position between birth and adult life. (A) The position of the infant mandible relative to that of the adult jaw. The arrow shows the direction of shift of the temporal region. (B) the theoretical position of the original infant mandible as carried forward and downward from the temporal region by mandibular growth.

occlusal relations of the upper and lower teeth established during mastication and swallowing. The forward and downward displacement of the mandible can still occur after removal of the condyles, probably due to a translatory action by the muscles of mastication.

Accompanying and keeping pace with this growth at the condyle, membrane bone is laid down along the posterior border of the ramus so that the ramus is built backward and maintained in relationship to the condyle. A similar growth takes place along the upper edge of the ramus and the coronoid process. The increase in area of the ramus accompanying the lengthening of the mandible provides the greater area necessary for muscular attachment throughout growth. In some cases the alveolar process of the mandible may be lengthened anteriorly by surface deposition but in others this is a site of bone resorption (Fig. 128).

During fetal life growth at the symphysis is mainly concerned with producing an increased separation of the anterior ends of the two halves of the mandible, just as condylar growth as well as lengthening the mandible is responsible for the increasing separation of the posterior condylar ends of the mandible (Fig. 114). This growth ceases before the end of the first year with the union of the two halves of the mandible at the symphysis.

The general increase in the dimensions of the body of the mandible that occurs throughout growth is due to surface deposition of bone. Though some increase in its height is produced by the deposition along

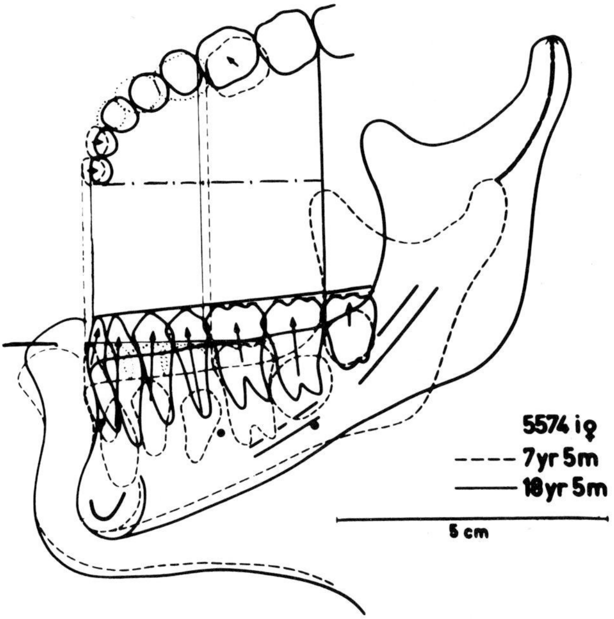

Fig. 127 Growth of the mandible and dento-alveolar development, analysed by means of implants. (*By courtesy of Prof A. Björk and Trans. Europ. Orthodont. Soc.*)

its lower border this is of small amount; by far the greatest increase is produced by alveolar growth. This occurs throughout the whole growth period and is of course closely associated with eruption of the teeth and their attainment of the occlusal plane (Figs. 127, 128).

Since the mandible, under normal conditions, is continually being carried forward by its growth the lower teeth are also carried bodily forward throughout the whole growth period. There may be in some individuals a small amount of actual movement of the teeth forward and outward with the alveolar bone in relation to bone deposition at the facial surface of the mandible. Thus the lower teeth are kept in relation to the upper teeth mainly through the forward positioning of the lower jaw. Room for the permanent molars is in part produced by the lengthening of the body of the mandible through the cutting back of

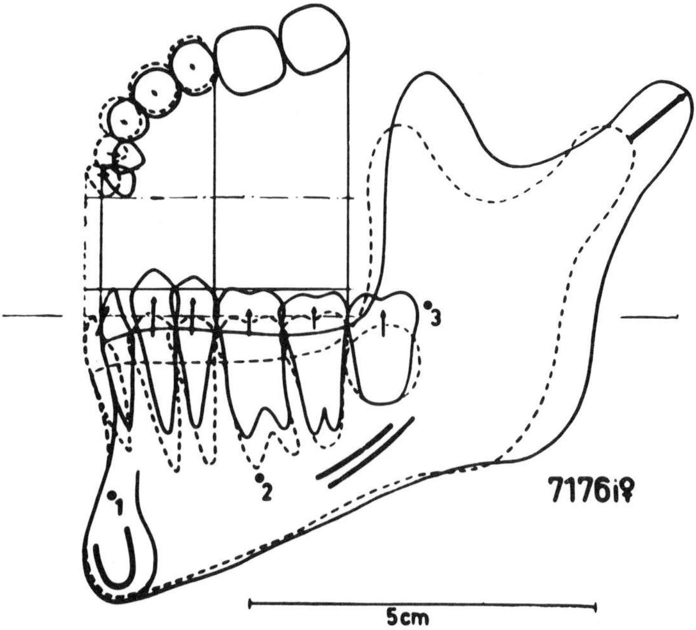

Fig. 128 Growth of the mandible and dento-alveolar development, analysed by means of implants. The three implants are numbered. The radiographic tracings of the two stages of mandibular growth are superimposed by means of the implants.---- 10 yr 6 m --- 15 yr 6 m. (*By courtesy of Prof. A. Björk and J. dent. Res.*)

the anterior border of the ramus, although this process is also related to the maintenance of the origin and insertion of the temporal muscle.

Apart from the major areas of bone deposition and resorption already described the mandible also shows smaller areas associated with a more localised remodelling growth and resorption. As the head of the condyle is progressively added to there is an accompanying resorption at the neck of the condyle which narrows down this region. At the coronoid process there is some deposition on its medial aspect whereas some resorption takes place on its lateral aspect (Fig. 129). On the lingual aspect of the body of the mandible certain localised remodelling resorptions take place.

CHANGES IN THE PROPORTIONS OF THE FACE AND SKULL DURING CHILDHOOD

The facial skeleton can be divided into a neural region related to the growing eyeballs and lying above the Frankfurt plane and a masticatory region lying below the level of the Frankfurt plane. The upper olfactory region of the nasal cavities lying between the orbital cavities and bounded by the ethmoid bone is related in its growth to the neural

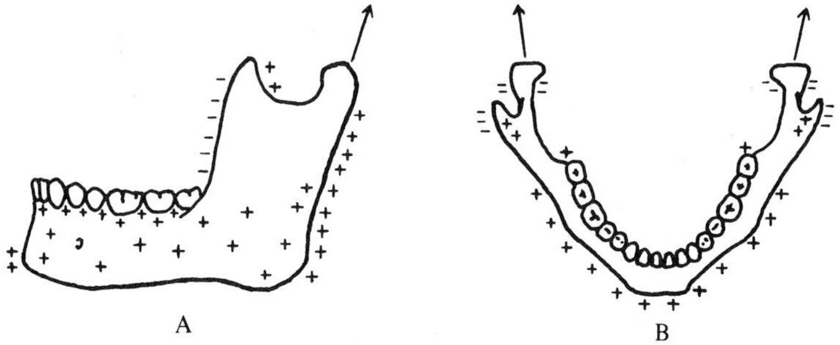

Fig. 129 Diagrammatic representation of the mandible showing the major sites of surface deposition and resorption. Deposition, +; resorption, −. (A) Lateral aspect of the mandible. (B) The mandible as seen from the occlusal aspect. The arrows represent the direction of condylar growth.

region, whereas the lower respiratory part of the nasal cavity grows with the masticatory region of the face.

Proportions of neural and facial parts of skull to one another at different ages

Age	Neural Skeleton	Facial Skeleton
Birth	8	1
Second year	6	1
Fifth year	5	1
Adult	3	1

At birth the cranial part of the skull and the neural region of the face, which is related to the growth of the brain, the eyes, and the organs of hearing and balance, is about eight times as large as the masticatory part of the face which is built around the teeth, the tongue, and the respiratory region of the nasal cavity including the maxillary sinuses. In the adult the masticatory face is about a third of the size of the neural part of the skull. Between birth and adult life the cranium increases four times and the face about twelve times in volume (Fig. 130).

Most of the postnatal cranial growth, however (80 per cent), takes place during the first two years. During this period, while the deciduous teeth are erupting, both the cranial and facial parts of the skull are growing very rapidly, but after this time growth of the face, although continuing at a slower pace than previously, is more extensive than that of the cranium. By the end of the first decade brain growth and eyeball growth is very nearly complete. Facial growth and development of the dentition continue until about the twentieth year.

Growth of the skull is intimately associated with the growth of three groups of structures:

1. The brain and eyeballs.
2. The teeth.
3. The muscles of mastication.

These structures affect the growth of the skull at different periods.

The brain and eyeballs exert their main influence during the rapid growing period of early infancy (birth to the end of the second year). The teeth exert their main influence on facial growth during two periods:

1. During the time of eruption of the deciduous teeth. This period coincides with the period of most rapid postnatal growth of the neural structures.

2. Between six and twelve years of age, when the permanent teeth replace the deciduous teeth and the first and second permanent molars erupt.

The muscles (including the muscles of mastication) exert their main influence in later childhood and after the onset of puberty (twelve to eighteen years), but the facial muscles because of their activity in suckling are relatively well developed at birth.

The brain and eyeballs exert their chief influence upon the cranial part of the skull and upon the upper part of the face. The teeth exert their main influence upon the development of the alveolar processes of the maxilla and mandible, and also upon the buttress systems of the face whereby the stresses of mastication are transmitted to the cranial base. Muscular processes such as the coronoid process of the mandible, the angle of the mandible, the zygomatic arches, and lateral pterygoid plates reach their full development with the establishment of the adult musculature.

The growth of the individual. Much of the data on which the analyses of facial growth are based comes from the measurements of numerous individuals in each age group and the mean value of all the cases in each group is then taken as representative of the stage of growth reached at that age. This gives an impression of a steady rate of growth from year to year. If, however, the same individuals are measured at yearly intervals or less, it is obvious that every individual has his or her own growth pattern; so that similar adult dimensions may be reached by very different growth histories and children with similar dimensions at birth may reach very contrasting adult dimensions. The majority of children show a growth spurt during adolescence which involves the long bones, vertebral column and facial skeleton, but not the neural elements of the skull.

Cephalometric planes. In the analysis of facial growth by the use of orientated skull X-rays (cephalograms), a number of planes are used. The more important standard planes are as follows (Fig. 131):

1. Bolton plane: between basion (anterior margin of foramen magnum) or the deepest point on the notch behind the occipital condyle (Bolton point) and nasion, the point on the facial profile between the nasal and frontal bones.

2. Anterior cranial base plane: between the middle of the pituitary fossa and nasion.

3. Frankfurt plane: between upper margin of external auditory meatus (porion) and lower margin of orbital rim (orbitale).

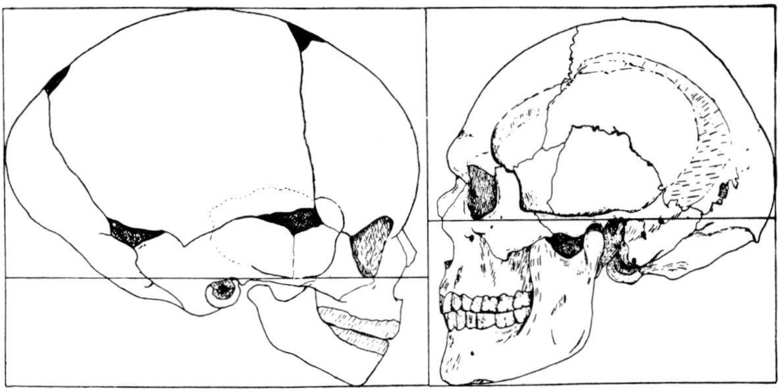

Fig. 130 Skulls of new-born child and adult compared in lateral view. The skulls are orientated on the Frankfurt plane. Relative to the adult skull that of the child has been magnified twice in all dimensions. (*By courtesy of Prof J. C. Brash and the Dental Board of the United Kingdom.*)

4. Palatal plane: from anterior to posterior nasal spine through the hard palate.
5. Mandibular plane: a line tangent to the lower border of the mandible.
6. Anterior facial plane: line from nasion tangent to the most anterior part of the mandible.
7. Occlusal plane.

The backward extension of the mandibular plane meets the backward extension of the Frankfurt plane at mandible plane angle No. 1.

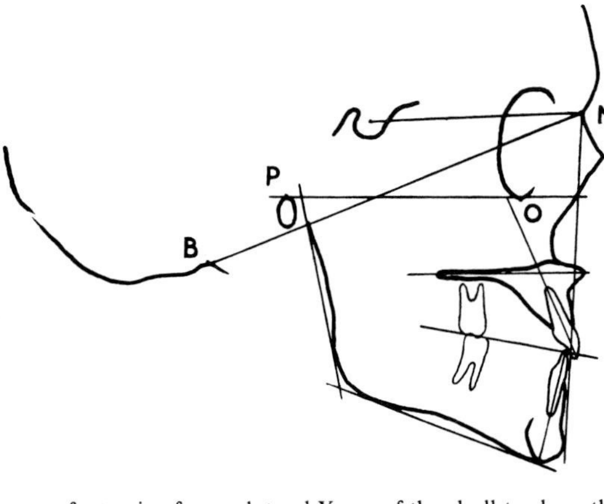

Fig. 131 Diagram of a tracing from a lateral X-ray of the skull to show the arrangement of certain cephalometric planes. (B) Bolton point; (N) nasion; (O) orbitale; (P) porion.

The backward extension of the mandibular plane meets the backward extension of the anterior cranial base plane at mandibular plane angle No. 2.

The backward extension of the mandibular plane meets the backward extension of the palatal plane at the palato-mandibular angle.

There are two chief facial angles: between the anterior facial plane and the anterior cranial base plane at nasion, and between the anterior facial plane and the Frankfurt plane.

There are two chief mandibular angles: between the mandibular plane and the facial plane at the chin, and between the mandibular plane and a line along the posterior border of the ramus.

The angles between the lower central incisors and the mandibular plane and between the upper incisors and the Frankfurt plane are also commonly used.

For each angle there is a normal range of variation at different periods of facial growth, but the range is very wide between individuals. These planes and angles are best used for the analysis of facial form and malformation in individual cases.

Clinical considerations. Though any part of skull growth may become insufficient or abnormal, naturally those sites of growth which persist throughout the whole growth period produce the greatest effects when damaged by trauma or disease, or when their growth becomes abnormal as in certain dysfunctions of the ductless glands or hereditary disturbances.

The main sites of growth which actively persist until the third decade are the synchondrosis at the base of the skull, between the basi-occipital and basi-sphenoid; the secondary cartilage of the condyle of the mandible; and the generalised surface deposition of bone on the facial and alveolar surfaces of the jaws and on the hard palate.

The most vulnerable of these growth sites to trauma is that at the condyle of the mandible; also by its proximity to the mandibular joint it may be involved in acute arthritis in childhood. Due to the damage, or even destruction of the secondary cartilage produced by trauma or inflammation, the mandible on the affected side fails to grow equally in length with the unaffected side.

In acromegaly, where growth occurs in adult life at a time when normally it has ceased, both jaws become abnormally large, due to continued surface deposition of bone; the mandible is also lengthened by the over-prolonged activity of the condylar growth centre.

In achondroplasia, which is a hereditary condition affecting the growth of cartilage, the base of the skull is the primary part involved. Other changes in the skull, such as the enlarged vault and the depressed upper face, are secondary effects due to the shortened cranial base and failure of growth of the cartilage of the nasal septum. The secondary cartilage of the mandibular condyle appears to be unaffected.

The whole skull is naturally involved in pituitary dwarfism or gigantism, conditions affecting the skeleton generally and commencing in early life.

Less drastic deformities of cranio-facial growth produce the common major malocclusions found in orthodontic practice such as prenormal and postnormal relationship between the upper and lower jaws and the conditions of open and close bite. Many of these conditions are due to failure of growth which may be limited to one or other of the jaws or the alveolar processes, or may involve the whole of the facial skeleton. In other cases the underlying abnormality is a disproportion between various elements of the facial skeleton. Such conditions may be due to hereditary factors or may be produced by abnormal habits such as thumb-sucking. In many cases they appear to be related to abnormal patterns of behaviour on the part of the muscles of the cheeks, lips and tongue, while sometimes the whole of the cranio-cervical musculature may be involved. Another possible factor in the aetiology of certain forms of malocclusion may be inadequate masticatory function. These matters are dealt with in textbooks of orthodontics.

BIBLIOGRAPHY

Baume, L. J. (1961). The postnatal growth activity of the nasal cartilage septum. *Helv. odont. Acta* **5**, 9.

Baume, L. J. (1968). Patterns of cephalofacial growth and development. *Int. dent. J.* **18**, 489.

Björk, A. (1963). Variations in growth pattern of the human mandible. *J. dent. Res.* **42**, 400.

Björk, A. (1964). Sutural growth of the upper face studied by the implant method. *Trans. Europ. Orthodont. Soc.* 49.

Brash, J. C., McKeag, H. T. A. & Scott, J. H. (1956). *The Aetiology of Irregularity and Malocclusion of the Teeth.* 2nd ed. London: Dental Board of the United Kingdom.

Dixon, A. D. (1961). Autoradiographic studies of jaw growth. *J. dent. Res.* **40**, 204.

Enlow, D. H. (1975). *Handbook of Facial Growth.* Philadelphia: Saunders.

Enlow, D. H. & Bang, S. (1965). Growth and remodeling of the human maxilla. *Amer. J. Orthodont.* **51**, 446.

Ford, E. H. R. (1958). Growth of the human cranial base. *Amer. J. Orthodont.* **44**, 498.

Koski, K. (1968). Cranial growth centres. Fact or fallacies? *Amer. J. Orthodont.* **54**, 566.

Latham, R. A. & Burston, W. R. (1966). The postnatal pattern of growth at the sutures of the human skull. *Dent. Practit.* **17**, 61.

Lebret, L. (1962). Growth changes of the palate. *J. dent. Res.* **41**, 139.

Meredith, H. V. (1960). Changes in form of the head and face during childhood. *Growth* **24**, 215.

Melsen, B. (1967). Craniometric study of dimensional changes in the nasal septum from infancy to maturity. *Acta odont. Scand.* **25**, 541.

Moore, W. J. & Lavelle, C. L. B. (1974). *Growth of the Facial Skeleton in the Hominoidea.* London: Academic Press.

Moss, M. L. (1968). A theoretical analysis of the functional matrix. *Acta Biotheor.* **18**, 195.

Müller, G. (1963) Growth and development of the middle face. *J. dent. Res.* **42**, 385.

Sarnat, B. G. (1963). Postnatal growth of the upper face; some experimental considerations. *Angle Orthodont.* **33**, 139.

Sarnat, B. G. & Wexler, M. R. (1967). Rabbit snout growth after resection of central linear segments of nasal septal cartilage. *Acta oto-laryngol.* **63**, 467.

Scott, J. H. (1954). Growth of the human face. *Proc. R. Soc. Med.* **47**, 91.
—— (1959). Further studies on the growth of the human face. *Proc. R. Soc. Med.* **52**, 263.
Symons, N. B. B. (1951). Studies on the growth and form of the mandible. *Dent. Rec.* **71**, 41.
Zollor, R. M. & Laskin, D. M. (1969). Growth of the zygomaticomaxillary suture in pigs after sectioning the zygomatic arch. *J. dent. Res.* **48**, 573.

9. Dental Development at Different Ages as shown in X-ray Examination

In this chapter it is proposed to give a summary of the development of the dentition and of facial growth as seen in the examination of X-rays. A series of radiographs of the jaws at intervals between birth and adult life provides an invaluable adjunct to a study of the development of the dentition and its relationship to the bone of the jaws. For in this way it is possible to see all the teeth, both erupted and unerupted, at the same time, and to examine the details of their relative arrangement. It should be remembered, however, that there is a considerable degree of individual variation in dental development and facial growth. The X-rays illustrating this chapter are from different individuals in which the heads have been bisected in the sagittal plane. Since the introduction of modern cephalometric techniques, it is possible to study the growth of the same individuals over a period of years. A disadvantage of this method is the superimposition of the shadows of structures on the two sides.

The literature on facial growth and dental development is now very extensive, but a considerable amount of research remains to be done on the variations in the growth of normal and abnormal facial skeletons, on the sites of growth in the cranio-facial skeleton, and on the relationship between dental development and skeletal growth.

Neo-natal period (Fig. 132). The calcifying crowns of the deciduous teeth lie in their alveoli in the alveolar bone of the mandible and maxilla. The roofs of the alveoli are covered over by the oral mucous membrane (gum pads) to which the follicles of the teeth are attached. Two-thirds of the crowns of the deciduous incisors are calcified, and about one-third of the crowns of the canines. In the first deciduous molars the individual cusps are calcified and united to one another so that the occlusal surface is almost complete. In the second deciduous molars the tips of the cusps are calcified but are still isolated from one another. The mesio-buccal cusp of the first permanent molar is calcified. In the lower jaw the crypt of the first permanent molar occupies the lower alveolar bulb which lies in the substance of the ramus and reaches almost as far back as the opening of the inferior dental canal. The upper first permanent molar occupies the upper alveolar bulb, which faces backward into the lower part of the pterygo-palatine fossa. The developing tooth germs of the permanent incisors, canines, and premolars lie to the lingual side of the developing deciduous teeth in the same alveoli but they have not yet begun to undergo calcification. In the upper jaw the developing teeth lie close beneath the orbital cavity, and the maxillary sinus lies on their inner side but has not yet grown outward over the teeth.

The temporo-mandibular joint is at about the same level as the upper alveolar margin. The glenoid fossa is flat or only slightly concave. There is no eminentia articularis. The bone which has replaced the secondary cartilage in the mandibular condyle shows as a wedge-shaped area running through the developing ramus to end below the crypt of the first permanent molar. The posterior and lower borders of the mandible meet at an angle opening upward of about 140 degrees; the coronoid

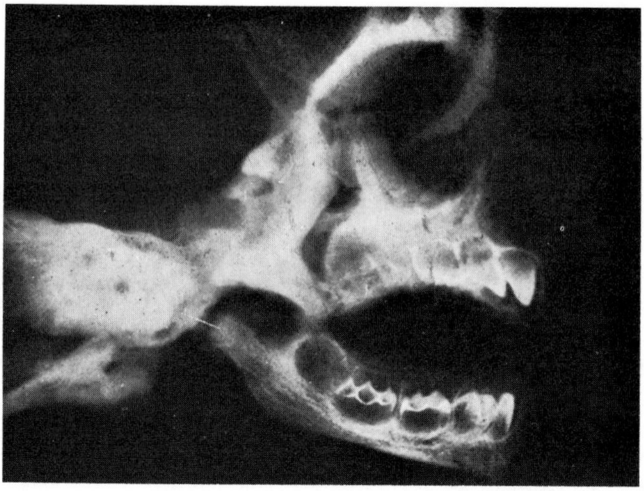

Fig. 132 Right side of male infant one month old.

process is poorly developed. The pterygoid plates slope markedly forward to meet the maxillary and palatine tuberosities; the pterygo-palatine fossa is wide but of limited vertical extent; with the mouth closed the upper and lower gum pads are usually in contact in the molar region. There is usually a space in front between the upper and lower pads in the incisor region through which the tongue protrudes; the lower jaw is often in postnormal relationship to the upper.

One year of age (Fig. 133). The deciduous incisors have erupted but their roots are not yet fully formed; the first deciduous molars are about to appear in the mouth and two-thirds of the roots are formed. The crowns of the second deciduous molars are fully formed and the occlusal surfaces of the first permanent molars are complete. In the upper jaw the first permanent molar occupies the alveolar bulb in the lower part of the pterygo-palatine fossa and its occlusal surface faces backward as well as downward; in the lower jaw the occlusal surface of the first permanent molar may face inward or outward as well as upward. Cal-

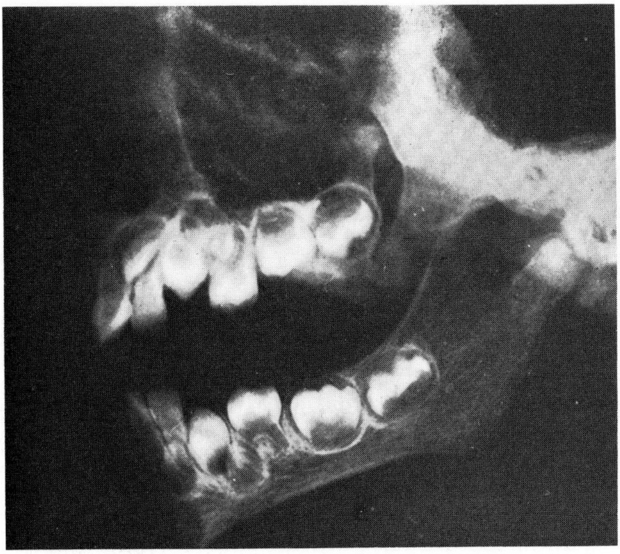

Fig. 133 Left side of female infant one year old.

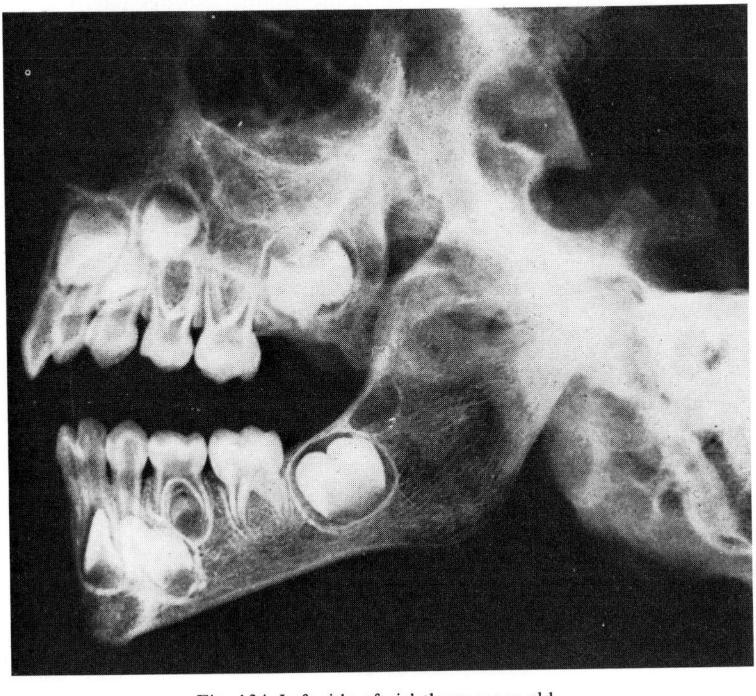

Fig. 134 Left side of girl three years old.

cification has commenced in the upper permanent central incisor, the lower incisors, and in the canines, and is just about to begin in the upper lateral incisor. The permanent replacing teeth now occupy separate crypts on the lingual side of the roots of the deciduous teeth, and their follicles begin to develop a separate attachment to the oral mucous membrane. In the upper jaw the developing sinus has begun to grow outward over the roots of the deciduous molars and the crypt of the permanent molar, separating them from the floor of the orbital cavity. The upper alveolar margin is now at a lower level than the mandibular joint. The ramus of the mandible has increased greatly in height by growth at the condylar cartilage and by bone deposition extending the coronoid process. It has also increased in width by bone deposition along the posterior border, which now joins the lower border at a more acute angle. During the first year the two halves of the mandible unite at the symphysis.

Three years of age (Fig. 134). The crowns of the permanent incisors are almost complete; that of the canines about two-thirds completed; and calcification has just commenced in the premolars, which are embraced by the roots of the deciduous molars. The crowns of the first permanent molars are virtually complete and their crypts have reached their full size. The crypt of the second permanent lower molar occupies the alveolar bulb in the substance of the ramus, but lies partly above the crypt of the first molar. The crypt of the second permanent upper molar lies at the back of the upper alveolar bulb, and the first permanent molar has moved forward and also rotated so as to face more downward and less backward. The bulge of the upper alveolar bulb into the pterygo-palatine fossa is reduced as the first molar moves forward, but it expands again as the second molar grows within its crypt. The roots of all the deciduous teeth are complete; their pulp chambers are large and the root canals wide. At about this time the eminentia articularis develops and the glenoid fossa acquires the typical convex-concave outline as the individual's occlusal relationship is established by the complete deciduous dentition.

Six years of age (Fig. 135). The first permanent molars have undergone a rapid development and have erupted behind the deciduous dentition; their roots are now more than half formed. The second permanent molar has now taken the position formerly occupied by the first molar at the end of the second year, the base of its crypt lying in close relationship to the inferior dental canal. Resorption of the deciduous incisors and canines is in progress; the crowns of the permanent canines are fully formed. The deciduous molars have become lifted away from the crypts of the premolars with further growth of the alveolar bone. In the upper alveolar bulb, the second molar has moved forwards and the posterior bulge of the bulb into the pterygo-palatine fossa is again less marked. The occlusal level of the teeth is now well below that of the glenoid fossa.

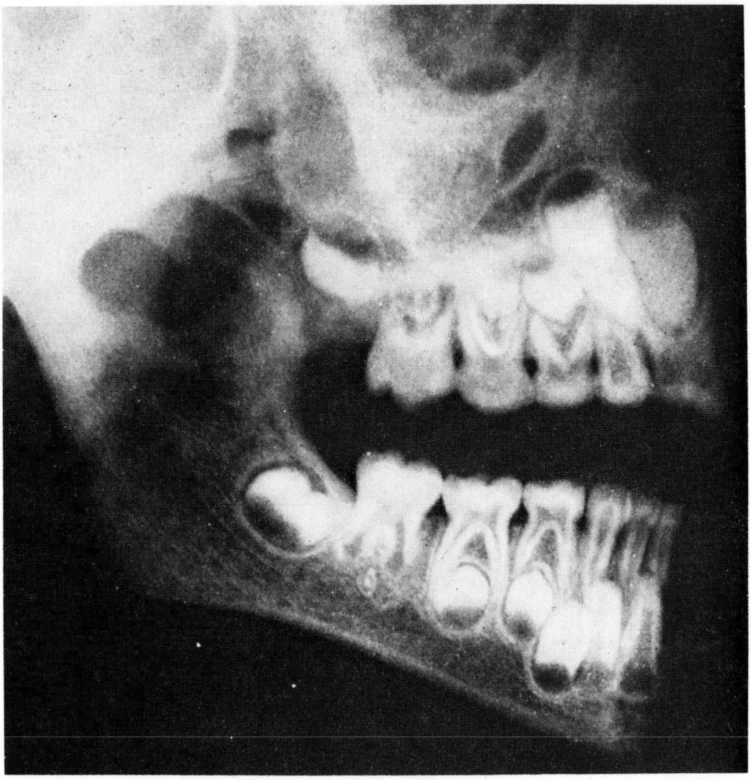

Fig. 135 Right side of boy six years old.

Seven years of age (Fig. 136). The permanent incisors have erupted or are erupting, resorption is commencing in the roots of the deciduous molars: the crowns of the premolars are almost fully formed and the crowns of the second permanent molars are almost complete; the apical foramina of the first permanent molars are still wide open; the permanent canines are lying at a deeper level in the jaws than the other teeth. The level of the upper alveolar border is now well below that of the temporo-mandibular joint; the maxillary sinus lies over the crypts of the second premolar, and the second permanent molar, as well as over the incomplete roots of the first permanent molar. The developing upper canine is related to the front wall of the sinus, the lateral wall of the nasal cavity and to the nasolacrimal duct. In the lower jaw note the space between the crypt of the second permanent molar and the distal root of the first molar. The apices of the developing and erupting upper permanent incisors are closely related to the floor of the nasal cavity. At this time the cranial and orbital cavities have reached more than 90 per cent of their adult dimensions, and growth in the cranial

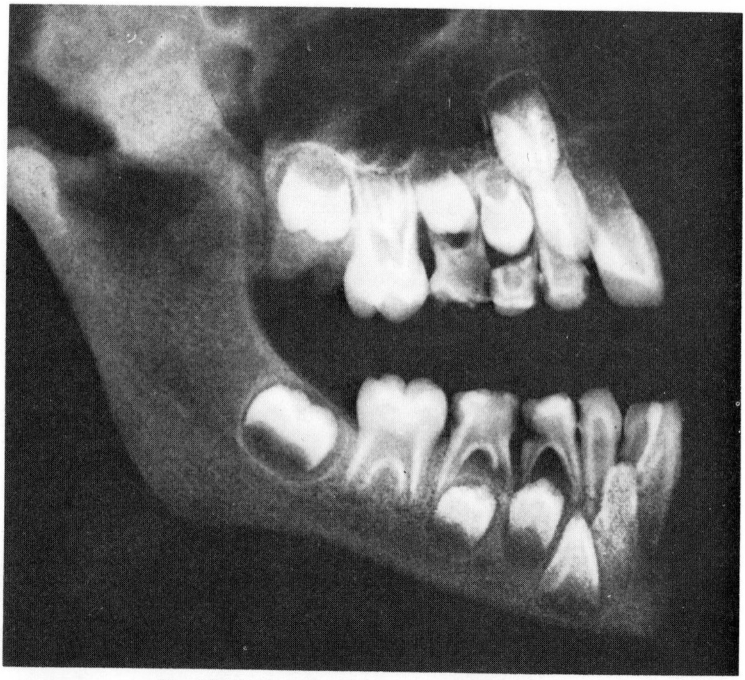
Fig. 136 Right side of boy seven years old.

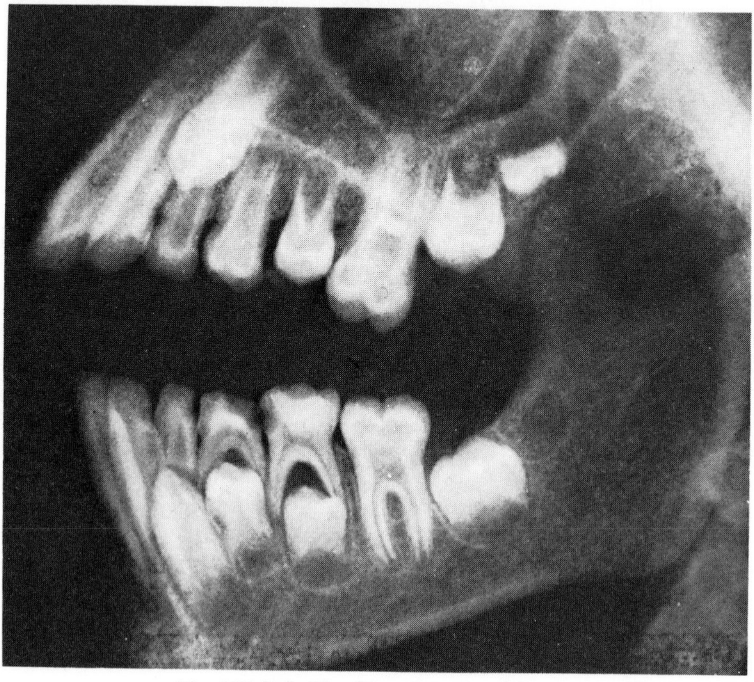
Fig. 137 Left side of boy ten years old.

part of the skull and neural part of the face is nearing completion. Growth in the facial skeleton below the Frankfurt plane is still far from complete.

Ten years of age (Fig. 137). The permanent incisors are fully erupted, the roots of the deciduous canines are undergoing resorption, and root formation has commenced in the permanent canines. In some cases at this age the permanent canines have cut the gum. The deciduous molars are in the process of being shed, and one or more of the premolars are usually present in the mouth. The second permanent molars are erupting and breaking through the roofs of their crypts. Calcification has begun in the third molars.

Thirteen years of age (Fig. 138). The canines and premolars have erupted or are erupting. The second permanent molars are erupting, and the crowns of the third permanent molars are fully formed and have reached the stage of development reached by the first molars at three years and the second molars at seven years. The floor of the sinus lies above the second premolar and the three permanent molars. At this time or soon afterwards the permanent dentition is complete except for the third molars. The muscles of mastication are growing rapidly to

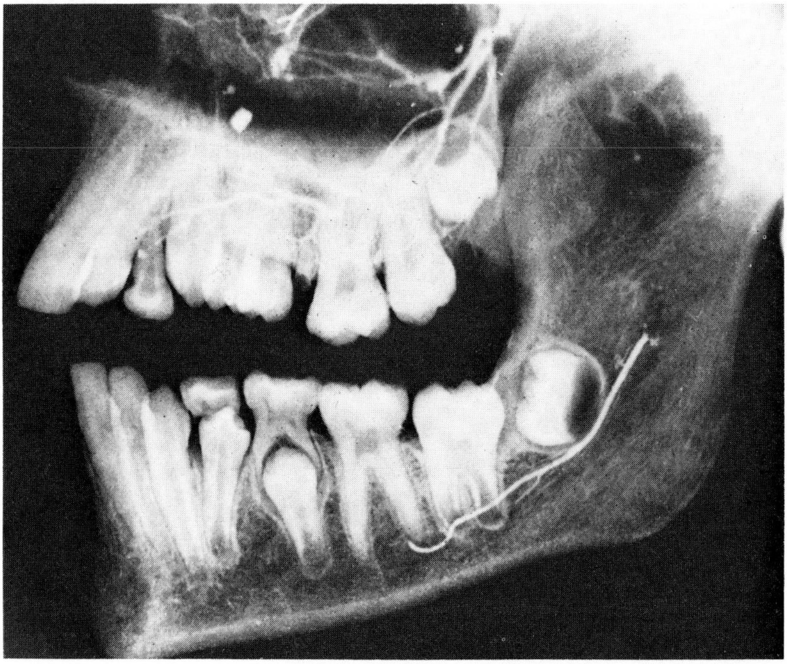

Fig. 138. Left side of girl thirteen years old. Note the retained deciduous upper canine and disto-buccal root of the second upper deciduous molar also the unusually tilted position of the lower third molar in its crypt.

meet the requirements of the adult dentition and the part of the skeleton to which they are attached, the pterygoid plates, the zygomatic arch, the coronoid process and the region of the mandibular angle, are increasing in size. The bone forming the buttress systems of the face is attaining adult dimensions and strength. The glenoid fossa and articular eminence are reaching their adult form as is the head of the mandibular condyle.

Clinical considerations. It will be appreciated that a proper co-ordination between tooth development, tooth eruption and jaw growth is necessary to produce a well formed dentition in which the teeth are in normal occlusion. Disharmony can be produced by:

1. Disproportion between tooth size and the size of the supporting alveolar bone and jaws.
2. Early loss of deciduous teeth with drifting of adjacent teeth and lack of space for the erupting successional teeth.
3. Extra teeth or missing teeth in one or both the deciduous and permanent dentitions.
4. Abnormal relationships between the upper and lower jaws and growth deformities of one or both jaws.

If the teeth erupt too early there may not be as yet enough room available in the jaws to avoid crowding; if they erupt too late there may be inadequate space for the last members of the series, the third permanent molars. These teeth are especially liable to occupy abnormal positions in the dental arches, to erupt late, to be impacted as a consequence of failure of rotation during eruption especially in the lower jaw and to give trouble during their eruption. They are absent in about 10 per cent of individuals among the white race, but agenesis is much less frequent among African and Asiatic peoples. They also vary more in form and size than any of the other teeth.

BIBLIOGRAPHY

Lewis, A. B. & Garn, S. M. (1960). The relationship between tooth formation and other maturational factors. *Angle Orthodont.* **30**, 70.

Symington, J. & Rankin, J. C. (1908). *An Atlas of Skiagrams.* London: Longmans, Green.

SECTION III

The development and histology of the dental and parodontal tissues

10. The Basic Structure of the Dental and Parodontal Tissues

All tissues in the body are made up of three constituents, cells, extracellular substance, and fluids. The proportions of these vary greatly with each tissue, and this accounts for much of the different nature of the various kinds of tissue. Epithelium, which consists almost entirely of cells, contrasts with the connective tissues in which the cells are generally much fewer in number with a considerable amount of extracellular material. Epithelial tissues do not contain blood vessels, unlike the connective tissues, and so are dependent for their nutritional supply on the connective tissues, which are adjacent to them.

The extracellular substance, known sometimes as intercellular substance, is itself a product of cells and has two components, fibres and an amorphous material. The fibres are composed of proteins and may be either collagenous, reticular, or elastic. The amorphous part of the extracellular substance contains a considerable amount of mucopolysaccharides and in it the fibrous element is embedded. Depending on its consistency the amorphous material is divided into two varieties, soft ground substance and firm cement or cementing substance. In certain tissues, namely bone, dentine and cement, the amorphous extracellular substance is modified by being mineralised (calcified); inorganic material in the form of crystallites is deposited in the amorphous substance, and in and around the collagen fibres which are found there. In the case of these mineralised tissues, the term organic matrix is commonly used to refer to the extracellular substance less its mineral content.

Cells. Within recent years a good correlation between the details of cell structure and function has been established as a result of investigations particularly with the electron microscope. Cells which produce and secrete protein can be readily distinguished from those which form protein but retain it. In the dental and parodontal tissues the former type of cell is very common, and examples include the odontoblast, the ameloblast, and the osteoblast. Each of these cells shows certain typical organelles, particularly large prominent mitochondria, a rough surfaced endoplasmic reticulum, and a well marked Golgi apparatus(Fig. 177).

Both the mitochondria and the ribosome particles are concerned in protein synthesis. Ribosomes, in such cells, are found on the outer surface of the membranes which form the cisternae of the endoplasmic reticulum and give its 'rough' surface. The ribonucleoprotein of the ribosomes is responsible for the well-known basophilia of the cytoplasm of these cells. Apart from the protein synthesis carried out by the ribosomes the endoplasmic reticulum is concerned in transporting substances from one part of the cell to another. The Golgi complex is related to the accumulation, and transport of the synthesised protein for eventual secretion outside the cell. It is also associated with the formation of carbohydrate and its attachment to certain protein secretions. Thus the Golgi apparatus is responsible for the incorporation of the carbohydrate component of mucus and of zymogen granules.

The keratin forming cells of the oral epithelium provide an example of a situation where although protein is formed it is not exported, and instead is retained within the cells. This difference in function compared with that of the protein secreting cells is reflected in the minute structure of the cells. In the stratum germinativum groups of mitochondria are noticeable but the Golgi body is inconspicuous. The endoplasmic reticulum is scanty and although ribonucleoprotein particles are present they are not associated with it but lie free in the cytoplasm. The fine filaments which make up structures known as tonofibrils are numerous; they represent the first stage in the synthesis of the protein, keratin. As the cells move towards the surface they become progressively flattened, the ribosomes, mitochondria and nuclei gradually disappear and the tonofibrils become more obvious. The latter become associated with an amorphous intracellular matrix which first appears as the keratohyaline granules in the stratum granulosum. Finally the cells become no longer distinguishable and are represented by a structureless mass of horny material, the stratum corneum. During keratinisation there is a loss of fluid from the cells. This starts in the deeper cell layers and so is not simply a surface desiccation, but is a controlled process.

The presence of lysosomes has been demonstrated within ameloblasts and odontoblasts, using a positive reaction for acid phosphatase as the criterion for the recognition of such bodies. Lysosomes are membrane bound vesicles of varying morphology which contain hydrolytic enzymes. It seems possible that the lysosomes are concerned in the regulation of the secretion of enamel and dentine. This may happen either by the extracellular breakdown of secretion products or by the destruction of secretion granules within the cells.

Lysosomes have been described in keratinising oral epithelium. In the deeper layers they are found within the cells and may be related to the gradual destruction of organelles. In the superficial layers lysosomal enzymes are situated intercellularly and may be concerned in the loosening and desquamation of the cells.

Collagen fibres. Collagen fibres are found widely distributed throughout the body and they have great tensile strength. They are the product of certain specialised cells, the fibroblasts. At rest they show a wavy conformation which disappears when the fibres are stretched. They form an important element of bone, dentine, cement, periodontal membrane, the lamina propria of the oral mucosa, and are also present in pulp tissue and the submucosa. In haematoxylin and eosin stained sections collagenous fibres do not show up well since the pinkish colour which they take is the same as the general background staining. Consequently certain fairly specific stains such as Mallory's connective tissue stain or Masson's trichrome, are used to display them; with these stains, the collagenous fibres are stained a different colour from the other tissue components. In the mineralised tissues, however, these stains are not very effective unless the tissue is first decalcified. With the PAS (periodic acid–Schiff) technique collagenous fibres are coloured a pale pink; which suggests the presence of a small amount of carbohydrate.

Collagen fibre bundles which are visible with low magnifications of the light microscope are made up of finer fibres about 0.3–0.5 μm in diameter, and these in turn are seen with the electron microscope to be composed of still finer fibrils. The fibrils are about 425–600 Å in diameter and show a characteristic cross banding with a periodicity of 640 Å. They in turn are composed of filaments, the collagen macromolecules, each of which consists of three polypeptide chains.

Collagen is characterised by the presence of the amino acid, hydroxylysine and by its high content of the amino acids, glycine, alanine, proline, and hydroxyproline. The latter four amino acids occupy two thirds of the places in collagen; so the remaining fourteen amino acids of collagen are present in rather small amounts. Hydroxyproline is virtually unique to collagen in the animal kingdom.

Reticular fibres (reticulin). Reticular fibres are much finer than collagenous fibres and unlike collagen fibres they show branching. They are commonly found at the junction between connective tissue and other kinds of tissues, such as at the border between the lamina propria and the epithelium of the oral mucosa. As these fibres are almost impossible to see in routinely stained sections it is usual to demonstrate them in silver stained preparations where they appear black, and so they are described as being argyrophilic. Collagen fibres by contrast are stained a brownish colour with silver though young collagen fibres, precollagen, are stained black. With the PAS technique reticular fibres stain red indicating the presence of a carbohydrate material; the fainter pink staining of collagen fibres with this method suggests that a lesser amount of carbohydrate is associated with them. With the electron microscope reticular fibres appear to be made up of microfibrils, some of which show the same 640 Å cross-banding as collagen fibrils and others which are unbanded.

Elastic fibres. Elastic fibres, unlike collagenous and reticular fibres, are not composed of fibrils, they are homogeneous. They are made up of a protein which is called elastin; it is very resistant to chemical change. Elastic fibres are very refractile, unlike collagenous and reticular fibres. The most common site of elastic fibres is in the wall of arteries. Elastic fibres have been demonstrated in the disc and the articular fibrous tissue of the temporomandibular joint. Recently a special type of fibre known as oxytalan fibres have been described. They show some of the characteristics of elastic fibres.

Extracellular amorphous substance. Although the nature of the amorphous extracellular substance is far from fully worked out, it has been established that it contains considerable amounts of protein-carbohydrate complexes, sometimes collectively referred to as mucosubstances. One group of mucosubstances, contains mixtures of hexosamines and often hexuronic acids; those containing hexuronic acid are frequently described as acid mucopolysaccharides, and some of these may be sulphated. A common example of the non-sulphated type is hyaluronic acid. This is a viscous substance which is widely distributed in the extracellular substances of the body. It is depolymerised by hyaluronidase and is thereby made less viscous. Chondroitin sulphates are examples of the sulphated type of mucopolysaccharide; they are generally more viscous than hyaluronic acid and tend to be associated with the firm cement substances.

As the name implies one of the chondroitin sulphates is an important constituent of the extracellular amorphous substance of cartilage; they are also present in the amorphous substance of bone, and in dentine and cement of teeth. The acid mucopolysaccharide content of these extracellular substances is largely responsible for the basophilia which is found with the basic dyes, such as haematoxylin. Since no other extracellular substances stain below pH 4·0 with methylene blue this intense basophilic quality can be used to indicate areas rich in acid mucopolysaccharide. Metachromatic staining with toluidine blue has commonly been taken as another indication of acid mucopolysaccharide.

Basement membranes. At the junction between an epithelium and the adjacent connective tissue there is commonly a layer of extracellular substance which is known as a basement membrane. These membranes are deeply stained with the PAS method but do not show metachromasia. For this reason the presence of acid mucopolysaccharide is excluded, but there would appear to be some other carbohydrate material present, probably neutral muccopolysaccharide. As well as this material reticular fibres can be demonstrated as a closely related network which acts as a support to the membrane.

With the electron microscope a layer of amorphous material, not more than a few hundred Å thick, the lamina densa, has been shown to lie beneath the epithelium of skin and oral mucosa, and separated from the basal epithelial cells by a less dense interval of similar dimensions, the lamina lucida (Fig. 252). This layer is called the basal lamina to distinguish it from the basement membrane of light microscopy. Clearly it cannot correspond to the basement membrane of light microscopy as a layer of such small dimensions could not be resolved by this technique.

Attached to the lamina densa are fibrils, called anchoring fibrils, forming loops through which run some of the collagen fibrils of the connective tissue. The methods used to demonstrate the basement membrane probably stain the anchoring fibrils and some of the associated collagen fibrils as well as the basal lamina.

Connecting the epithelium and the underlying connective tissue there are numerous hemidesmosomes. These consist of a dense cytoplasmic plaque on the inner aspect of the plasma membrane from which tonofilaments spread out into the cytoplasm; opposite the cytoplasmic plaques there are electron dense areas in the lamina lucida, from which fine filaments pass into the connective tissue.

Epithelium. Epithelial tissues are characterised by the close arrangement of their constituent cells so that there is a minimum of extracellular substance. The cells are linked together by structures known as desmosomes. In electron micrographs desmosomes show as localized thickenings of the plasma membranes of adjacent cells (Fig. 254). Between these attachment plaques there is a condensation of the extracellular substance to form several distinct layers. Fine filaments within the cells, the tonofibrils, are related to the desmosomes.

Lining the whole of the mouth cavity is the epithelial layer of the oral mucous membrane; it is of the stratified squamous variety. As has been described in Chapter 3 epithelium is of great importance in the development of the teeth. In the completed tooth there is one tissue of epithelial origin, the enamel. As a mineralised tissue of epithelial origin the enamel is unique in the human body. It is probably more correct to regard it as a calcified secretion than as a tissue.

Keratin. Keratin is produced by the epithelium of the skin and the oral mucous membrane. Keratin is made up of very long and closely packed polypeptide chains. These are held together by the disulphide bond of the amino acid cystine. Owing to the tight packing of the chains keratin is highly resistant to solvents and enzymes. It is insoluble in dilute alkalis, water, and organic solvents.

The organic matrix of the enamel was at one time thought to be similar to keratin, but it is now realised that it differs from the true keratins in a number of respects, notably in its very low content of cystine. The virtual absence of hydroxyproline and hydroxylysine distinguish it clearly from collagen.

Dental connective tissues. All the dental tissues, apart from enamel, are connective tissues and so contain collagen fibrils. Dentine and cement show little cellular element and the extracellular substance is mineralised. The pulp is the only part of the completed teeth which is not mineralised. In it the cells are numerous, and as the amount of collagen fibres is small the tissue is delicately constructed.

The parodontal tissues, with the exception of the epithelial layer of the gingival mucosa, are all connective tissues. The alveolar bone is a mineralised connective tissue. The periodontal membrane and the lamina propria of the gingivae contain many densely arranged bundles of collagen fibres and so may be described as dense fibrous connective tissue. In the periodontal membrane, however, in the intervals between the main bundles of collagen fibres, which are known as the principal fibres, there are areas of loose connective tissues in which the blood vessels and nerve fibres run. Recently oxytalan fibres have been described in the periodontal membrane.

The structure and function of bone. It is not intended that this section on Bone should be a comprehensive account of the tissue; it is expected that for this the student will already be familiar with one of the detailed descriptions given in the standard works of general histology. The intention here is simply to concentrate on certain aspects of the functions of bone in their relationship to its structure.

The major functions of bone are twofold, firstly a supportive and/or protective function and secondly a homeostatic function in which bone serves as a storehouse for certain mineral ions which are in equilibrium with those in the tissue fluids and the blood. Both functions are closely related to and are subserved by the remodelling and turnover activities which takes place in the skeleton throughout life.

The relationship between the supportive / protective function of bone and its structure is well seen in a section through an adult bone (Fig. 241). In such a cross-section there appear to be two distinct parts, an outer densely formed zone which is alternatively called cortical bone because of its position as a cortex to the bone or compact bone because of its dense appearance. Internal to the cortical bone is a bony network surrounding marrow spaces and this network constitutes the cancellous bone. The width of the compact bone and the thickness of the individual bars of bone, the trabeculae, which constitute the cancellous tissue are intimately related to the functional requirements of the particular bone. For example, a cross-section through the body of the mandible shows a greater development of both cortical and cancellous areas than does the maxilla and this is due to the fact that in the mandible the forces of mastication transmitted through the teeth to the jaw have inevitably to be taken up and dissipated in the structure of the jaw itself, whereas in the upper jaw these same forces can be carried away from the jaw by the attachment of the maxilla to the rest of the cranium (see p. 290). In both jaws individual changes in the functional activity of the masticatory apparatus are reflected in changes in the internal architecture of the jaws. Where teeth have been lost in one jaw the bone of the other jaw which now carries unopposed teeth shows a gradual reduction in the thickness of the trabeculae of the cancellous tissue and in their number. On the other hand increased stress, such as that falling on an isolated tooth, can produce a strengthening of the cancellous tissue. These changes are mediated through the remodelling activity of bone, bone being added by deposition or removed by resorption as necessary.

Although when examined at a naked-eye level compact and cancellous bone have a different arrangement, when examined microscopically it can be appreciated that they have the same basic structure. Both compact and cancellous bone are made up of layers of bone, the lamellae. Lamellae are distinguished from each other by the arrangement of their collagen fibres. The fibres in adjacent lamellae tend to be orientated in different directions and the fibres in one lamella do not usually cross into other lamellae. Although the arrangement of the collagen fibres is only to be properly appreciated in specially stained sections the lamellar pattern can still be made out in sections stained with routine stains such as haematoxylin and eosin. In cortical bone there are a great number of constituent lamellae, whereas in cancellous bone the trabeculae are composed of usually only a few superimposed lamellae. The arrangement of the lamellae appear to be related to the nutritional supply of the bone. In the case of the trabeculae of the cancellous bone or the most superficial lamellae, the circumferential lamellae, of the cortical bone, which are close to the blood-vessel of the marrow spaces and the periosteum respectively the pattern of the lamellae is simple. These lamellae which make up only a narrow zone of bone are arranged roughly parallel to the bony surface. Here the nutritional requirements of the bone can be met by diffusion from the blood-vessels on the surface of the bone. Where however a considerable thickness of bone is encountered as in the deeper parts of the bony cortex, then a simple diffusion process from the surface would not suffice alone. In this case the substance of the bone is permeated by a system of ramifying blood-vessels which are surrounded by concentrically arranged lamellae, which constitute the Haversian systems, or osteones (osteons). In this way diffusion of nutrient fluid from the contained blood-vessels of the osteones can reach all parts of the bone. The diffusion of nutrients to the bone is facilitated by the existence of a well-defined system of microscopic spaces, the lacunae, and their inter-connecting channels, the canaliculi. The canalicular system opens on the surface of the bone or on the walls of the central canals, containing the blood-vessels, of the osteones. The osteocytes which are contained within the lacunae are seldom further than 100 μm from blood capillaries.

Any drop in the level of plasma calcium from the normal 10·4 mg per 100 ml leads to the stimulation of the parathyroid glands. The action of the parathormone produced brings about a resorption of bone through the action of osteoclasts. The action of parathormone is opposed by calcitonin, which is produced as a response to a rise in the level of plasma calcium. In this way the structure of bone is related to the maintenance of the plasma calcium. It can be argued that the functional aspects of bone are related to this as well if it happens that areas of bone which are no longer required functionally are those which are preferentially resorbed.

During infancy, childhood and adolescence when the skeleton is growing rapidly both bone formation and resorption are active, but as formation outstrips resorption there is a net increase in the amount of bone. In the elderly resorption outstrips formation so that osteoporosis is produced. It has been estimated that even in the healthy adult skeletal resorption amounts to 10 per cent a year and formation to 9·3 per cent a year so that an annual skeletal loss of the order of 0·7 per cent takes place.

The homeostatic function of bone is also reflected in certain features of its microscopic structure. It has been shown by microradiographic studies that the osteones when first formed are not fully mature and their final level of mineralisation is only gradually attained. Such immature osteones are preferential sites for the uptake of radioactive isotopes. Since increasing levels of mineralisation involve a progressive diminution of the water content of the matrix of mineralised tissues and decreased pathways for diffusion through the tissues it follows that the newly formed immature osteones with a lower mineral content but higher water content will be the areas principally involved in ionic exchange between bone on the one hand and tissue fluid and blood serum on the other.

The osteocytes also appear likely to be directly involved in this mineral exchange. In electron photomicrographs it is evident that there is a narrow zone surrounding the osteocyte which is constituted of unmineralised connective tissue. With microradiography it has also been shown that in mature bone there is a perilacunar area of matrix which is more highly mineralised than the rest of the interlacunar bone. This perilacunar zone is formed by the osteocyte after it has been surrounded by bone matrix. These observations combined with others which indicate that there is a form of internal bone resorption or osteolysis which affects the walls of the lacunae suggest that there can be a mineral interchange which is controlled by the osteocyte. Certainly the involvement of the lacunae would provide a vast surface area of crystallites for this purpose.

Mineralisation (Calcification). Mineralisation, in mammalian tissues, is the process of deposition of inorganic material, consisting of calcium salts, in the amorphous substance around the fibrils of the mineralising tissue. In bone, dentine, and cement the fibrils are collagenous. Enamel may represent an exception to this arrangement as it is possible that there are no fibrils in its organic matrix which instead may have an entirely gel-like nature. In all these tissues the inorganic material is built up into apatite crystals; the formula for hydroxyapatite, the most commonly found variety is $Ca_{10}(PO_4)_6(OH)_2$. In bone and dentine the apatite crystals are arranged with their long axis parallel to the fibrils. When first formed both the fibres and the amorphous substance of the organic matrix contain a large amount of water. During mineralisation a considerable quantity of this water is replaced by the inorganic material.

It has recently been suggested that the mineral in the calcified tissues may not all be in the form of apatite. Evidence from X-ray diffraction studies indicates the possibility that a large proportion of non-crystal-line or amorphous calcium phosphate is contained in bone. In young animals the amorphous content is estimated as 70 per cent but this declines with age to 40 per cent or less and is replaced by apatite. The mineralising front in a bone is richer in amorphous content than the older parts. With the electron microscope the amorphous particles are rounded or doughnut shaped granules which range in diameter from 60 to 250 Å.

Theories of mineralisation of the calcified tissues fall into three groups (1) those that postulate a mechanism whereby the Ca x PO_4 solubility product is exceeded locally so that the mineral can precipitate spontaneously, (2) those that suggest the presence of nucleating sites or the removal of barriers at these sites, so that apatite can form from tissue fluid levels of calcium and phosphate, (3) those that propose that apatite is not formed initially, but is produced by hydrolysis from a less basic calcium phosphate.

The alkaline phosphatase theory is an example of the first group. According to this theory alkaline phosphatase released phosphate ions from organic phosphates and so produced a precipitation of calcium phosphate from the local tissue fluid which was already nearly saturated with calcium and phosphate. Although alkaline phosphatase is commonly present at sites of mineralisation it also occurs widely in the body in situations where mineralisation does not normally take place, such as in the kidney. A further objection is that the amounts of organic phosphate in blood or tissue fluid are low; though this difficulty was countered by the suggestion that hexose phosphates could be produced by the action of phosphorylase on glycogen already stored in the area.

The second type of theory is now represented chiefly by the concept of epitaxy. This means the induction of crystallisation of the mineral material by contact with a foreign solid. It is most likely to occur when the dimensions of the structural features of the foreign solid are similar to those of the mineral crystals that are formed. It may be that the collagen fibrils of bone, dentine, and cement act as such a template and ions are attracted by electrostatic forces which hold them in positions similar to their arrangement in the structure of apatite. Support for this idea has been provided by the observation of a close physical relationship between the collagen fibrils of bone and the crystallites at the beginning of mineralisation. It has also been found that *in vitro* only native collagen with the 640 A periodicity will mineralise. A difficulty also arises with this concept in that collagen is widely distributed in regions where mineralisation does not normally take place. The presence of mucopolysaccharides in considerable quantities at sites of mineralisation has been thought possibly to play some part in conjunction with the epitactic phenomenon. In one view calcium could be bound by the strongly acidic sulphate groups of these substances and so act as a 'local factor' together with collagen in initiating mineralisation. In an opposite view this property of binding calcium has been thought of as inhibiting mineralisation by reducing the quantity of calcium available for mineralisation and so preventing the phenomenon of epitaxy at sites where it otherwise might occur.

In the third concept of mineralisation the calcium phosphate is first formed as an amorphous calcium phosphate and not as apatite. Once formed the amorphous calcium phosphate becomes the controlling source of ions for the formation of apatite crystallites, and it could fulfil this role since it is more soluble than apatite. The collagen fibrils of the local matrix could act as the site for the initial seeding of the apatite crystals, but would only do so where a prior formation of the amorphous calcium phosphate had already taken place. The controlling factor in the production of the amorphous salt might well be the formative cells involved at the mineralisation site for there is some indication that certain cell organelles such as mitochondria or Golgi vesicles can form amorphous granules of calcium phosphate.

Some workers have demonstrated the presence of extracellular membrane bound bodies in the early stages of the mineralisation of bone, dentine and cartilage; the electron-dense material contained by them is calcium phosphate and this can be released at nucleating sites by the breakdown of the surrounding membrane. These bodies have been called matrix vesicles. It is not known if they are formed intracellularly or by the pinching-off of small processes of the cell membrane of the osteoblasts and odontoblasts.

BIBLIOGRAPHY

Anderson, D. J. *et al.* (Editors) (1967). *The Mechanisms of Tooth Support.* Bristol: Wright.

Bourne, G. H. (Editor) (1972). *The Biochemistry and Physiology of Bone.* 2nd ed. New York: Academic Press.

Cohen, B. & Kramer, I. R. H. (Editors) (1976). *Scientific Foundations of Dentistry.* London: Heinemann.

Eastoe, J. E. (1968). Chemical aspects of the matrix concept in calcified tissue organisation. *Calc. Tiss. Res.* **2**, 1.

Fullmer, H. M. (1967). Connective tissue components of the periodontium. In *Structural and Chemical Organization of Teeth.* Ed. Miles, A. E. W. New York: Academic Press.

Hancox, N. M. (1972). *Biology of Bone.* London: Cambridge University Press.

Melcher, A. H. & Bowen, W. H. (1969). *The Biology of the Periodontium.* London: Academic Press.

Moyers, R. E. & Krogman, W. M. (Editors) (1971). *Cranio-facial Growth in Man.* Oxford: Pergamon Press.

Osborn, J. W. & Ten Cate, A. R. (1976). *Advanced Dental Histology.* 3rd ed. Bristol: Wright.

Posner, A. S. (1969). Crystal chemistry of bone mineral. *Physiol. Rev.* **49**, 760.

Sognnaes, R. F. (Editor) (1960). *Calcification in Biological Systems.* Washington: American Association for Advancement of Science.

Squier, C. A. & Waterhouse, J. P. (1970). Lysosomes in oral epithelium: The ultrastructural localization of acid phosphatase and non specific esterase in keratinised oral epithelium in man and rat. *Archs. oral Biol.* **15**, 153.

11. Enamel

DEVELOPMENT OF ENAMEL (AMELOGENESIS)

There are two major processes concerned in the development of the enamel, namely, matrix formation and the subsequent calcification (mineralisation) of the matrix. When first laid down the enamel matrix is completely organic, but it very quickly begins to calcify. The production of the highly calcified, definitive, enamel is associated not only with the influx of large amounts of mineral salts but with changes in the nature of the organic matrix itself. The late stages in enamel formation are often referred to as maturation of the enamel.

It is only after the internal enamel epithelium undergoes further differentiation, during which fully formed ameloblasts are produced, that formation of the enamel begins. Before these changes take place the internal enamel epithelium initiates two other functions. The first of these is the mapping out of the form of the crown of the tooth; the second is to induce the formation of dentine. Under the influence of the internal enamel epithelium certain of the cells on the surface of the dental papilla are induced to form an odontoblast layer. The cells of this layer immediately begin to deposit a layer of dentine on the pulpal aspect of the basal lamina which separates the dental papilla (pulp) from the enamel organ. When some dentine has been deposited formation of enamel commences, and this only takes place in the coronal part of the tooth. Before any deposition of enamel occurs, however, the basal lamina is disrupted and disappears.

The formation of ameloblasts by the internal enamel epithelium is a secondary and limited function, for this only happens after the shape of the coronal part of the tooth has been mapped out and the development of an odontoblast layer induced. Moreover, these functions are also carried out by the internal enamel epithelium of Hertwig's sheath over the root area of the tooth, and in this area the internal enamel epithelium does not proceed to differentiate into an ameloblast layer and no formation of enamel takes place.

Cellular changes. When the enamel organ is fully differentiated into its four component layers, and before formation of dentine and enamel has started, the internal enamel epithelium is composed of a layer of cells, low columnar in shape, with oval nuclei (Figs. 139, 63). These cells are separated from the dental papilla by a basal lamina and at their other, basal, ends are adjacent to the cells of the stratum intermedium. At this stage the nuclei of the internal enamel epithelial cells are not uniformly arranged, for the nucleus may be found at any point between the two ends of the cell. During this phase cell division still occurs for mitotic figures may be observed. The approach of dentine formation is indicated by a lengthening of the cells of the enamel epithelium; at the same time their nuclei become uniformly arranged, close to their basal ends.

As the cells of the internal enamel epithelium reach their maximum length the odontoblast layer begins to appear on the adjacent surface of the pulp. At this stage the cells of the internal enamel epithelium are very highly columnar with elongated oval nuclei (Fig. 14). The Golgi apparatus having migrated from its former position at the basal end of the cell has come to lie in the distal half in preparation for enamel formation. The now highly differentiated cells of the internal enamel epithelium show no cell division, and mitotic figures are therefore never seen at this stage.

Very soon after their first appearance the cells of the odontoblast layer begin to form dentine; as this happens the cells of the internal enamel epithelium shorten again (Figs. 139, 141). With the start of enamel formation, which quickly follows, the internal enamel epithelium is known as the ameloblast layer. In the ameloblasts, as in the later

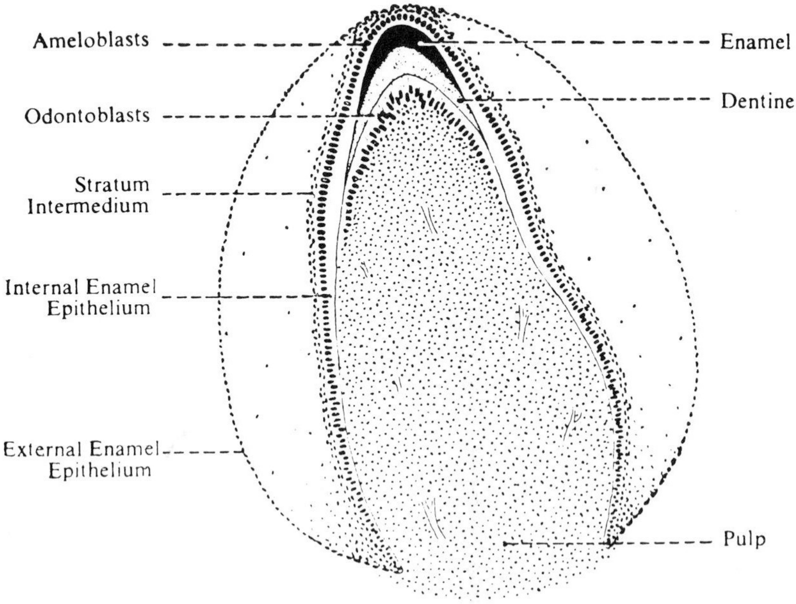

Fig. 139 Diagrammatic illustration of a developing human tooth after the commencement of dentine and enamel formation. Note the lengthening of the cells of the internal enamel epithelium during their differentiation before odontoblast formation beings. Note also the subsequent shortening of these cells in becoming ameloblasts and starting the formation of enamel.

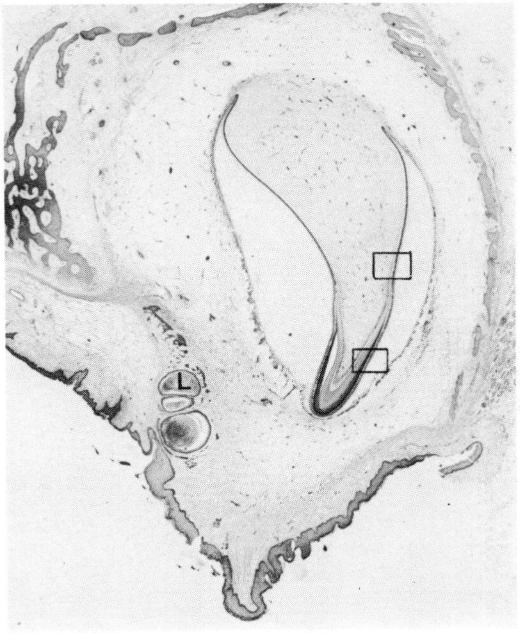

Fig. 140 Developing deciduous upper central incisor in its follicle in the alveolar bone. Formation of dentine and enamel has well begun. Lingually there is an artifact space between the layers of dentine and enamel. The dental lamina shows degenerative changes. Figs. 141 and 142 are high power views of the boxed areas of the labial aspect of the developing tooth. Human fetal of 210 mm. C.R. length. L. dental lamina. ×14.

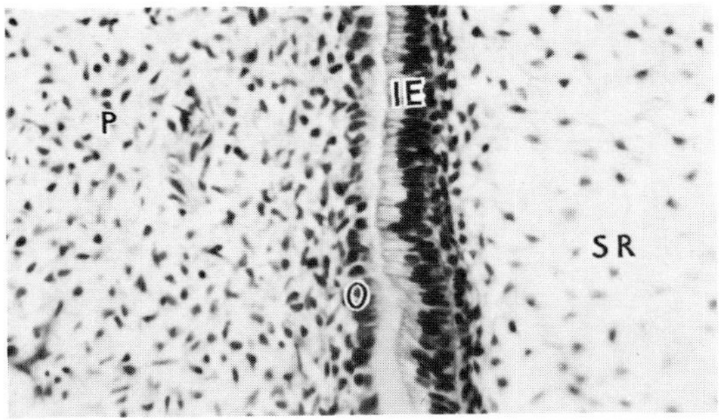

Fig. 141 Differentiating cells of the internal enamel epithelium, the associated appearance of odontoblasts, and the beginning of predentine formation. (I.E.) internal enamel epithelium; (O.) odontoblast layer; (P.) pulp; (S.R.) stellate reticulum. H. & E. ×200.

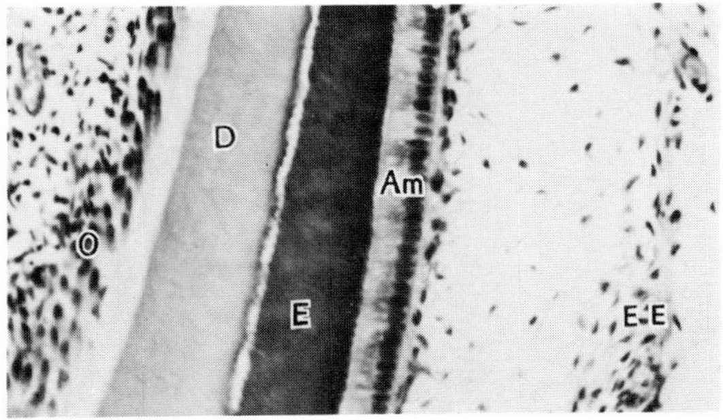

Fig. 142 Dentine and enamel formation (Am.) ameloblast layer; (D.) dentine; (E.) enamel; (E.E.) external enamel epithelium; (O.) odontoblast layer. H. & E. ×200.

stages of the internal enamel epithelium, the nuclei are uniformly arranged, close to the basal ends of the cells (Fig. 142). The ameloblasts are even more uniform in length and arrangement than the cells of the internal enamel epithelium (Figs. 141, 142).

In certain other animals there are differences of detail in these events. In the rat, for example, the approach of enamel formation is not indicated by a shortening of the cells of the internal enamel epithelium for there is a continued increase in height which only reaches its maximum after enamel formation has well begun. The height of the cells is maintained until the full thickness of the enamel matrix has been laid down.

Ameloblasts. With the electron microscope numerous organelles are to be seen in the ameloblasts(Fig. 143). Between the basal or non-formative end of the cell and the nucleus there is a heavy concentration of

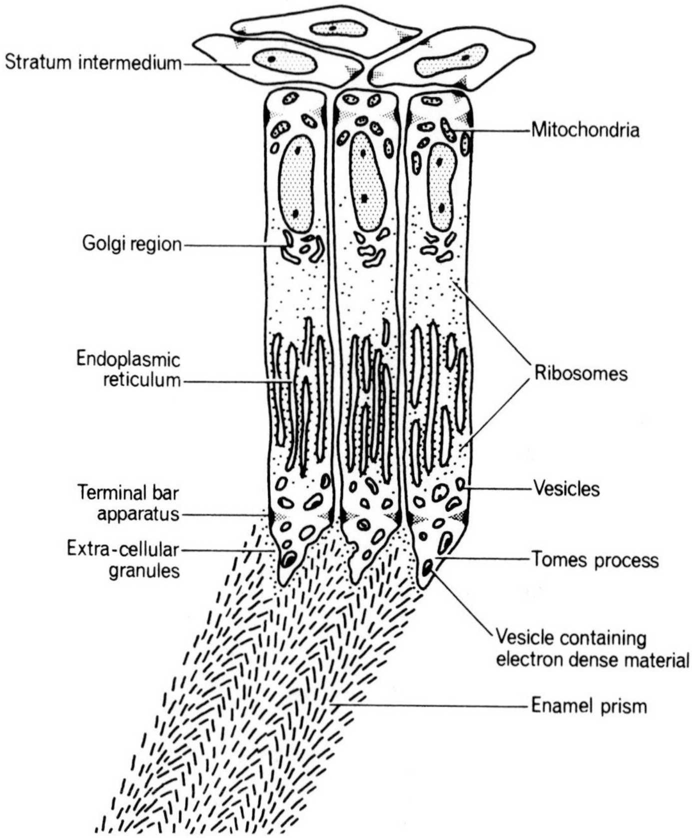

Fig. 143 Composite diagram of the essential features of enamel formation based on the electro microscopy of developing enamel. For clarity the distance between adjacent ameloblasts has been exaggerated. (*Modified from Fearnhead*, 1960.)

mitochondria. Adjacent to the nucleus on its distal aspect lies the Golgi complex. The central part of the cell is occupied by the endoplasmic reticulum; this consists of a complex arrangement of granula membranes. Throughout the cytoplasm are numerous ribosomes or RNA granules. Towards the distal or formative end of the cell are large numbers of vesicles containing dense granules of about 500 Å in diameter. The plasma or cell membrane covering the distal end of each ameloblast shows long narrow processes that extend towards the dentine; these appear just before enamel formation begins and remain only during the initial deposition of the enamel.

Tomes processes. The Tomes process is a small pyramidal cytoplasmic extension at the distal end of each ameloblast, and it is marked off from the rest of the cell by the terminal bar apparatus (Fig. 143). In electron micrographs this shows as a thickening of the cell membrane with associated microfibrils or tonofilaments. The latter pass a short distance into the cell so giving the appearance of an incomplete septum between the Tomes process and the rest of the ameloblast. With the light microscope the Tomes process seems to be marked off from the rest of the ameloblast by condensations of intercellular substance and this appearance has been described as a terminal bar (Fig. 144). However, electron microscope studies show that the ameloblasts are very closely packed so that their plasma membranes are only separated by a very nar-

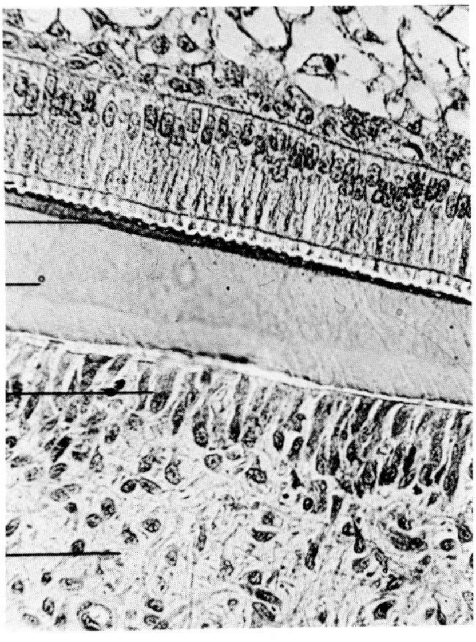

Fig. 144 Early enamel formation showing Tomes processes of the ameloblasts. These can be seen clearly due to the pulling away of the ameloblasts from the enamel during the preparation of the section. 'Terminal bars' are present at the basal and distal ends of the ameloblasts. × 300.

row interval of not more than 100-200 Å in width which is below the resolving power of the light microscope. The 'terminal bar apparatus' of the ameloblasts represents a form of junctional complex which is commonly found at the free margins of epithelial cells. At the proximal end of the ameloblasts a similar 'terminal bar apparatus' is found with the electron microscope.

The Tomes processes are embedded in the forming enamel. In some sections where the ameloblast layer has been detached from the enamel

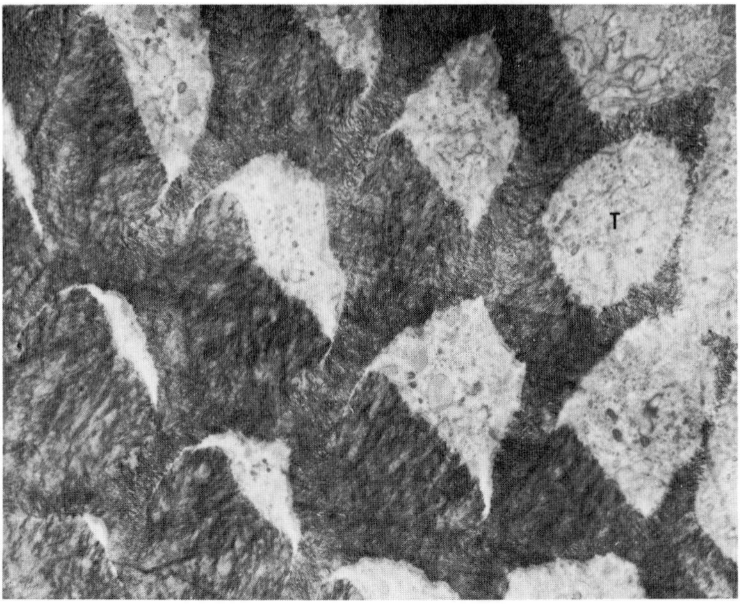

Fig. 145 Electron micrograph of a section through newly formed human enamel surrounding the Tomes processes of the ameloblasts. At the bottom left-hand corner of the field the prism pattern is almost complete. T. Tomes process. Original magnification × 16000. (*By courtesy of Dr A. Boyde.*)

the Tomes process can be seen to project from it (Fig. 144). The layer of newly formed enamel, when seen in oblique or cross-section, gives the appearance of a honeycomb-like network. The intervals in the network are occupied by the Tomes processes (Figs. 145, 147). In the cytoplasm of the Tomes process there are vesicles which contain dense granules of about 500 Å in diameter.

Using tritiated proline it has been shown that a high level of radioactivity occurs quickly in the Golgi region during amelogenesis. From the Golgi region the labelled protein diffuses through the body of the ameloblast to reach the Tomes process (Fig. 146).

Amelogenesis. The formation of enamel takes place extracellularly, and it begins after a narrow layer of mineralised dentine has appeared. A little enamel is deposited in the region of the amelodentinal junction before the Tomes processes appear, but subsequent to their formation the material for the enamel is secreted through them. Around the formative ends of the cells the extracellular area becomes slightly widened and filled with masses of granules (Figs. 143, 146). Apart from the earliest stage of enamel formation there is only a thin seam, of about 500 Å

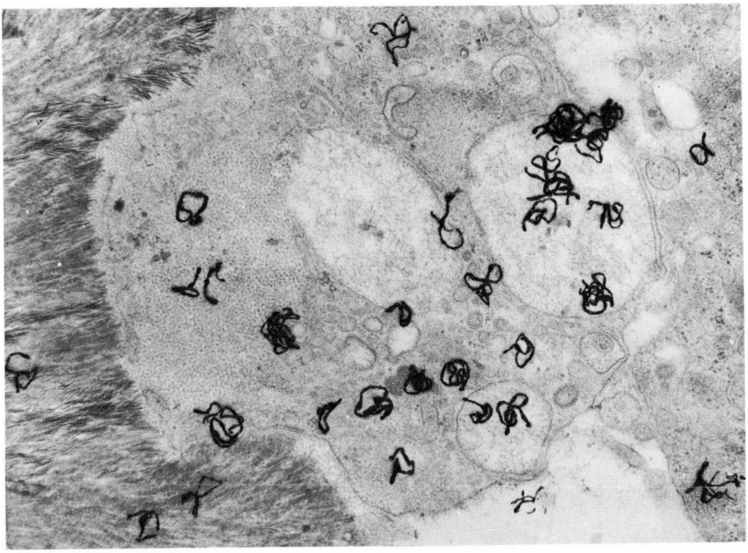

Fig. 146 Developing cat enamel. Labelling in the Tomes process one hour after intravenous injection of tritiated proline. Original magnification × 15600. (*By courtesy of Dr R. M. Frank and the Archs. oral Biol.*)

thick, in which hydroxyapatite crystallites are not present. The crystallites are deposited in this organic matrix secreted by the ameloblasts and when first formed look like fibres. They soon reach the length and width of mature crystallites but initially have a thickness of about 15 Å (see p. 190). The full thickness of the mature crystallite is only gradually attained.

Apart from the very earliest deposit of enamel a prism pattern can be distinguished in the enamel and this pattern is produced in relation to the Tomes processes. The long axes of the ameloblasts lie at a considerable angle to the prism direction so that the junction of the ameloblasts and the forming enamel is like the edge of a saw when seen in sections cut parallel to the long axes of the ameloblasts. Each Tomes process occupies a depression in the surface of the forming enamel and is orientated so that one of its surfaces is in line with the direction of

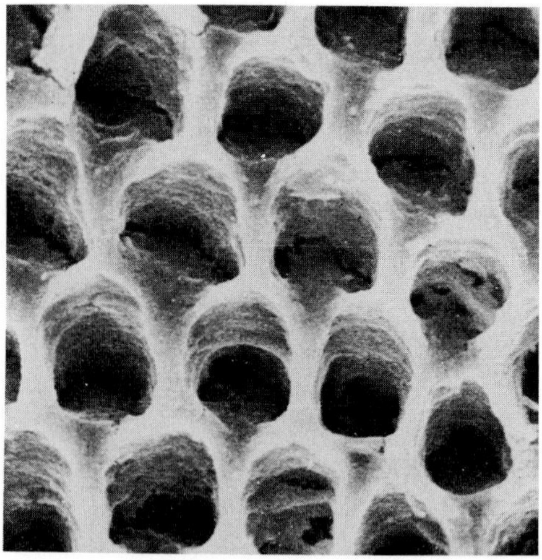

Fig. 147 Pits in the developing enamel surface caused and occupied by the Tomes processes of the ameloblasts. Human deciduous molar. (*By courtesy of Dr A. Boyde and Proc. Roy. Soc. Med.*)

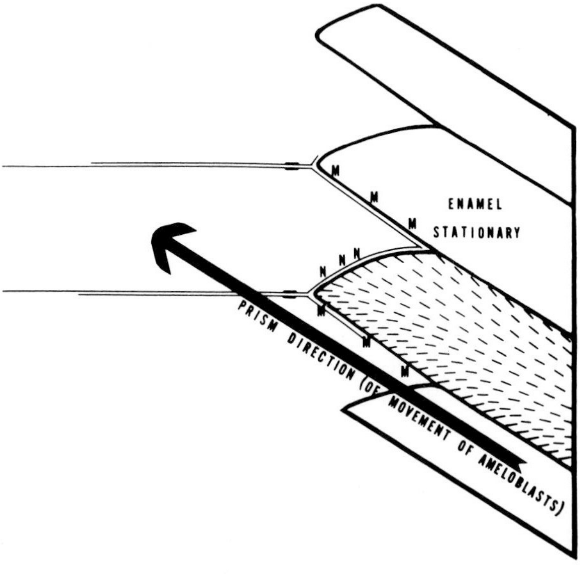

Fig. 148 The relationship of crystallite orientation to the shape and orientation of the mineralising front and the direction of movement of the ameloblasts. A maximal relative sliding movement between the surface of the ameloblast (Tomes process) and the mineralising front must occur in the regions marked M M M; a minimal movement at N N N. (*By courtesy of Dr A. Boyde and Messrs. John Wright & Sons Ltd.*)

movement of the ameloblasts as they retreat in the process of laying down the enamel (Figs. 147, 148). The enamel crystallites are formed with their long axes perpendicular to the plasma membrane of the Tomes process and on certain aspects of the Tomes process this orientation is modified by the sliding movement of the ameloblasts relative to the mineralising front (Fig. 148). Thus the arrangement of the ameloblasts and their Tomes process produces abrupt changes in the orientation of the crystallites at certain planes in the enamel (Fig. 148). These planes represent the boundaries of the prisms (see p. 183). This arrangement means that no one prism is related to a single ameloblast. Indeed it is now believed that three or possibly four ameloblasts are related to the formation of each prism (Fig. 149).

In sections stained with Mallory's connective tissue stain and examined with the light microscope a narrow blue stained layer is found

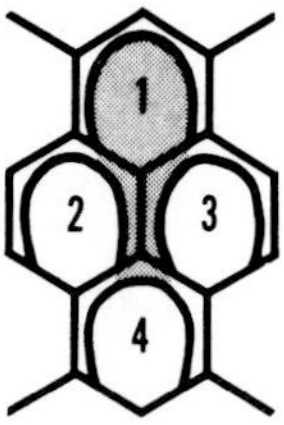

Fig. 149 Shows the relationship between the secretory territories of individual ameloblasts (hexagonal area), 'prism sheaths' (horseshoe-shaped lines) and the regions which may be defined as belonging to individual prisms (dotted areas). (*By courtesy of Dr A. Boyde and Messrs. John Wright & Sons Ltd.*)

adjacent to the formative ends of the ameloblasts, whereas the older formed enamel, next to the dentine, is coloured a brilliant orange red. Because of this the blue stained layer has been taken to represent a separate entity and has been called pre-enamel in distinction to the orange-red stained layer which is known as young enamel. However, with the electron microscope the pre-enamel is seen to represent merely the part of the forming enamel in which the Tomes processes are embedded; the difference in staining is probably due to this interdigitation.

During the deposition of the enamel the cells of the ameloblast layer retreat from the enamel-dentine junction. As this happens the stellate reticulum disappears. By the time that some thickness of enamel matrix has been laid down the cells of the external enamel epithelium are in contact with those of the stratum intermedium. As a result the capillaries of the dental follicle are very close to the ameloblast layer. No doubt this facilitates the passage of material necessary for the elaboration of the enamel to the ameloblast layer.

After some thickness of young enamel has formed the orange-red colour, found in association with this stage on staining with Mallory, begins to fade out and is replaced for a time by a blue or bluish-pink colour. In this stage the enamel is often described as transitional. Whereas the young enamel is so dense that no structural detail can be distinguished in such sections, in the transitional enamel the prism pattern shows very clearly (Fig. 150). Following this the matrix becomes increasingly difficult to stain. About the time the transitional enamel appears the enamel organ shows certain changes. There is a great development of prominent but irregular papillae on its surface and the

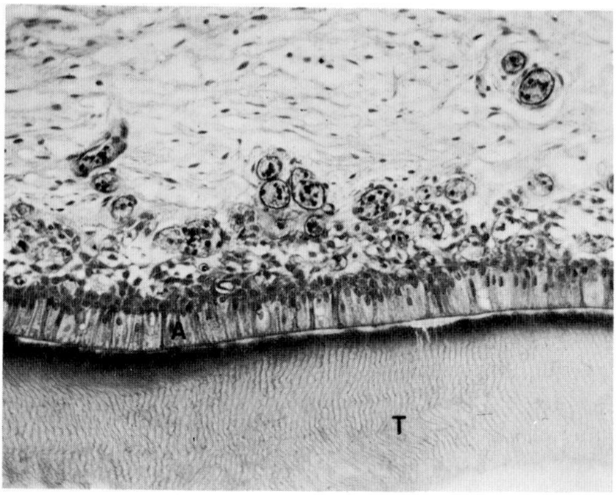

Fig. 150 Advanced enamel formation. The deep staining associated with the young enamel has disappeared except in a narrow zone adjacent to the ameloblasts. The bulk of the enamel is in the transitional form and the prism pattern is clearly visible. The stellate reticulum has completely disappeared, and the cells of the enamel organ external to the ameloblasts form papillae which interdigitate with numerous capillaries. Human fetus of 290 mm. C.R. length (ninth month of fetal life). Mallory. A, ameloblasts; T, transitional enamel. × 140.

disappearance of the stratum intermedium as a distinct layer; all the cells external to the ameloblasts become similar in appearance (Fig. 150).

The late stages of enamel formation are indicated by a disappearance of the enamel with routine decalcification in the preparation of histological sections; the organic matrix of the pre-enamel, and the young and transitional forms is large enough to remain after decalcification.

Although the successive changes which are seen with Mallory may represent changes in the composition of the tissue, it is more likely that they indicate alterations in the texture and permeability of the tissue which produce a selective entrance of the various dye molecules depending on their size. The acid dyes of this stain have an affinity only for amino groups.

The changes which take place in the internal enamel epithelium prior to the formation of the enamel do not occur over the whole of the enamel organ at the same time. These changes first appear at the deepest part of the concavity of the enamel organ; that is, at the region which in an anterior tooth corresponds to the incisive edge, and in a posterior tooth to a cusp. From these regions the differentiation of the internal enamel epithelium, leading to the appearance of an ameloblast layer, gradually spreads to the rest of the enamel organ, in a cervical direction or across the occlusal surface towards the other cusps. Formation of the enamel also starts at the same places and similarly spreads over the rest of the crown. Enamel formation takes place in a rhythmic fashion, periods of activity alternating with periods of quiescence. Thus the enamel is laid down in a series of layers which surround the initial area formed. Each layer is more extensive than the previous one, for the ameloblast layer, which has already been active, not only contributes to it but additional areas of ameloblast layer come into function with the spread of cellular differentiation.

Calcification (mineralisation). There are two phases in the calcification of the enamel. An initial one in which each increment of the organic matrix is partially mineralised immediately after its deposition. This is quickly followed by the second phase in which the final heavy mineralisation of the enamel takes place. This starts at the amelo-dentinal junction, initially in the region of the incisive edge or a cusp, and spreads cervically and also peripherally towards the enamel surface (Fig. 151).

The advancing edge of this mineralisation is at first parallel to the amelodentinal junction but later is parallel to the enamel surface. Sometimes a heavy mineralisation appears at the surface of the enamel before that spreading from the amelo-dentinal junction reaches the surface.

The two phases of mineralisation occur simultaneously over a long

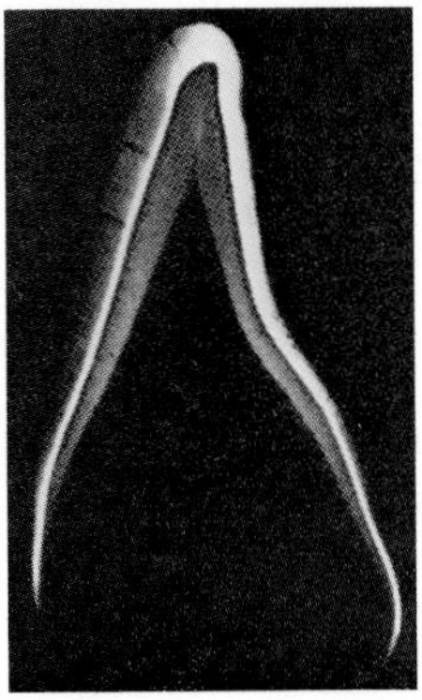

Fig. 151 Microradiograph of a ground section of a lower deciduous central incisor from a full-term fetus. The distribution of the highly radio-opaque zone indicates that mineralisation of the lingual enamel is in advance of the labial enamel. ×8·5. (*By courtesy of Prof H. S. M. Crabb and the Proceedings of Royal Society of Medicine*.)

period, for the second phase begins well before the whole of the enamel matrix is laid down.

The first formed crystallites are ribbon-shaped and have a thickness of only 15 Å. Although their width and length rapidly attain the dimensions of the crystallites of mature enamel, 400 and 1600 to possibly as much as 10 000 Å respectively, their thickness increases much more slowly. It would seem that the final heavy calcification of enamel may be equated with the thickening of the crystallites to the mature size of about 250 Å.

Maturation. There is evidence that during the later stages of enamel formation there is a withdrawal of a considerable amount of soluble protein and water from the organic matrix. This, in addition to the massive influx of mineral salts during the secondary phase of calcification, increases the relative amount of the inorganic element. The withdrawal of organic material is clearly a selective one for the matrix of developing enamel shows different proportions in its constituent amino acids from that of mature enamel (see p. 195).

The cellular mechanism behind these changes is not well understood, but the retention during this phase of a definite ameloblast layer and the formation of prominent papillae by the external layers of the enamel organ all suggest that the cells of the enamel organ play a considerable part in maturation of the enamel. The presence of the papillae, which are surrounded by capillaries, provides a large surface through which material could pass in either direction.

The presence of an extensive system of lysosomes in the cytoplasm of the ameloblasts, including the Tomes process, suggests that it may be through the agency of the hydrolytic enzymes contained in the lysosomes that the partial degradation of the organic matrix of the enamel takes place. The products of this degradation would then pass outward through the enamel. There are certain difficulties, however, in the concept of an enzymatic diffusion through the peripheral zone of young enamel, which is still mineralising, to reach a deeper zone of enamel.

This difficulty is avoided in an alternative view in which the loss of protein from the enamel matrix is regarded as brought about by the growth of the enamel crystallites during maturation. The organic matrix may act as a thixotropic gel, flowing as a direct result of the pressure of the growing crystal surfaces.

It is possible that the prism sheaths are produced during maturation. In developing enamel there is no more organic material at the prism boundaries than in the surrounding enamel. As organic material flows backwards towards the ameloblasts during maturation, more of it may be left in the regions between the prisms where there are few or no crystallites.

In the rat the whole of the enamel matrix is in the young enamel form at the time when its full thickness has been deposited. The subsequent change to the transitional form is associated with a distinct change in the ameloblast layer. The cells though remaining columnar shorten to about a half of their former length (Fig. 152). These changes in matrix and ameloblasts have generally been taken to indicate the beginning of the process, described as maturation of the enamel, whereby the lightly calcified matrix is converted into the highly calcified form of adult enamel.

In man, however, the transitional stage of the enamel matrix has already been reached by the time that the full width of the matrix has been laid down and there is only a slight and very gradual reduction in length of the ameloblasts which occurs over the whole of this period.

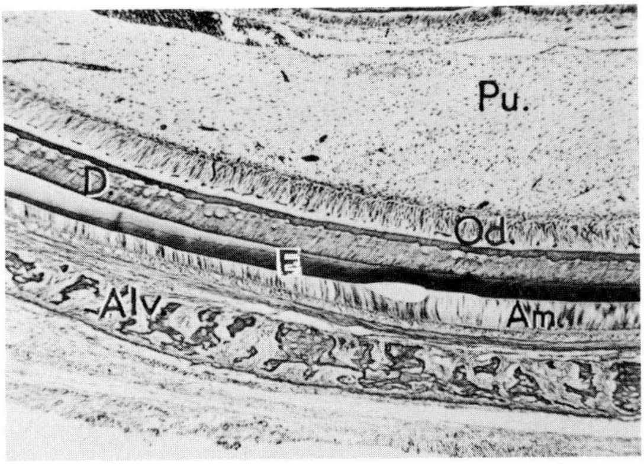

Fig. 152 Sagittal section of lower incisor of seven-day-old rat. To the right of field is the region of tall ameloblasts and the terminal phase of enamel matrix formation; to the left the shortened ameloblasts. In the latter area there is a change in staining of the enamel indicating the appearance of 'transitional' enamel. At the junction of shortened and unshortened ameloblasts there is a gap between ameloblast layer and the enamel; an artifact which commonly occurs there. (Alv.) alveolar bone; (Am.) ameloblast layer; (D.) dentine, (E.) enamel; (Od.) odontoblast layer; (Pu.) pulp. × 45.

Histochemical considerations. A considerable amount of information has already been accumulated on the distribution of various substances in the enamel organ and in the developing enamel. Exact knowledge of the part taken by these substances in the formation of the enamel is, however, still very incomplete.

During matrix formation the heaviest concentration of alkaline phosphatase is found in the stratum intermedium, whereas the cells of the ameloblast layer are practically devoid of the enzyme (Fig. 186). This suggests that the cells of the stratum intermedium are active in elaborating some substance which is then passed on to the ameloblast layer. The nature of the material is uncertain. Originally it was thought that the alkaline phosphatase was related to calcification of the enamel; it is now generally held to be concerned in the synthesis of proteins which are needed for the building up of the organic matrix.

The pre-enamel and the young enamel are believed to contain a protein-carbohydrate complex since they are positive with the periodic acid–Schiff reaction. The finding of a certain degree of metachromasia in the same tissues suggests the presence of a limited amount of acid mucopolysaccharide, probably chondroitin sulphate. This has been postulated by some authorities as being the 'local factor' essential for calcification, binding the calcium ions to the organic matrix.

The glycogen which is found in the enamel organ, particularly in the internal enamel epithelium and the stratum intermedium, could possibly be related to the synthesis of the acid mucopolysaccharide by serving as the initial source of hexose phosphates. It is significant that the disappearance of glycogen from those layers coincides with the beginning of enamel matrix formation, the reduction of the stellate reticulum, and the approximation of blood vessels to the ameloblasts. The later supply of hexose phosphates could come from the red blood cells. The ground substance of the stellate reticulum is PAS-positive and strongly metachromatic.

Throughout enamel formation the ameloblast layer is rich in ribonucleic acid, the content being of a level equal to that of active osteoblasts. This is in the form of free ribosomes in the cytoplasm and as the ribosomes of the rough-surfaced endoplasmic reticulum.

The reduced enamel epithelium. At the end of the formation of the enamel the ameloblasts have been described as depositing a very thin organic covering on the surface of the enamel. This layer, which is said to be about 1 μm thick, is known as the enamel cuticle, or frequently as the primary enamel cuticle. At the same time the cells of the ameloblast layer gradually lose their columnar shape and become indistinguishable from the outer cells of the enamel organ. This shrunken enamel organ is referred to as the reduced enamel epithelium. The cells of the reduced enamel epithelium are polyhedral and are very similar in appearance to the cells forming the stratum spinosum of the oral mucous membrane. The functions of this epithelial covering are:

1. To protect the surface of the enamel from the adjacent mesodermal vascular tissue of the follicle prior to the eruption of the crown of the tooth in the mouth cavity.
2. To provide an epithelial-lined pathway for the eruption of the tooth into the mouth cavity. This is brought about by the fusion of the reduced enamel epithelium with the oral epithelium during eruption.
3. To attach the gingival epithelium to the surface of the tooth.

In electron micrographs no structure is to be found in unerupted teeth which can be equated with the enamel cuticle. The cells of the reduced enamel epithelium are united to the surface of the enamel by hemidesmosomes and a basal lamina (Fig. 153). This lamina has a thickness of about 400 Å and so is much too slender to correspond to the enamel cuticle of light microscopy. This suggests that the enamel cuticle is an optical phenomon possibly produced by a combination of section thickness and an oblique plane of cut.

Clinical considerations. Disturbances may occur during the development of the enamel, the effects of which are encountered clinically on examination the erupted teeth. These disturbances can affect either the formation of the enamel matrix or its calcification. Disturbance of matrix formation results in hypoplasia; disturbance of calcification in a hypocalcification of the enamel.

Hypoplasia of the enamel may range from a small localised defect

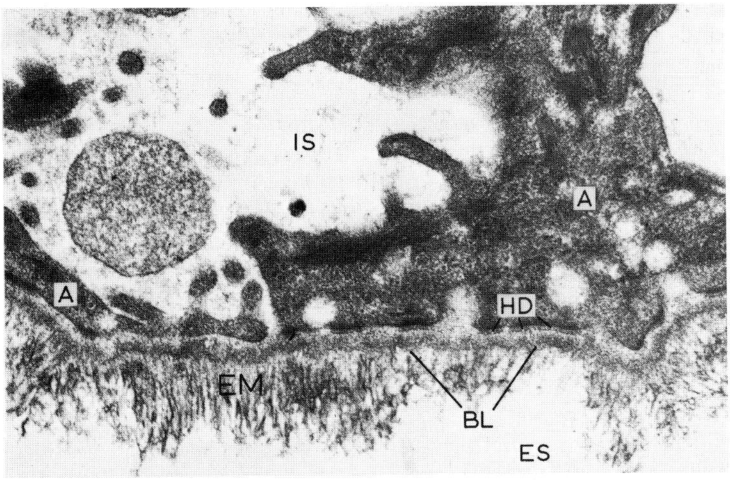

Fig. 153 Junction of ameloblasts (A) with enamel. The cell membrane is attached by hemidesmosomes (HD) to a basal lamina (BL) consisting of a dense layer separated from the ameloblasts by a clear zone. Patches of enamel matrix (EM) are attached to the basal lamina. ES, enamel space; IS, intercellular space. Original magnification ×38 000. (*By courtesy of Dr M. A. Listgarten and Archs. oral Biol.*)

to multiple defects or even the whole enamel may be affected. When a single tooth shows a hypoplastic defect the most likely cause is sepsis: usually of a deciduous tooth, which then affects the formation of the underlying permanent successor. The most common variety of hypoplasia involves a number of teeth in which formation of the enamel matrix takes place over the same period. The causative agent affects that zone of the enamel of each of these teeth which was being produced during its onset. A variety of conditions have been suggested as the aetiological factor, particularly the exanthematous fevers, hypoparathyroidism, and vitamin-D deficiency. Whatever the aetiology, hypoplasia can only be produced if the disturbance coincides with a period of active enamel matrix formation. The enamel of all the teeth is affected in the condition known as amelogenesis imperfecta. This a hereditary condition in which the enamel is everywhere very thin or entirely absent.

The most important known cause of hypocalcification is an excessive amount of fluorine in drinking water. The condition is frequently described as 'mottled enamel'.

COMPOSITION AND STRUCTURE OF ENAMEL

Physical characters. The enamel is the most highly calcified and hardest tissue of the body. Unlike dentine, cement, and bone it is produced by cells of ectodermal origin. In the human tooth the enamel normally forms a covering layer for the whole of the crown, but varies considerably in thickness over different parts of it. It is thickest at the incisive edges and cusps of the teeth reaching to as much as 2·5 mm, whereas at the cervical margin it thins down to a very fine edge. The density and hardness of the enamel also vary in different parts of the crown. The density decreases from the surface of the enamel to the dentine-enamel junction, and from the incisive edge to the cervical margin. The hardness is greatest at the incisive edge and decreases steadily towards the cervical margin. In permanent teeth, according to some authorities, the hardness is greatest at the surface, but decreases close to the surface and then remains relatively constant until just before reaching the dentine-enamel junction, when it drops considerably. In deciduous teeth the enamel is less hard than in the permanent teeth; the hardness is also greatest at the surface and decreases gradually towards the dentine-enamel junction.

The average value of the elastic modulus of enamel is 19×10^6 pounds per square inch; the breaking stress has an average value of 11 000 pounds per square inch. The fracture of enamel takes place along planes which are determined by the distribution of stresses rather than by the structure of the material.

The colour of the enamel varies considerably, from yellow to shades of grey or grey-blue. This depends on the translucency of the enamel; the more translucent the enamel, the more the yellow of the underlying dentine can show through. The shades of blue are most evident at the incisive edges, where there is no underlying layer of dentine. The translucency is probably associated with a high degree of calcification and homogeneity of the enamel, and is influenced by the thickness of the enamel layer.

Chemical composition. The inorganic content of mature enamel amounts to 96–97 per cent by weight, the remainder consisting of organic matter and water. The actual organic content is extremely small, being only 0·4–0·8 per cent in permanent enamel, and 0·5–0·9 per cent in deciduous enamel. A considerable part of this organic content is to be found as ribbon-like entities, the lamellae and tufts, mainly in the inner part of the enamel. The organic content is made up of soluble protein, peptides, insoluble protein, and citric acid. The soluble protein represents the fraction of the enamel protein which goes into solution when enamel is demineralised with EDTA or weak organic acids. The soluble and insoluble proteins are present in about equal amounts.

When first formed by the ameloblasts the organic matrix is much greater in amount, and can represent as much as 19 per cent of fetal enamel. Fetal enamel has a protein content which shows a number of features distinguishing it from other tissues. It contrasts with the keratins in its huge proline content and in the virtual absence of cystine,

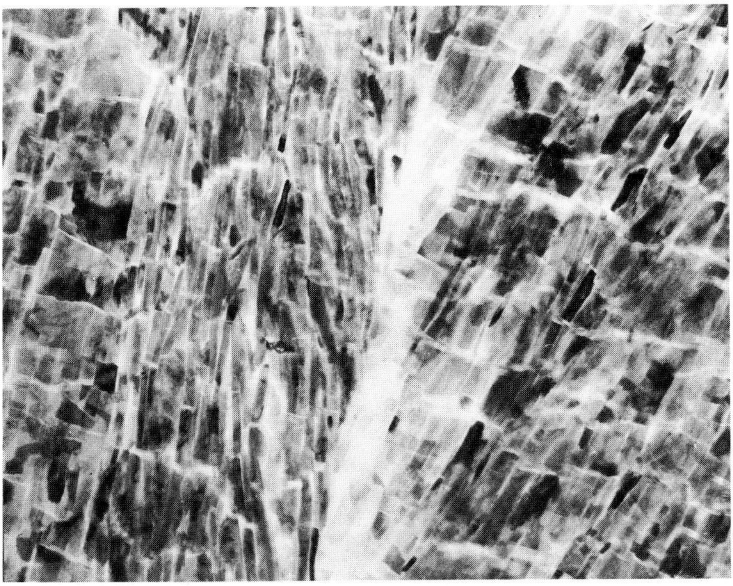

Fig. 154 Parts of two enamel prisms sectioned lengthwise and separated by a 1000–2000 Å wide organic sheath. The longitudinally cut crystallites show a change of orientation on either side of the sheath. Electron micrograph. Original magnification. × 54 000. (*By courtesy of Dr J.-E. Glass and Dr M. N. Nylen and Arch. oral Biol.*)

and its low glycine content and the virtual absence of hydroxyproline and hydroxylysine separate it from collagen. As the enamel matures certain remarkable changes take place in its content of amino acids. There is a very considerable loss of proline and histidine, which suggests that the fraction of the organic matrix containing these amino acids is of importance in enamel formation, and so the term 'amelogenins' has been used to describe them.

The composition of enamel matrix is difficult to determine with exactness due to the small quantity of purified material which can be readily prepared and to the complex mixture of proteins which is present. Moreover samples of enamel are liable to be contaminated by the adjacent dentine and cement, and as these contain a much higher protein content serious errors in the estimations are then introduced.

The inorganic element of mature enamel has the following approximate composition: Ca, 37 per cent; Na, 0·5 per cent; Mg, 0·5 per cent; PO_4, 55·5 per cent; CO_3, 3·5 per cent; with water of constitution and traces of other components. X-ray diffraction patterns indicate that the mineral material of enamel has an apatite structure. It is generally accepted that enamel apatite is the hydroxyapatite $Ca_{10}(PO_4)_6(OH)_2$, although its Ca:P ratio is slightly lower than that of hydroxyapatite. The relation of the carbonate of the enamel to the hydroxyapatite is still unclear.

Since the percentage of organic material in enamel is generally expressed in terms of weight, an incorrect impression of its amount may be given. It should be remembered that mineral material has a weight which is about three times that of organic material. In terms of volume the organic matrix of enamel constitutes a much greater percentage than in terms of weight.

It has been estimated that about 86 per cent of the volume of fresh mature enamel is occupied by inorganic material, the remaining volume being filled by organic material and water. About 2 per cent of the total volume is taken up by the organic matrix so that the remaining 12 per cent is occupied by water. Some of the water occurs as a loosely-bound fraction whereas the remainder is firmly bound to the crystallites as a hydration shell. Between the crystallites and their hydration shell there is a zone of adsorbed ions. The loosely bound water between the crystallites seems to be freely moveable and can be exchanged rapidly. Assuming that this narrow interval between the crystallites with their hydration shells is of the order of a few Å thick sizable molecules could not penetrate through the enamel. This concept would explain the limited permeability of mature enamel.

Submicroscopic structure. Since the introduction of the electron microscope it has been possible to obtain much greater and more exact information about the minute structure of the enamel, though the technical difficulties presented by the extremely dense, calcified material still leave much to be discovered. Previously information of this kind could only be obtained by more indirect methods, for such minute structures are beyond the resolution of the light microscope.

The mineral element of the enamel is arranged in the form of submicroscopic crystallites (Fig. 154). In mature enamel the crystallites can be described as slightly flattened hexagonal rods of fairly uniform size, though irregular forms are found in human enamel (Fig. 155). Their dimensions are large compared with the crystallites of bone or dentine. The average width is about 400 Å and the average thickness about 250 Å, though some authorities would place their width at 400–1200 Å. Definite statements about the length are not yet possible as it is difficult to decide whether the crystallites seen with the electron microscope are

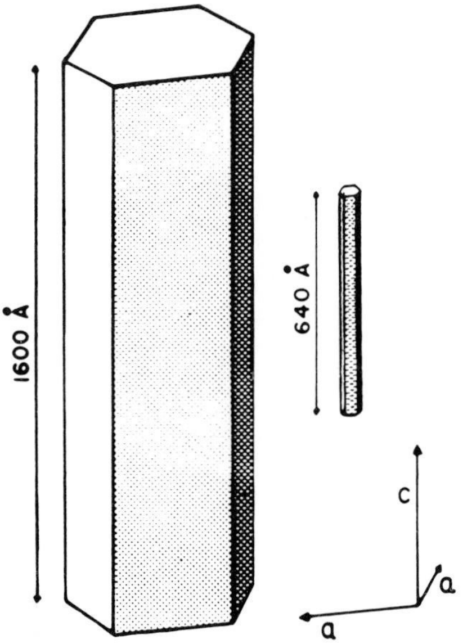

Fig. 155 The relationship in shape and size between the apatite crystallites of enamel (left) and bone or dentine (right). The optic axis (crystallographic *c*-axis) coincides with the long dimension of the crystallites. (*By courtesy of Dr D. Carlström and the Academic Press.*)

complete or are fragments of longer units. Estimates of length have varied between 1600 Å and as much as 10 000 Å. Enamel crystallites show a high degree of preferred orientation. They are mainly arranged with their long axis, which is the *c* or optic axis, parellel to that of the enamel prism. There is, however, a spread of orientation away from this which occurs in passing to that aspect of the prism which is situated towards the cervical part of the enamel (Fig. 161).

Apart from the arrangement of their long axes there is no other preferred orientation shown by the enamel crystallites. Thus the crystallites are not completely tightly packed and intervals exist between them even when the crystallites are touching (Fig. 156). It should be realised that even the degree of the preferred orientation varies considerably, it is highest in the central part of the enamel thickness and is usually least shown in the inner part.

The enamel crystallites are embedded in an organic matrix but so far no certain information about the structure of this organic element has appeared. In some preparations it appears as a delicate network which seems to be composed of submicroscopic fibrils, but this appearance may be produced by the procedures used in preparing such sections (Fig. 157). It may exist as a gel-like material in which the crystallites are embedded.

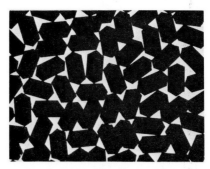

Fig. 156 Close packing of enamel crystallites randomly orientated with regard to their *a*-axes. The long dimension of the crystallites is perpendicular to the plane of the drawing. (*By courtesy of Dr D. Carlström and the Academic Press.*)

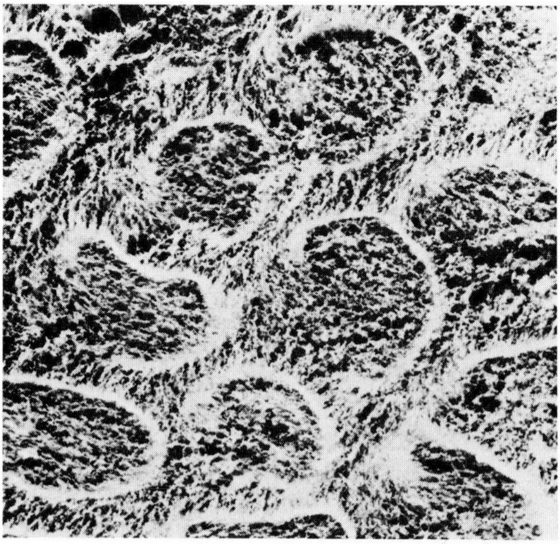

Fig. 157 Electron microscope picture of developing enamel showing as well as the prism sheaths the more delicate organic network which is present throughout the whole tissue. Plastic embedded material. Original magnification × 10 000. (*By courtesy of Dr K. Little.*)

The repeating pattern of the hydroxyapatite molecules or unit cells builds up the so-called lattice structure of the crystallites. Substitution of ions can take place in the lattice structure. The substitution may be either isoionic such as the replacement of a Ca ion by a Ca ion, or heteroionic when a Ca ion is replaced by a different ion such as a Mg ion. The substitution of a F ion for the centrally situated hydroxyl group of the hydroxyapatite unit cell in the lattice structure produces fluorapatite and this entails changes in the apatite structure which render it less soluble than the original hydroxyapatite. The decrease in solubility of fluorapatite as compared with hydroxyapatite may account for the increased resistance of fluorosed teeth to dental caries as compared with those with little or no fluorapatite in their structure.

Surface enamel. Considerable evidence has accumulated which indicates that the surface layer of enamel differs from the rest of the enamel in certain physical and chemical characteristics. The surface enamel is highly radio-opaque, harder, and less soluble compared with subsurface

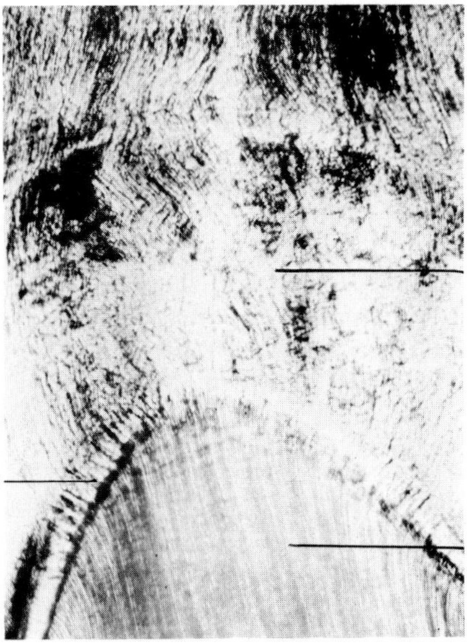

Fig. 158 Gnarled enamel. Cuspal region of premolar. Ground section. × 70.

enamel; it contains five to ten times more fluoride, and a much higher concentration of carbohydrate. Some of these features exist in the surface enamel of unerupted teeth. The difference may be further accentuated by post-eruptive adsorption from the saliva.

In deciduous teeth and in about 70 per cent of permanent teeth the outermost layer of the enamel is devoid of the usual prism structure. In this layer, which is about 30 μm wide, the crystallites are arranged with their *c* axis almost perpendicular to the surface of the enamel. Their orientation is therefore somewhat different from that of the crystallites of the underlying enamel. This layer is of great interest for in early carious lesions it appears to resist the spread of the lesion much more than the rest of the enamel.

Enamel prisms. On examination with the light microscope the enamel appears to be composed of structures which are described as enamel prisms or rods. There are some millions of prisms to each tooth and they pass from the dentine-enamel junction to the surface of the tooth. As a rough approximation it may be taken that the general direction of the prisms is perpendicular to the dentine surface. In a deciduous tooth the prisms lie roughly in a horizontal plane except for those in the incisive or occlusal third of the crown, where they gradually become more obliquely placed until they are almost vertical below the incisive edge of the apices of the cusps. In permanent teeth the arrangement is similar, except that in premolars it has been ascertained that 25 per cent show a rootward inclination of the prisms as they pass outward. The individual prisms do not follow a straight course but have a wavy arrangement. In some areas of the enamel, especially in the regions of the cusps, this is marked, the prisms becoming very twisted. Such areas are known as 'gnarled enamel' and are associated with an increased strength of the enamel (Fig. 158).

Since the outer surface of the enamel is greater than its dentinal surface it follows that the size of the prisms must increase towards the surface of the tooth so that although the average width of the prisms is often taken to be about 4–5 μm there must be a considerable variation along the course of the prisms.

When ground sections are examined in which the prisms have been cut perpendicularly to their course the prisms show a shape and

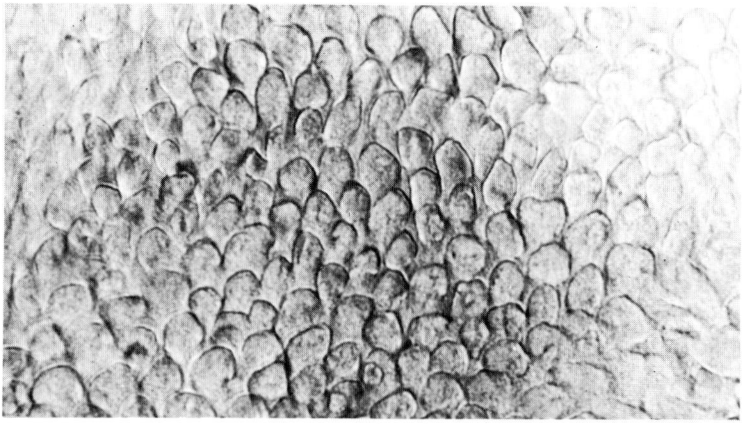

Fig. 159 Ground section of mature enamel, showing 'fish-scale' appearance of the prisms. Etched with van Gieson. × 1170. (*By courtesy of Prof E. B. Manley.*)

arrangement which resemble that of fish scales (Fig. 159). A prism boundary is readily defined on the convex side of each prism but on the opposite aspect this boundary appears to be deficient. This outer bounding layer of each prism is known as the prism sheath or prism cortex and is thought to contain a higher content of organic material than the rest of the prism. If decalcified sections are studied this would appear to be the case, for deeply staining structures remain which outline the prism pattern. This apparent sheath has a considerable thickness, of somewhere in the region of 0·5–1·0 μm (Fig. 160).

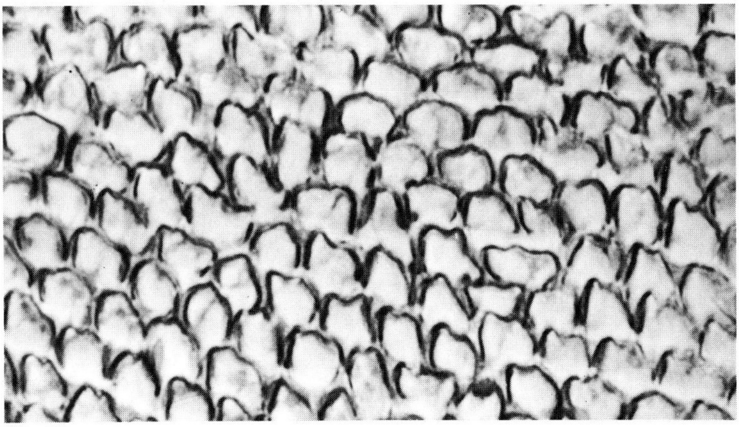

Fig. 160 Decalcified paraffin section of *mature* enamel showing 'fish-scale' appearance of the prisms. The deeply stained line at the periphery of each prism is the prism sheath. Stained with methyl blue. × 1300. (*By courtesy of Prof E. B. Manley.*)

From recent electron microscope work, however, it seems that no prism sheath of such dimensions can be distinguished, though there may be a certain concentration of organic material in this region of the order of 0·1–0·2 μm in thickness (Fig. 154). It may be that the thickness of the sections used for light microscopy together with changes produced in the organic matrix of the enamel by the decalcification procedures account for the appearance seen in sections of decalcified enamel.

Studies with the electron microscope have made it clear that the appearances seen in ground sections with the light microscope are due primarily to the arrangement of the minute crystallites which compose the inorganic part of the enamel. In cross-section each prism shows a rounded 'head' and a narrower 'tail' region (Fig. 161). The rounded 'head' of each prism fits closely into the concavities between the 'head' and 'tail' of the prisms on either side. In the 'head' region of each prism the crystallites are arranged with their long axes parallel to the long axis of the prism but passing towards the 'tail' of the prism the crystallites show a progressive inclination away from this until they are orientated about 65°–70° away from the long axes of the prisms. This means that the boundaries of the prisms represent planes where there are abrupt changes in orientation of the crystallites. In sections examined with the light microscope the transmitted light is diffracted at these planes and shows up the prism boundaries (see also pp. 185–187). The greatest change in orientation of the crystallites is found in passing from the 'tail' of one prism to the 'head' of the prism immediately beneath, and it is precisely in this region that the prism boundaries are seen most distinctly (Fig. 161).

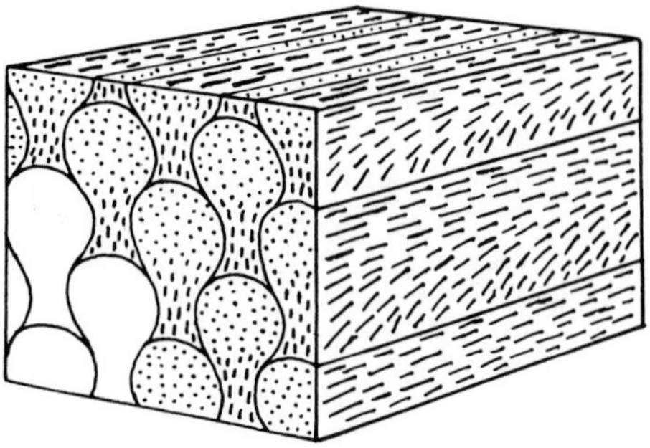

Fig. 161 Model of enamel prisms showing their arrangement and that of the crystallites as found commonly in human permanent teeth. The 'heads' of the prisms which appear in transverse section are directed towards the cusps and the 'tails' towards the cervical region. (*After Meckel, Griebstein & Neal.*)

Though this shape and arrangement of the prisms is the one generally found throughout human enamel there are some divergences from it, notably at incisive edges, cuspal tips and close to the amelo-dentinal junction. In cuspal regions the prisms may take a more circular shape in cross-sections and be separated from each other by interprismatic enamel. The composition and structure of such interprismatic enamel is not different in any essential way from that of the prisms.

In longitudinal section seen with the light microscope the prisms are given the appearance of being composed of a series of segments by dark lines, the cross striations, which cross the prisms at intervals of about four micrometres (Fig. 162). Each striation has been thought to represent a rest phase during the formation of the enamel. The striations are well marked in sections which have been etched with dilute acid. In fractured enamel examined with the scanning electron microscope the striations can be seen to represent variations in width of the prisms (Fig. 163).

Hunter–Schreger lines. It has already been stated that the enamel prisms do not pass in a straight direction from the dentine-enamel junction to the crown surface but follow a wavy course. The basic pattern made by the prisms in their course can best be understood if the enamel is imagined as being constituted of a series of horizontal plates or discs.

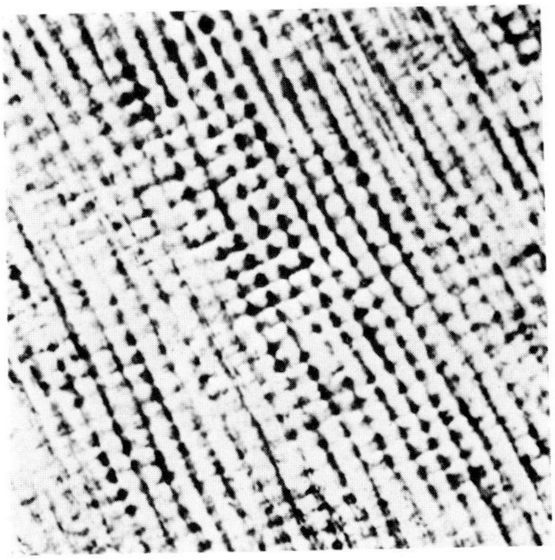

Fig. 162 Cross-striation of the enamel prisms. Ground section. × 300.

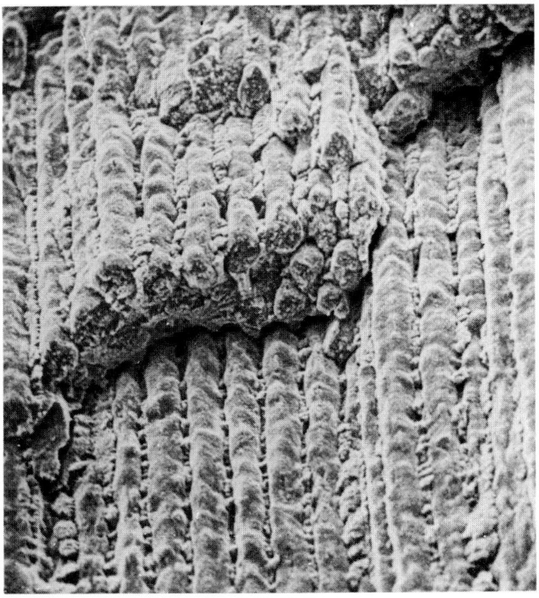

Fig. 163 Fractured enamel showing that enamel does fracture along the prism boundary planes (prism sheaths) and that the cross-striations of the prisms are variations in the width of the prisms. Original magnification × 1500. (*By courtesy of Dr A. Boyde.*)

In each disc the prisms commence by running out from the dentine-enamel junction at right angles for a short distance, then they turn to the left or to the right, the direction of the turning alternating in each disc. In the outer part of the enamel all the prisms again run straight to the surface (Fig. 164). This arrangement of the prisms is responsible for an optical phenomenon, the appearance of the Hunter-Schreger lines or bands (Figs. 165, 166). When a longitudinal ground section of the enamel is examined with the light coming down on the surface of the section obliquely from one side, the surface shows a series of alternating light and dark bands. The bands commence near the dentine-

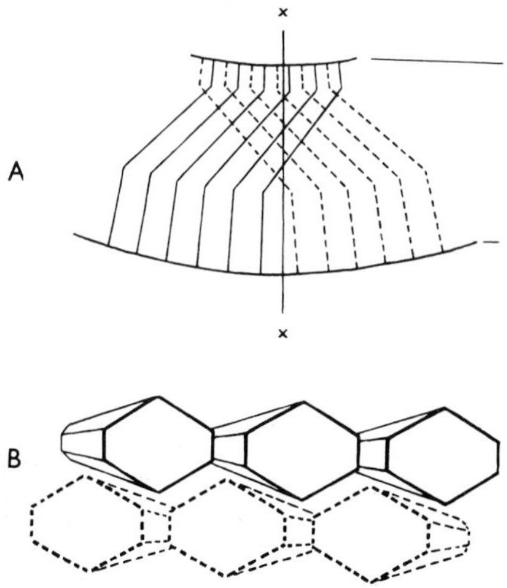

Fig. 164 Diagram to show the formation of the Hunter-Schreger bands. (A) A cross-section through the crown by a tooth indicating the direction taken by the prisms in passing from the enamel-dentine junction to the surface of the tooth. In one layer indicated by continuous line, in another layer by broken line. (B) The appearance to be seen in a vertical section if made along the line x–x in (A). The cut surfaces of the two layers of prisms are represented and the prisms running away at different angles in the two layers.

enamel junction and occupy usually about the inner two-thirds of the thickness of the enamel, disappearing as the outer part of the enamel is approached. They are curved with the convexity of the curve always facing rootwards (Fig. 166). In such a section the prisms in the middle part of their course are cut obliquely; the prisms passing from the cut surface to the right and to the left in alternating discs. In those discs where the direction of the prisms coincides with that of the obliquely directed light, the light passes along the prisms, *i.e.*, it is absorbed, and so these areas appear as dark bands. In those discs where the prisms run in the opposite direction the light is reflected from the sides of the prisms, so producing the light bands (Fig. 164). If the light is allowed to fall from the opposite side, the position of these light and dark bands

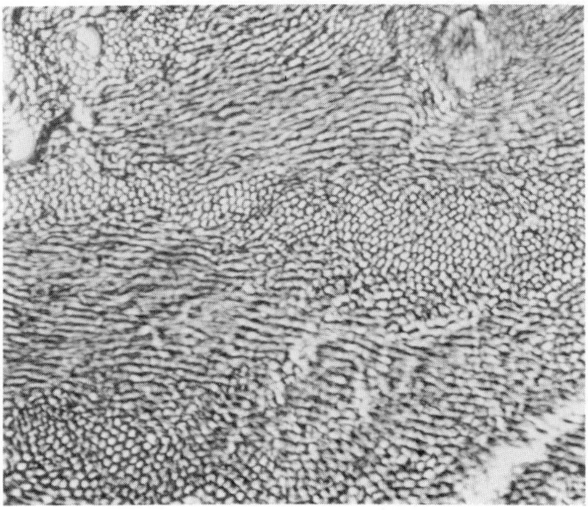

Fig. 165 Photomicrograph of developing human fetal enamel showing the structural basis of the Hunter-Schreger band phenomenon. The enamel prisms in alternate bands are arranged almost at right angles to each other. Decalcified section. × 250.

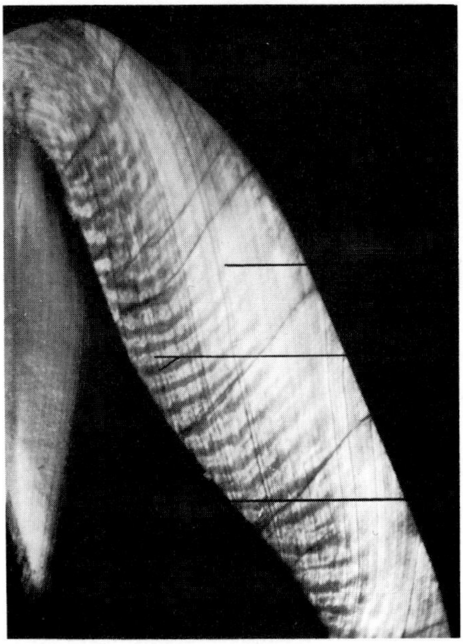

Fig. 166 Hunter–Schreger bands. A photomicrograph of enamel taken by reflected light. The Brown Striae of Retzius can also be seen as fine lines running in almost the opposite direction to the Hunter–Schreger bands. × 20.

is reversed as the light is now absorbed or reflected by the prisms of opposite sets of discs from that in the previous arrangement.

Brown striae of Retzius. A further series of bands appears in ground sections of the enamel; these are the brown striae or incremental lines of Retzius. In longitudinal sections they appear as bands of

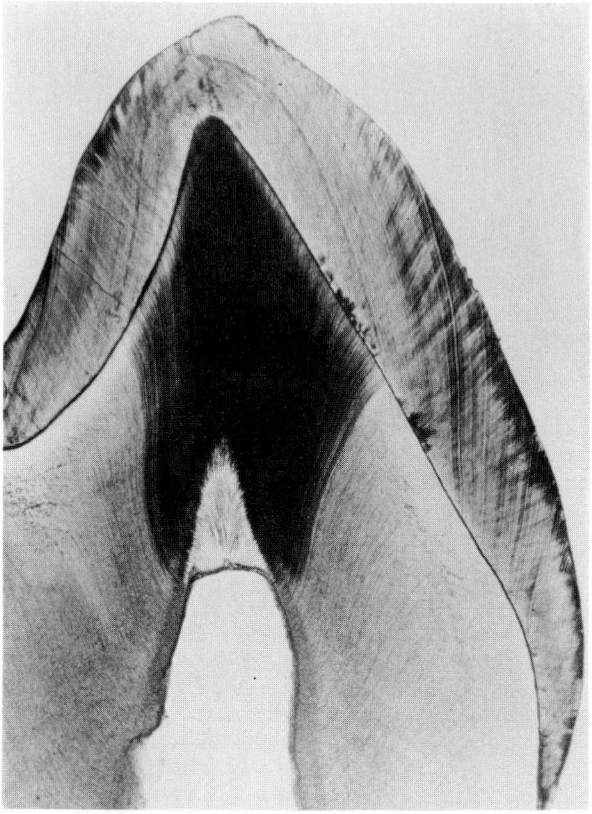

Fig. 167 Brown striae of Retzius. Longitudinal ground section of premolar. Note the difference in the orientation of the incremental lines in the cuspal region as compared with the rest of the enamel. × 12.

apparently brown pigmented enamel running obliquely from the dentine-enamel junction upward and outward to the surface of the enamel. They are most numerous and close together in the cervical region (Fig. 167). Towards the incisive edge or cusps of the tooth they do not reach the surface and surround the tip of the dentine (Fig. 167). Each band represents the former outline of the enamel at succeeding stages in its formation, from the first layer deposited on the dentine-enamel junction at the cusps, or incisive edge, to the cervical margin where the last layer is deposited (Fig. 168). Since the enamel is formed in a rhythmic manner each band corresponds with one of the phases of quiescence that alternate with periods of active enamel formation. A concentration of submicroscopic spaces occurs along each band and this by altering the optical qualities of the enamel gives the effect of a brown pigmentation in ground sections. In transverse ground sections of a tooth the brown striae of Retzius appear as concentric circles similar to the growth rings seen on the cut surface of a tree trunk, with which indeed they correspond, being true incremental lines in the pattern of enamel formation (Fig. 169).

In those parts of the crown where the incremental lines of Retzius reach the surface there are a series of transverse ridges (known as perikymata) separated by slight furrows which correspond with the incremental lines. These ridges are most numerous in the cervical part of the crown and are naturally absent over the incisive edges and tips of the cusps, that is in those areas where the incremental lines do not reach the surface. They are most marked in the newly erupted tooth, gradually disappearing through wear of the enamel surface. They are sometimes referred to as the imbrication lines of Pickerill and can be demonstrated by rubbing graphite on the surfaces of the teeth.

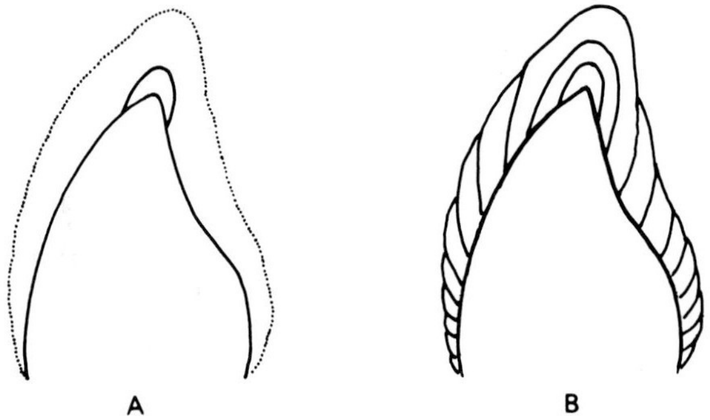

Fig. 168 Diagram to illustrate the arrangement of the Brown Striae (incremental lines) of Retzius. (A) The first deposit of enamel above the tip of the dentine giving the characteristic outline to the incremental line in this area of the enamel. The final surface of the enamel is indicated in dotted line. (B) The arrangement of the incremental lines in the fully formed enamel.

Neo-natal line. In the deciduous teeth and in the first permanent molars an accentuated incremental line appears between the enamel which is formed before birth and that which is formed after birth (Fig. 170). This line is known as the neo-natal line and is associated with the disturbance in enamel formation produced at birth, due to changes in nutrition and environment. The prenatal enamel is more homogeneous than the postnatal enamel, due probably to the more constant surrounding and nutrition of the fetus.

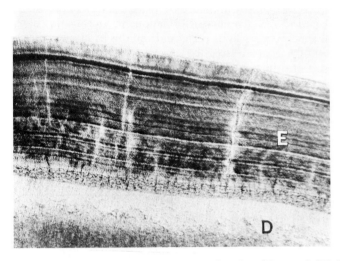

Fig. 169 Brown striae of Retzius. Transverse ground section. (E) enamel; (D) dentine. × 25.

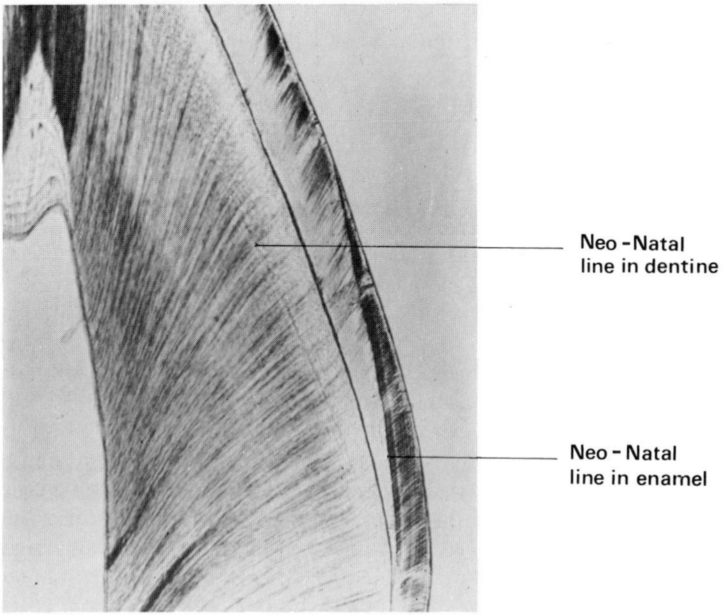

Fig. 170 Neo-natal lines in enamel and dentine. Ground section of deciduous central incisor. × 25.

Amelo-dentinal junction. The dentinal surface of the enamel is formed by a series of dome-shaped elevations which are closely arranged. In a section these elevations give the familiar scalloped appearance to the enamel-dentine junction, so that the surface of the dentine appears to be formed by a series of bays (Fig. 171). Occasionally the elevations seem to be absent, for in some sections stretches of the enamel-dentine junction are smooth and regular. The irregular shape of the junction helps to strengthen the union between the dentine and the enamel. This irregularity is most marked in the cusps of the tooth.

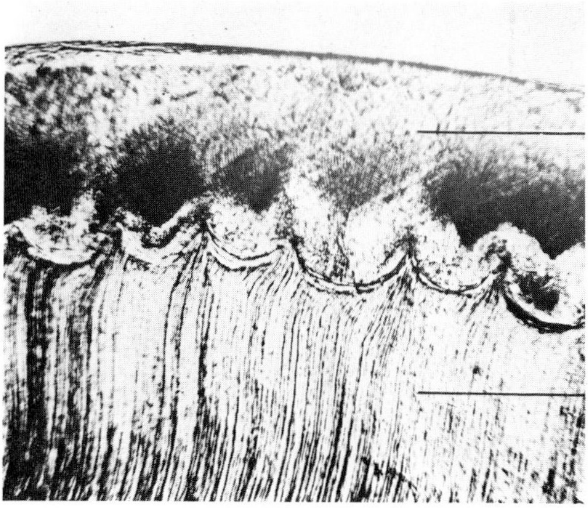

Fig. 171 Amelo-dentinal junction. Longitudinal ground section. ×80.

Enamel spindles. In some areas dentinal tubules pass into the enamel for short distances and are surrounded by the interprismatic substance of the enamel. They may terminate as pointed or rounded processes or may have a noticeably thickened end; in the latter case they are known as enamel spindles (Fig. 172). They are found in greatest numbers in the region of the cusps (Fig. 159). They run at right angles to the dentine surface and have no definite relationship to the enamel prisms. The enamel spindles must presumably be produced by odontoblast process which insinuate themselves between the cells of the internal enamel epithelium of the enamel organ before either dentine or enamel is laid down. It has been suggested that the enamel spindles do not strictly enter the enamel but are exaggerated forms of the projections which alternate with the bays of the dentine-enamel junction.

Lamellae. The lamellae are thin sheet-like structures arranged radially and vertically in the enamel (Fig. 173); and so are seen best in transverse sections of the teeth (Fig. 174). They extend from the surface of the tooth, reaching a considerable distance into enamel, usually as far as the dentine-enamel junction. Lamellae are mainly found in

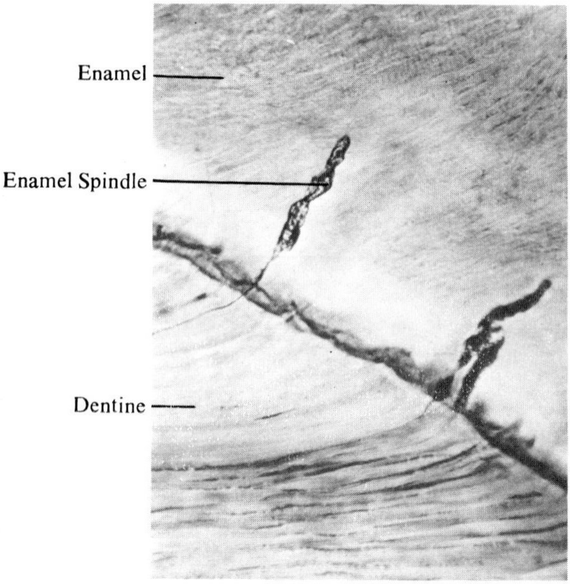

Fig. 172 Enamel spindles. Ground section. × 180.

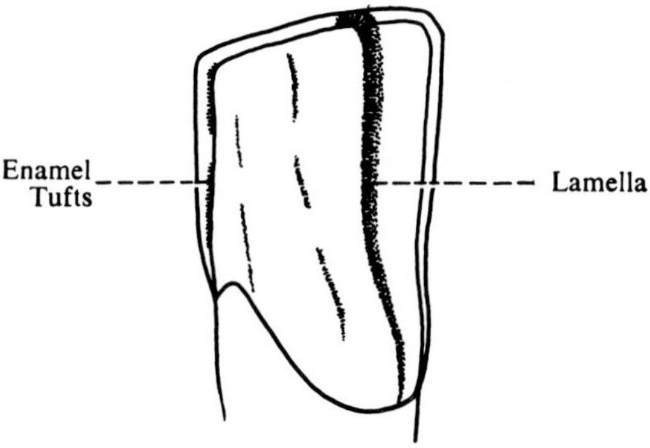

Fig. 173 Diagram of a permanent lower incisor, with the enamel shown as if it was transparent, to illustrate the arrangement of enamel lamellae and tufts.

the cervical half of the crowns and are more numerous on the interstitial surfaces than buccally or lingually; occlusally they are sometimes associated with the fissures. In general, however, throughout the enamel they do not occur in great numbers and have no regular distribution.

Lamellae are organic structures and are produced by cracks in the enamel which become filled with organic material. Since lamellae can be found in teeth which are in a pre-eruptive stage it is clear that some of them are developmental in origin, occurring as cracks in the partially calcified matrix. There is evidence which indicates that some lamellae occur after the teeth have erupted. The organic material of such lamellae

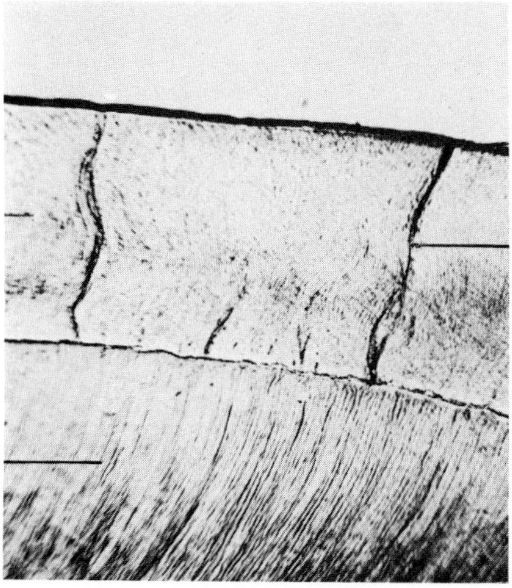

Fig. 174 Transverse ground section to show the appearance of lamellae. These features could alternatively be cracks in the enamel. Final proof could only be provided by the decalcification of the enamel. × 80.

may be derived from the saliva or the dentine. Sometimes bacteria are found in lamellae. Lamellae are commonly arranged quite independently to prism direction, since they can cross through prism substance. They have a thickness which ranges from about 3 μm in adult enamel to less than 1 μm in deciduous enamel.

Lamellae should not be confused with the cracks which can be produced in ground sections of the enamel during histological preparation. These look very like lamellae and can only be distinguished by a careful decalcification of the section. The organic material of the true lamellae is revealed by the decalcification.

Enamel tufts. The enamel tufts spring from the dentine-enamel junction and reach a short distance into the enamel, not usually farther than one-third of its thickness. The enamel tufts were so called since when viewed under low magnification they look like tufts of grass. They do not, however, arise from a single stem but are thin wavy ribbons attached by one side to the dentine-enamel junction (Fig. 173). When traced through the enamel their wavy course exactly parallels the change in direction of the prisms at succeeding levels in the enamel. Like the lamellae they are organic structures and have a vertical arrangement and so are best seen in transverse sections (Fig. 175). They are much more numerous than the lamellae. Both tufts and lamellae are relatively insoluble to weak organic acids and EDTA.

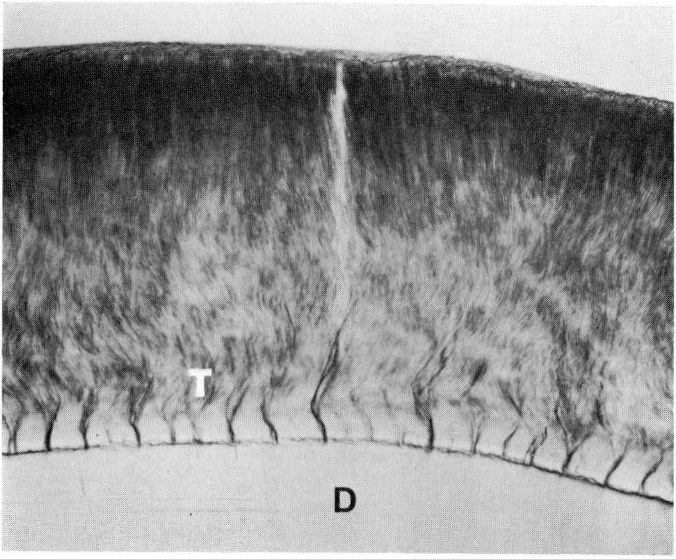

Fig. 175 Transverse ground section showing enamel tufts. D, dentine; T, tufts. × 65.

Permeability. Though the mature enamel is such a densely calcified tissue it has been shown by the use of radio-active isotopes that it has a certain degree of permeability. The main pathway is from the saliva into the outer part of the enamel, but there is a lesser degree of permeability from the pulpal blood supply across the dentine.

Earlier work employing osmotic and cataphoretic methods also indicated that the enamel was permeable, and not only to small inorganic ions but also to some extent to larger ions such as those of dyes. In contrast, however, this work suggested that whereas the enamel of teeth not long erupted was equally permeable from the dentinal and outer surfaces, in old enamel the permeability from the mouth disappeared, though it remained on the dentinal surface.

The importance of these results lies in showing that although there is no cellular mechanism by which the enamel of functioning teeth may undergo physiological change, yet changes on a chemical (ionic) level can take place. This means that in this respect the enamel comes into line with the other calcified tissues, though as yet the extent to which a turn-over of any of its organic or inorganic constituents can occur is unknown. Moreover it is conceivable that in this way some alteration in the composition of the enamel could take place. It has been suggested that final maturation of enamel may occur after the tooth appears in the mouth cavity by way of the ionic interchange between the enamel and the saliva.

Laboratory and clinical considerations. The features which are seen with the light microscope in the examination of a ground section of the enamel are produced either by variations in the mineral content of the tissue or by the arrangement of the enamel crystallites. Zones of non-mineralised enamel contrast with the translucent appearance of the surrounding enamel; thus lamellae and enamel tufts are seen as dark structures in the substance of the enamel. The pattern of the prisms is established by the abrupt changes in crystallite orientation which occur at the prism boundaries; though here too the greater amount of organic matrix which is present at these regions may also contribute to this effect (see p. 201). Even minute differences in mineralisation of the enamel can be appreciated with the light microscope for it is now widely accepted that the incremental lines, the Brown striae of Retzius, are produced by an increased number of sub-microscopic pores or defects in the mineral arrangement. In the early carious lesion in the enamel the several zones which can be distinguished, such as the 'dark' zone, are brought about by varying amounts of destruction and cavitation of the mineral content by the acids associated with the carious attack.

The very high mineral content of the enamel makes it hard but also liable to fracture. Enamel which is unsupported by dentine is very fragile and this must be taken into consideration in cavity preparation. No overhanging edges must be allowed to remain, and the enamel should be cut back to at least the vertical plane. Where the nature of the filling material permits it is preferable to bevel the edges of the cavity so that the margins are protected by the restoration.

Since enamel fractures along planes which are parallel to the line of the prisms a knowledge of the direction of the prisms in their course through the enamel is of value in cavity preparation. In general direction the prisms run perpendicular to the surface of the dentine. On occlusal surfaces the cleavage planes leave overhanging edges since the prisms on either side of the fissures are inclined towards each other.

The altered characteristics of the apatite structure of the enamel which occurs when fluorapatite replaces hydroxyapatite can be made use of in helping to lower the incidence of dental caries. The replacement of hydroxyapatite by fluorapatite can be produced either while the enamel of the teeth is being formed or after the teeth have erupted into the mouth cavity (see p. 199). Advantage of this is taken in prophylactic action to control the incidence of caries, either by adding 1 p.p. million of fluorine to the water supply so that it may be incorporated in the enamel of teeth during their formation, or by the topical application of fluoride solution, usually as 1·5–2·0 per cent sodium fluoride, to the surface of teeth in the mouth cavity. These measures form one of the most important aspects of preventive dentistry.

During the carious attack alternating phases of dissolution and remineralisation are believed to occur. The latter is favoured by the presence of fluorine. This may constitute a further mode of action of fluorine in the control of caries, in addition to the lesser solubility of fluorapatite as compared with hydroxyapatite.

BIBLIOGRAPHY

Allan, J. H. (1967). Maturation of enamel. In *Structural and Chemical Organization of Teeth.* Ed. Miles, A. E. W. New York: Academic Press.

Boyde, A. (1964). The structure of developing mammalian dental enamel. In *Tooth Enamel.* Eds. Stack, M. V. & Fearnhead, R. W. Bristol: Wright.

——(1976). Amelogenesis and the structure of enamel. In *Scientific Foundations of Dentistry.* Eds. Cohen, B. & Kramer, I. R. H. London: Heinemann.

Boyde, A. (1967). The development of enamel structure. *Proc. R. Soc. Med.* **60,** 923.

Carlström, D. (1964). Polarization microscopy of dental enamel with reference to incipent carious lesions. In *Advances in Oral Biology.* Ed. Staple. P. H. London: Academic Press.

Cooper, W. E. G. (1968). A microchemical, microradiographic and histological investigation of amelogenesis in the pig. *Archs. oral Biol.* **13,** 27.

Crabb, H. S. M. & Darling, A. I. (1962). *The Pattern of Progressive Mineralisation in Human Dental Enamel.* Oxford: Pergamon Press.

Elwood, W. K. & Bernstein, M. H. (1968). The ultrastructure of the enamel organ related to enamel formation. *Amer. J. Anat.* **122,** 73.

Eisenmann, D. R., Ashrafi, S. & Neiman, A. (1979). Calcium transport and the secretory ameloblast. *Anat. Rec.* **193,** 403.

Fearnhead, R. W. & Stack M. V. (Eds.) (1971). *Tooth Enamel* II. Bristol: Wright.

Frank, R. M. & Nalbandian, J. (1967). Ultrastructure of amelogenesis. In *Structural and Chemical Organization of Teeth.* Ed. Miles, A. E. W. New York: Academic Press.

Glas, J.-E. & Nylen, M. U. (1965). A correlated electron microscopic and microradiographic study of human enamel. *Arch. oral Biol.* **10,** 893.

Gustafson, G. & Gustafson, A.-G. (1967). Microanatomy and histochemistry of Enamel. In *Structural and Chemical Organisation of Teeth.* Ed. Miles, A. E. W. New York: Academic Press.

Hardwick, J. L. & Fremlin, J. H. (1959). Isotope studies on permeability of enamel to small particles and ions. *Proc. R. Soc. Med.* **52,** 752.

Helmcke, J.-G. (1967). Ultrastructure of enamel. In *Structural and Chemical Organization of Teeth.* Ed. Miles, A. E. W. New York: Academic Press.

Meckel, A. H., Griebstein, W. J. & Neal, R. J. (1965). Structure of mature human dental enamel as observed by electron microscopy. *Arch. oral Biol.* **10,** 775.

Newman, H. N. (1980). Ultrastructural observations on the human pre-eruptive enamel cuticle. *Arch. oral Biol.* **25,** 49.

Nylen, M. U. & Termine, J. D. (Eds.) (1979). *Tooth Enamel* III. *J. dent. R.* **58,** Special Issue B.

Osborn, J. W. (1968). Direction and interrelationship of enamel prisms from sides of human teeth. *J. dent. Res.* **47,** 223.

Palamara, J., Phaykey, P. P., Rachinger, W. A. & Orams, H. J. (1980). Electron microscopy of surface enamel of human unerupted and erupted teeth. *Arch. oral Biol.* **25,** 715.

Poole, D. F. G. & Brooks, A. W. (1961). The arrangement of crystallites in enamel prisms. *Arch. oral Biol.* **5,** 14.

Reith, E. J. (1967). The early stages of amelogenesis as observed in molar teeth of young rats. *J. Ultrastruct. Res.* **17,** 503.

Reith, E. J. & Butcher, E. O. (1967). Microanatomy and histochemistry of amelogenesis. In *Structural and Chemical Organization of Teeth.* Ed. Miles, A. E. W. New York: Academic Press.

Ripa, L. W., Gwinnett, A. J. & Buoncore, M. G. (1966). The 'prismless' outer layer of deciduous and permanent enamel. *Arch. oral Biol.* **11,** 41.

Stack, M. V. & Fearnhead, R. W. (Eds.) (1965). *Tooth enamel.* Bristol: Wright.

Stack, M. V. (1967). Chemical organization of the organic matrix of enamel. In *Structural and Chemical Organization of Teeth.* Ed. Miles, A. E. W. New York: Academic Press.

Ten Cate, A. R. (1962). The distribution of glycogen in the human developing tooth. *Arch. oral Biol.* **7,** 1.

—— (1962). The distribution of alkaline phosphatase in the human tooth germ. *Arch. oral Biol.* **7,** 195.

Tyldsley, W. R. (1959). The mechanical properties of human enamel and dentine. *Brit. dent. J.* **106,** 269.

Weinmann, J. P., Wessinger, G. D & Reed, G. (1942). Correlation of chemical and histological investigations on developing enamel. *J. Dent. Res.* **21,** 171.

12. Dentine

DEVELOPMENT OF DENTINE

Early Dentine Formation. At first all the cells of the dental papilla are similar in appearance; they are embryonic in form and mesodermal in origin. Distributed in random fashion among the cells of the dental papilla are a number of very fine fibres which are described as being argyrophilic since they stain black with silver. Under the influence of the internal enamel epithelium the cells on the adjacent surface of the dental papilla begin to differentiate. By this differentiation the odontoblast layer is produced. About the same time or a little before, those argyrophilic fibres which are related to the basal lamina between enamel organ and dental papilla (pulp) begin to show an orderly arrangement. Groups of these fibres become gathered together to form single thicker fibres which pass between the cells of the odontoblast layer and, deep to it, mingle with the fine fibres of the pulp.

The thicker fibres passing through the odontoblast layer are known as the fibres of von Korff, and they form the organic matrix of the first formed or mantle dentine (see p. 372). Each group of finer fibres spreading out from a von Korff fibre towards their attachment to the basement membrane has a fan-shaped appearance as seen in section (Fig. 176). With certain fixatives the fibres of von Korff show a marked spiralling along their course. This has earned them the name of corkscrew fibres, but the fibres are sometimes seen to be quite straight (Fig. 176). The electron microscope has shown that the von Korff fibres are composed of groups of fibrils; the constituent fibrils are 1000–2000 Å in diameter and show the 640 Å cross banding which is typical of collagen.

It has been suggested that the classical description of the von Korff fibres is based on an artifact produced by the staining with silver of the inter-cellular substance between the odontoblasts. It is admitted that radially arranged thick collagen fibres are to be found in the early stages of coronal dentinogenesis but there are believed to be confined to the region peripheral to the necks of the odontoblasts close to the forming dentine matrix. According to this view no fibres pass from the dental papilla between the odontoblasts and then fan out.

The odontoblast. The fully differentiated odontoblast layer is composed of a single layer of cells sharply defined from the rest of the pulp tissue. The odontoblast at this stage is a columnar cell with a large, distinct roundish or oval nucleus. The nuclei of the odontoblasts are situated towards the basal ends of the cells, that is remote from the enamel organ (Fig. 176).

With the electron microscope concentrations of rough-surfaced endoplasmic reticulum are found close to the nucleus and in the distal or formative end of the odontoblast; these concentrations are interconnected by strands of reticulum which run parallel and close to the cell membranes (Figs. 177, 178). The Golgi complex in the centre of the cell is surrounded by this arrangement of the endoplasmic reticulum. Mitochondria and ribosomes are scattered throughout the cytoplasm. The mitochondria contain dense calcium granules. Some globules lie amongst the subnuclear concentration of endoplasmic reticulum and as the cell becomes active similar globules appear in the distal concentration. At first the distal end of the odontoblast shows numerous foldings but with full differentiation these projections disappear and are replaced by a single process, the odontoblast process. Unlike the body of the cell which is filled with a variety of organelles the odontoblast process contains few and is occupied mainly by a finely stippled material and numbers of microfilaments, microtubules and

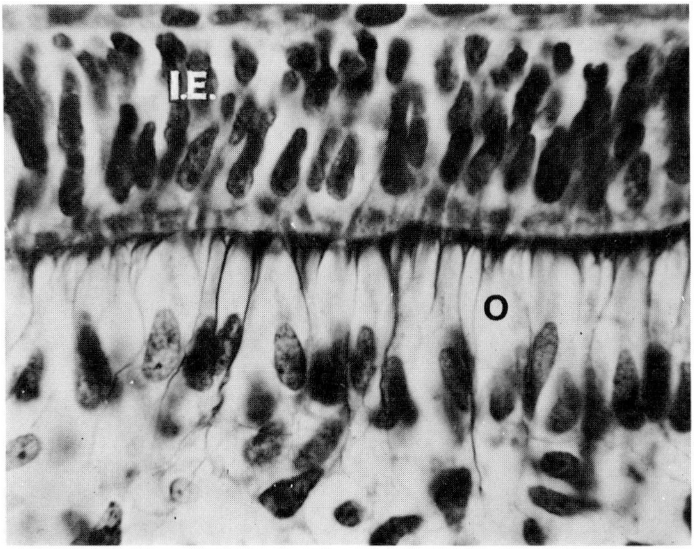

Fig. 176 Fibres of von Korff. I.E., internal enamel epithelium; O, odontoblast layer. Rat incisor. Wilder's silver stain. × 700.

some dense granules. The lateral surfaces of the odontoblasts are connected by desmosomes, but towards the predentine they are attached by a junctional complex.

Using tritiated proline it has been shown that the endoplasmic reticulum very quickly shows radioactivity indicating it as a site of protein

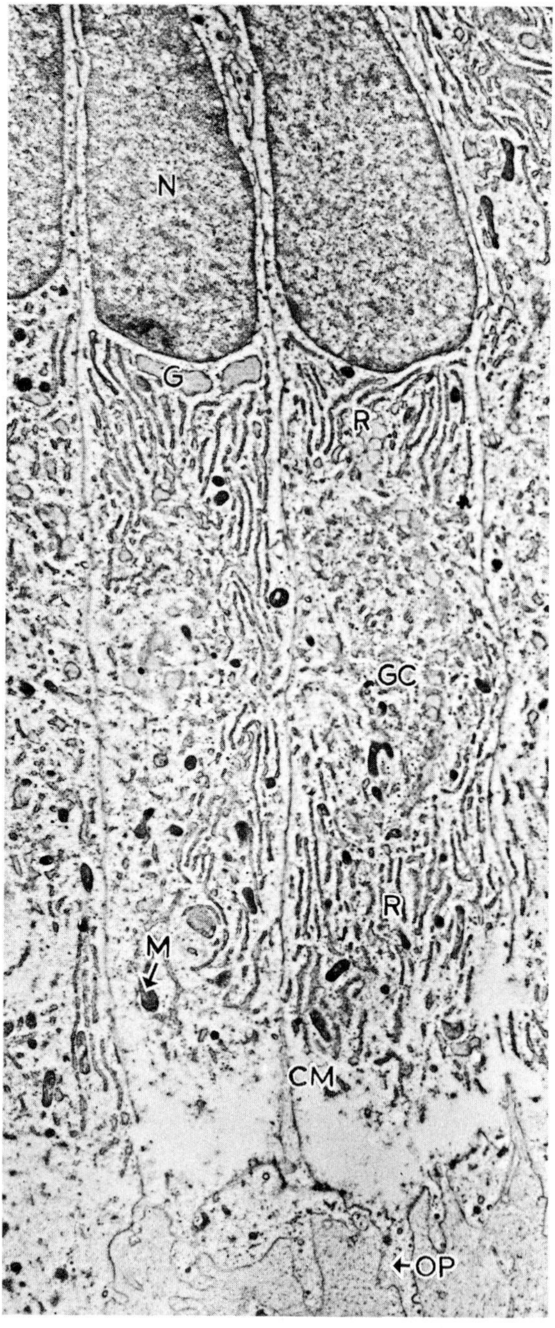

Fig. 177 Electron microscope picture of odontoblasts. CM. cell membrane; G. globule; GC. Golgi complex; M. mitochondrion. N. Nucleus; OP. odontoblast process; R. endoplasmic reticulum (*By courtesy of Dr M. U. Nylen and Dr D. B. Scott.*)

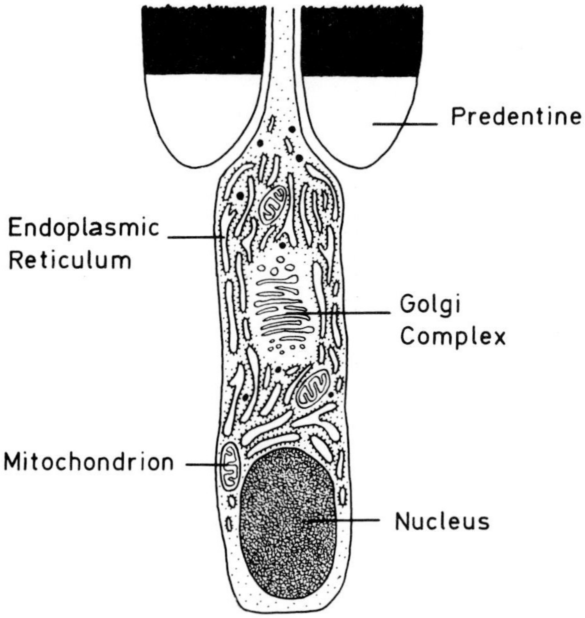

Fig. 178 Diagrammatic representation of an odontoblast as seen with the electron microscope, showing the major cell organelles. (*By courtesy of W. Heinemann Medical Books Ltd.*)

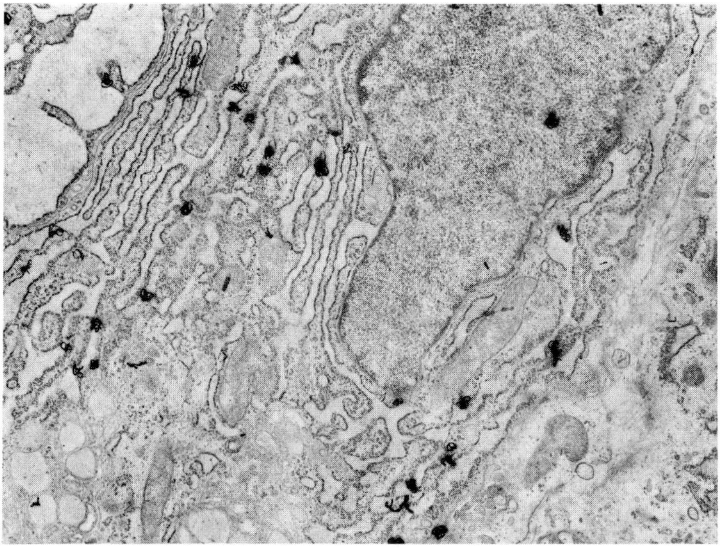

Fig. 179 Longitudinal section of odontoblast. Labelling is present in the endoplasmic reticulum 5 minutes after intravenous injection of tritiated proline. Original magnification × 7000. (*By courtesy of Dr R. M. Frank and the Archs. oral Biol.*)

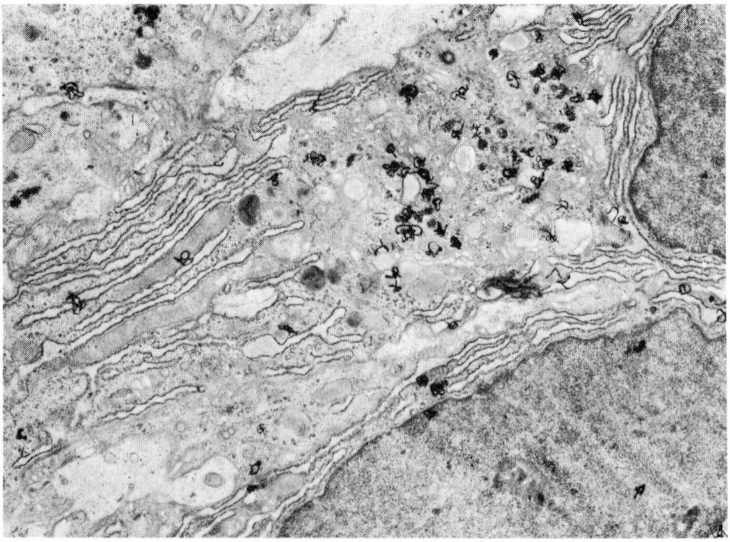

Fig. 180 Longitudinal section of odontoblast. Labelling has appeared in the Golgi region 1 hour after intravenous injection of tritiated proline. Original magnification × 5520. (*By courtesy of Dr R. M. Frank and the Archs. oral Biol.*)

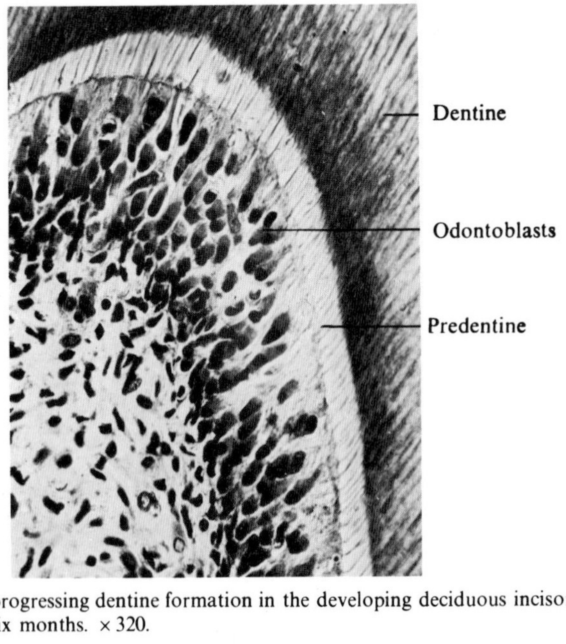

Fig. 181 Actively progressing dentine formation in the developing deciduous incisor of a human fetus of six months. × 320.

formation (Fig. 179). The labelled protein next appears in the region of the Golgi complex (Fig. 180). From there it passes to the odontoblast process from where it reaches the organic matrix of the predentine.

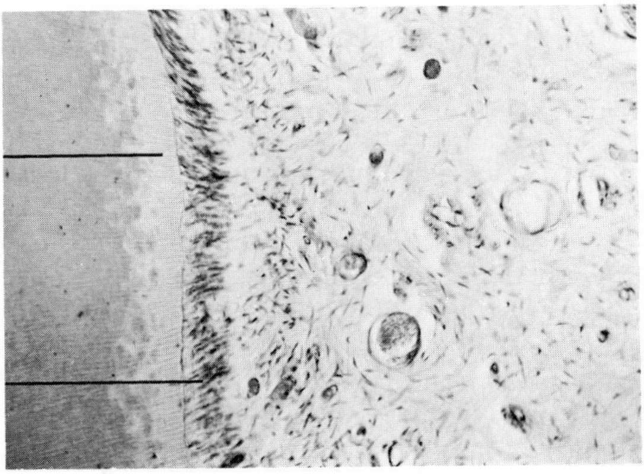

Fig. 182 Odontoblast layer and continuing dentine formation. At the junction between dentine and predentine there are numbers of calcospherites. Section through the crown of an extracted permanent human tooth. × 160.

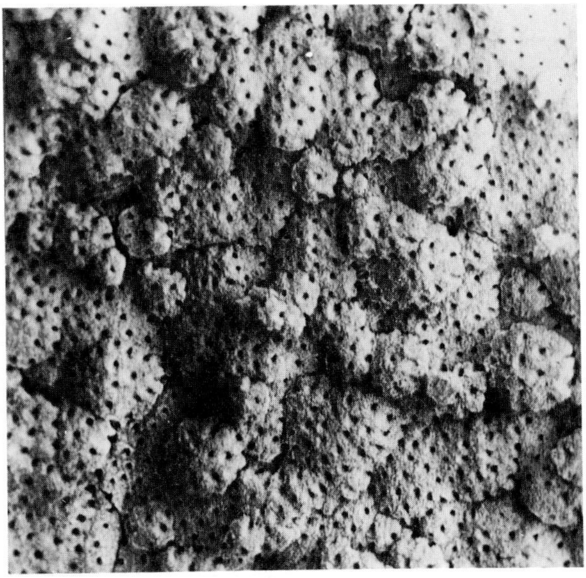

Fig. 183 Mineralising front in human dentine uncovered by removal of the organic matrix. The elevations on this surface correspond to calcospherites. Each of these is pierced by several tubules. Original magnification × 600. (*By courtesy of Dr A Boyde.*)

A definite layer of dentine matrix first appears at the light microscopic level as a deposition of a ground substance around the fan-shaped extensions of the von Korff fibres. As a result the pulpal surface of this layer of dentine shows a series of conical projections to each of which a von Korff fibre is attached. The fine fibres surrounded by the ground substance become less distinct and no longer stain black with silver. This dentine formation is completely organic, and it is only as the layer increases in width that the inorganic element is deposited. Calcification begins in the oldest part of this organic matrix; that is, adjacent to the basal lamina between enamel organ and pulp, now represented by the dentine-enamel junction. The layer of dentine on the advancing pulpal surface is always uncalcified and is known as the predentine or odontogenic zone. With continued dentine formation the cells of the odontoblast layer retreat farther from the dentine-enamel junction.

Later dentine formation. As the dentine increases in thickness certain changes take place in it and in the odontoblast layer. Whereas in the first formed narrow layer of dentine the fibres (of von Korff) in its substance are radially arranged, approximately at right angles to the dentine-enamel junction, in the later additions to the dentine the collagen fibres have a more transverse distribution (Fig. 191). These fibres are finer than the von Korff fibres and are produced by the odontoblasts. This later formed dentine is sometimes called circumpulpal dentine. The pulpal surface of the dentine begins to show, in sections, what may be described as a squarer edge. At the same time dentinal tubules appear and these become more obvious as the dentine continues to increase in width (Fig. 181). The dentinal tubules are minute canals traversing the dentine, each of which contains the protoplasmic process of an odontoblast.

The cells of the odontoblast layer become pyriform and as their basal ends are arranged at different levels an appearance of pseudostratification is produced. This altered arrangement of the odontoblasts is no doubt associated with the continued pulpward expansion of the forming dentine, the same number of cells being accommodated, in this way, opposite a smaller surface of dentine. At this time capillaries appear in the odontoblast layer, forming a network which ramifies amongst the cells.

This arrangement of the dentine matrix and the odontoblast layer persists during the rest of active dentine formation; that is, of the primary dentine. As in the first-formed narrow layer of dentine, calcification always lags behind the laying down of the organic matrix so that as long as dentine formation takes place the most recently formed layer on the pulpal surface of the dentine is uncalcified and is called predentine. The width of the predentine bears some relationship to the rate at which the dentine matrix is laid down; the more rapid the formation of dentine the broader is the layer of predentine.

The inorganic material deposited in the organic matrix during calcification becomes apparent as spherical masses which, at first discrete, become larger and gradually fuse together to produce the fully formed dentine. These spherical masses are known as calcospherites. At the advancing edge of calcification, between dentine and predentine, the calcospherites can frequently be seen, some still separate, others partially united with the calcified dentine (Figs. 182, 183). Even in normal teeth the dentine is frequently not equally well calcified. This is indicated in sections stained with haematoxylin and eosin by variations in the depth of staining. The better calcified areas stain more deeply with the haematoxylin. Sometimes alternate bands of darker and lighter stained dentine may be seen, or the globular form of the calcospherites may be distinguished within the mass of the dentine.

Within each dentinal tubule, and surrounding the odontoblast process, a zone of dentine is formed which is known as the peritubular dentine (Figs. 193, 196). It becomes more highly mineralised than the surrounding, or intertubular, dentine. Its pulpward development varies relative to the intertubular dentine at different stages of tooth formation (Fig. 184).

Dentine formation, like that of the enamel, first occurs at the deepest part of the concavity of the enamel organ; that is, at the region corresponding to the incisive edge in an anterior tooth and a cusp in a posterior tooth. The formation of the dentine, which starts before that of the enamel, gradually spreads from these regions until the whole of the dentine is produced. The cusps represent individual growth centres from which dentine formation spreads across the occlusal surface until

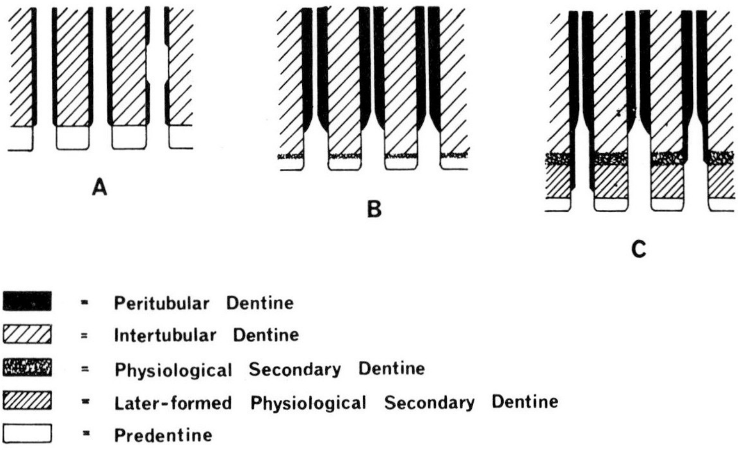

Fig. 184 Diagrammatic representation of three stages in the deposition of the coronal dentine. A, during the formation of the primary dentine; B, shortly after the tooth has appeared in the mouth; C, after the tooth has been present in the mouth for a considerable number of years.

eventually fusion takes place. As in the case of the enamel, dentine formation takes place in a rhythmic fashion; that is, there are alternating periods of activity and quiescence. Evidence of this rhythmical deposition of the dentine is indicated by incremental lines which can be seen in sections of the fully formed tooth (Fig. 185).

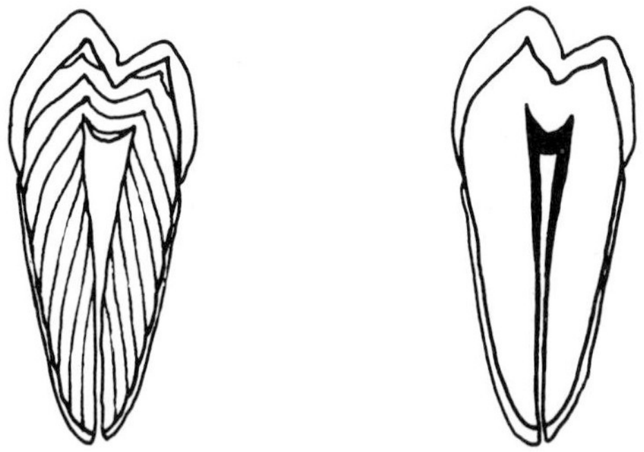

Fig. 185 Diagram to show the pattern of formation of primary dentine and the usual distribution of regular secondary dentine. (A) The arrangement of the incremental lines in the primary dentine. (B) The distribution of regular secondary dentine after the tooth has been present in the mouth for some time; regular physiological secondary dentine shown in solid black.

Unlike the enamel, the formation of dentine is not confined to the period before the tooth erupts but can take place throughout the whole life of the tooth. When eruption begins little more than the coronal part of the dentine is formed. As eruption proceeds the formation of the dentine for the root of the tooth takes place, but even when the tooth has attained its proper occlusal relationship only about two-thirds of the root has been formed. Formation of the root is not completed until about one to one and a half years after the tooth first appears in the mouth cavity in the case of a deciduous tooth, and two to three years after this time in the case of a permanent tooth.

In the same way as formation of the coronal dentine is initiated by the cells of the internal enamel epithelium of the enamel organ, so the formation of the dentine for the root is initiated by the epithelial sheath of Hertwig. On the commencement of eruption the sheath of Hertwig becomes active and proliferates, mapping out the shape of the root and at the same time inducing the differentiation of an odontoblast layer on the surface of the pulp (Fig. 66).

After the bulk of the dentine has been formed, a further but slower deposition of dentine takes place within the pulp cavity. This begins in the region of the pulpal cornua even before the tooth has emerged into the mouth cavity. Though found eventually over the whole pulpal surface of the coronal dentine it usually occurs most actively at the roof,

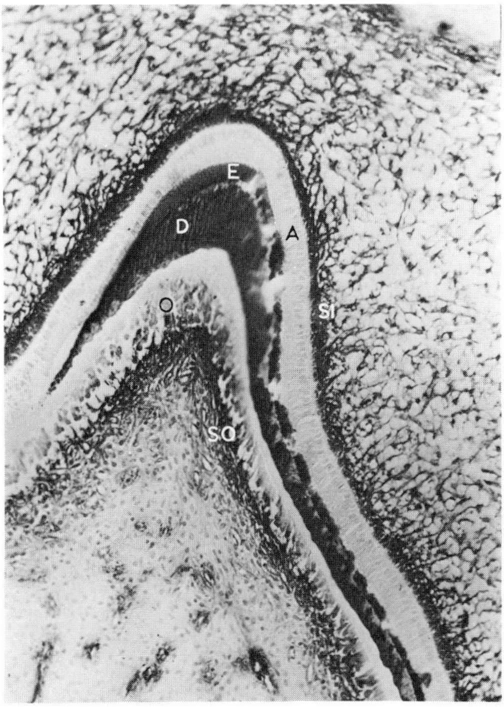

Fig. 186 Alkaline phosphatase activity in the developing human tooth. The heaviest activity is in the subodontoblast layer and the stratum intermedium. The black precipitate in the dentine and enamel is produced by calcium salts and does not represent enzyme activity. Gomori cobalt method. (A) Ameloblast layer; (D) dentine; (E) enamel; (O) odontoblasts; (S.I.) stratum intermedium; (S.O.) subodontoblast layer; × 300. (*By courtesy of Dr A. R. Ten Cate.*)

and in multi-rooted teeth on the floor of the pulp chamber. This slow, continued formation of dentine gradually diminishes the size of the pulp cavity. The dentine which produces the gross typical form of a tooth is known as primary dentine; that which is deposited more slowly as an age change and brings about a narrowing of an existing pulp cavity is distinguished as physiological secondary dentine (Fig. 185B).

Histochemical considerations. As in the case of the enamel, the significance of the available histochemical information related to dentine formation is not yet fully understood.

During active dentine formation the greatest concentration alkaline phosphatase is found in the narrow zone of pulp tissue immediately deep to the odontoblast layer and along the course of the von Korff fibres across the odontoblast layer. The odontoblasts and the general pulp tissue show a lower level of the enzyme. The heavy concentration of alkaline phosphatase in the subodontoblastic zone and along the course of the von Korff fibres is in keeping with the now widely accepted

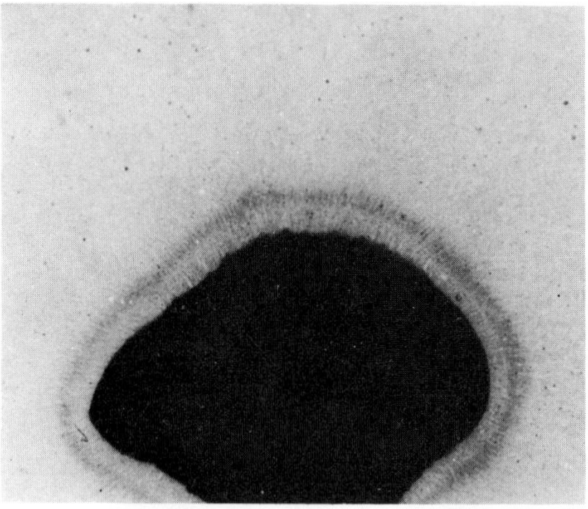

Fig. 187 Microradiograph of a horizontal ground section through the crown of a newly-erupted premolar. Surrounding the pulp cavity is a radiopaque zone separated from the bulk of the dentine by a narrow radiolucent zone. Original magnification × 16.

view that alkaline phosphatase is concerned in the formation of fibrous proteins, for the fibres of von Korff take part in the formation of the fibres of the matrix of the dentine and the cells of the subodontoblastic zone are related to the von Korff fibres (Fig. 186).

Throughout its course the peritubular matrix shows a content of acid mucopolysaccharide; this is especially marked near the pulp. In the predentine and in the dentine near the pulp the odontoblast process stains heavily and appears to be rich in an aldehyde containing lipid, and a carbohydrate-protein complex. This part of the odontoblast process also shows alkaline phosphatase activity. Although the odontoblast process shows little staining in the middle and outer parts of the dentine a strong basophilia and staining with alcian blue is found at the junction between the peritublar matrix and the contents of the dentinal tubule. Whether this represents the outer limit of the odontoblast process or the inner part of the peritubular matrix is uncertain, but since neither it nor peritubular matrix are found where the dentinal tubules pass through interglobular dentine it probably is related to the peritubular matrix.

In newly erupted teeth a narrow zone of dentine is found pulpally which is somewhat different from the rest of the coronal dentine. It shows a high generalised content of a carbohydrate-protein complex and of acid mucopolysaccharide and it is strongly radiopaque (Fig. 187). This zone of dentine probably constitutes the regular physiological secondary dentine for the tubules in it are as numerous and as regular as in primary dentine (Fig. 207). A layer with such morphological and histochemical characteristics cannot be distinguished in the root of the tooth.

COMPOSITION AND STRUCTURE OF DENTINE

Distribution. The dentine forms the bulk of the tooth substance and gives the basic shape to each tooth, though in the crown it is covered by the enamel and in the root by the cement(Fig. 188). The thickness of the enamel may considerably modify the shape of the tooth, especially over the cusps, which are accentuated.

Physical and chemical characters. Dentine is yellowish in colour. It has a high degree of elasticity; the average value of the elastic modulus of dentine is $1{\cdot}79 \times 10^6$ pounds per square inch. It is less hard than enamel, but is harder than either bone or cement. The average value of the breaking stress of dentine is 38 800 pounds per square inch.

Dentine has a considerably higher organic content than enamel. The content of organic material is about 19 to 21 per cent by weight. The organic material is made up of 18 per cent of collagen, 0·9 per cent of citric acid, and 0·2 per cent each of insoluble protein, mucopolysaccharide, and lipid, The inorganic content amounts to approximately 75 per cent, by weight, and the rest of the total weight is accounted for by water. It is generally accepted that the inorganic element is composed of apatite molecules, and chiefly in the form of hydroxy apatite, for which the approximate empirical formula is $Ca_{10}(PO_4)_6(OH)_2$. The apatite crystallites in dentine are much smaller than those in enamel, having a length of 200–1000 Å and a width of about 30 Å. They are of similar dimensions to the crystallites in bone and cement.

Structure. Dentine is composed of cells, the odontoblasts, and an intercellular substance. The latter is only intercellular in the sense that it lies between protoplasmic processes of the odontoblasts, the odontoblasts themselves always forming a layer on the surface of the dentine. This is different from bone, where the bone cells lie between the bone lamellae. The dentine is everywhere permeated by the minute tubes, dentinal tubules, which contain the protoplasmic processes of the odontoblasts (Figs. 189, 199). The dentinal tubules run parallel to each other and in the one direction, from the outer surface of the dentine to the pulp cavity (Fig. 188). The intercellular substance, apart from the peritubular dentine, is composed of fine collagenous fibrils which are embedded in a calcified cement substance. The fibrils are usually bound together in dense bundles or fibres (Fig. 190). The fibres are arranged in a lattice-like fashion, coursing in gentle curves between the tubules (Fig. 191). In the outer zone of the dentine, however, the fibres are coarser and they are arranged at right angles to the surface. This zone is considerably broader beneath the cement than beneath the enamel. Beneath the cement groups of the fibres form arcade-like arrangements.

Odontoblasts and odontoblast processes. The odontoblasts are normally found as a layer of closely arranged cells on the pulpal surface of the dentine. In the fully formed tooth the odontoblasts are elongated cells with their nuclei situated at the basal end (the end remote from

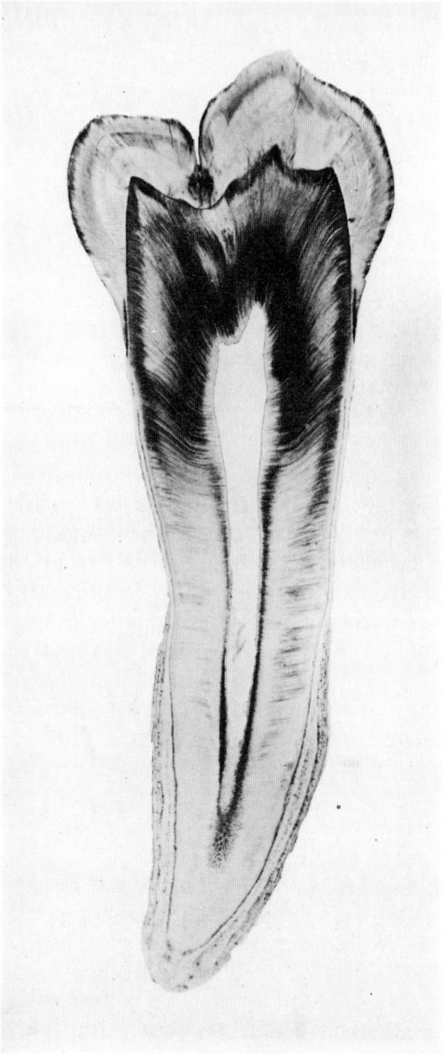

Fig. 188 Longitudinal ground section of a lower premolar to show the distribution of the enamel, dentine, and cement. Note the course of the dentinal tubules and the arrangement of the acellular and cellular cement.

the dentine) of each cell. As the odontoblasts are of variable length the nuclei appear at different levels in the odontoblastic layer. Each odontoblast possesses a protoplasmic process which, it is generally believed, passes through the full thickness of the dentine in a dentinal tubule. Each odontoblast process gives off fine branches along its course

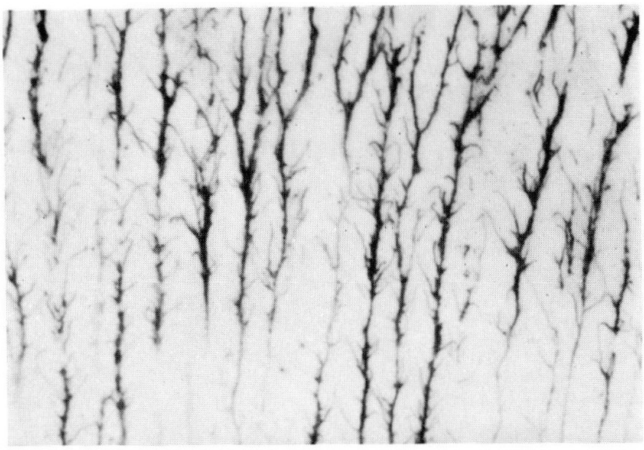

Fig. 189 Dentinal tubules and their lateral branchings. Human tooth stained with silver. × 475.

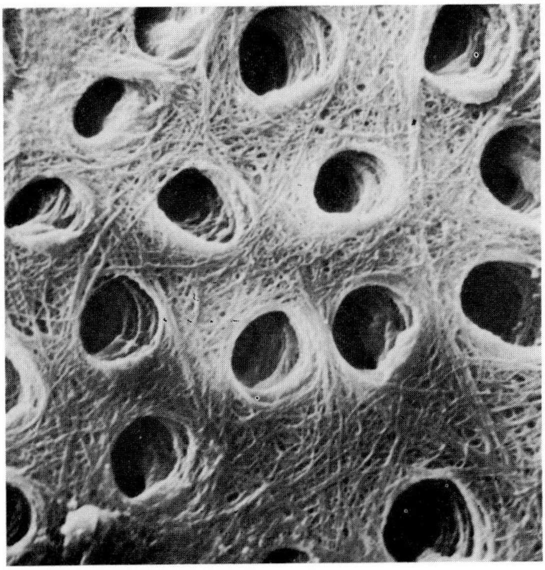

Fig. 190 Predentine surface showing the openings of the dentinal tubules and the dense network of collagen fibres which surround these and constitute the matrix of the intertubular dentine. Original magnification × 5600. (*By courtesy of Dr A. R. Boyde.*)

which are contained in lateral extensions of the tubule; many of these branches unite with those of adjacent processes (Fig. 189).

The odontoblast process does not fill the lumen of the tubule so that between the process and the tubular wall there is a periodontoblastic space. This space is filled with fluid, the dentinal fluid, which has a

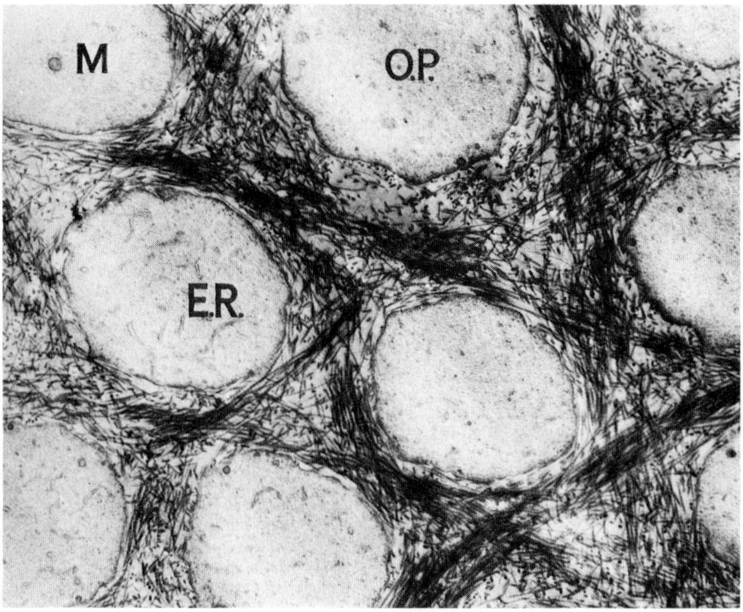

Fig. 191 Electron micrograph of a section cut transversely to the odontoblast processes (O.P.) in the predentine. The odontoblast processes are separated by numerous interlaced collagen fibres. E.R., endoplasmic reticulum; M, mitochondrion. Original magnification × 17 000. (*By courtesy of Dr R. M. Frank and Arch. oral Biol.*)

composition similar to tissue fluid. In the inner dentine, the periodontoblastic space also contains a few uncalcified collagen fibre bundles.

Recent work with the electron microscope has shown that, where it lies in the predentine, the odontoblast process displays a content of organelles which is similar to that of the distal end of the odontoblast. There are ribosomes, some endoplasmic reticulum and an occasional mitochondrion (Fig. 191). A fine network composed of numerous filaments of about 56–80 Å in thickness as well as large vacuoles with a finely granular content are also present (Fig. 192). These vacuoles appear to discharge their contents into the space immediately surrounding the odontoblast process. The retention of these various features in the odontoblast process indicates that the odontoblast process has a secretory function. It seems certain that the odontoblast process is responsible for the formation of the peritubular dentine.

In the calcified dentine at the level where a highly mineralised peritubular zone has not as yet appeared the odontoblast process still shows a ribosomal content, vacuoles, and a network of fine filaments, though any sign of endoplasmic reticulum and mitochondria has virtually disappeared. More peripherally a marked change in the ultrastructure of the odontoblast process becomes evident. The centre of the process is

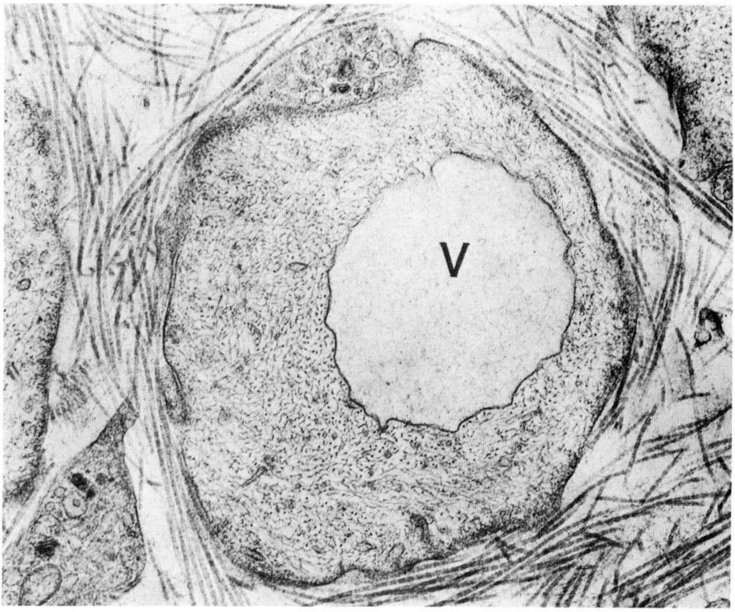

Fig. 192 Electron micrograph of a section cut transversely to an odontoblast process in the predentine. A vacuole (V), bounded by a membrane is present in the odontoblast process. Numerous collagen fibres surround the odontoblast process. Two non-myelinated nerve fibres are present, one of which lies in a concavity in the odontoblast process, the other at the lower left-hand corner of the field. Original magnification × 36 000. (*By courtesy of Dr R. M. Frank and Arch. oral Biol.*)

occupied by a large vacuole which compresses the cytoplasm into a peripherally placed ring(Fig. 193). Progressively this narrow cytoplasmic ring takes on a hyaline appearance.

Although the presence of an odontoblast process has been demonstrated with the electron microscope in the predentine and the inner or pulpal part of the mineralised dentine there is uncertainty as to whether an undoubted process extends more peripherally in the fully formed tooth. Although none has yet been shown there the failure may be due to the problems of rapid fixation in such a densely mineralised tissue. Support for the concept that only a limited part of the dentinal tubule is occupied by an odontoblast process is lent by the composition of the fluid in the dentinal tubules. This contains large quantities of sodium and chloride but very little potassium. This large Na/K ratio suggests that the dentinal fluid is extracellular.

Peritubular dentine. When routinely decalcified sections of dentine are examined a wide space is found between the process and the tubule (Fig. 194). This occurs because each odontoblast process is surrounded by a peritubular zone which is very highly calcified, much more so than

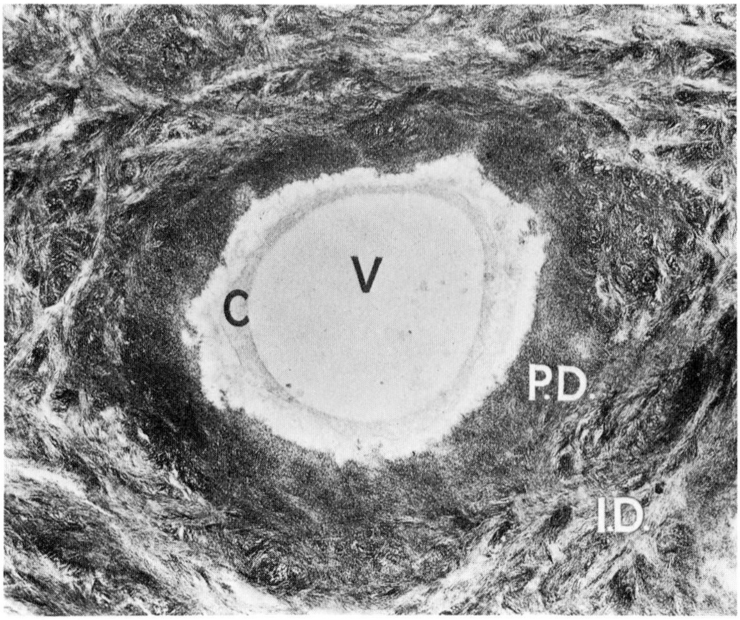

Fig. 193 Electron micrograph of a transverse section through a dentinal tubule. This is occupied by an odontoblast process, which is constituted by a central vacuole (V) which has condensed the cytoplasm (C) peripherally. P.D., peritubular dentine; I.D., intertubular dentine. Original magnification × 37 500 (*By courtesy of Dr R. M. Frank and Arch. oral Biol.*)

the rest of the dentine matrix. The delicate matrix of this hypercalcified zone is broken down in decalcification and shrinks on to the odontoblast process. This results in the appearance of an artifact space around the odontoblast process. Thus in a decalcified section the diameter of the odontoblast tubule appears greater than it is in reality, and what appears to be odontoblast process is the odontoblast process (if not destroyed by the histological technique) plus the shrunken remains of the matrix of the highly calcified zone (Figs. 194, 195). In ground sections of dentine which have been made transversely across the tubules the peritubular zones are readily seen as translucent areas (Fig. 196). In microradiographs the peritubular zones show as rings which are more radiopaque than the surrounding intertubular dentine (Fig. 197). The true diameter of the tubule is about 1·5 μm over the greater part of its length, though variations in diameter ranging from 1 to 2·5 μm do occur.

There is little organic matrix in peritubular dentine and so far no collagen fibrils have been demonstrated in it (Fig. 198). It has generally been assumed that the inorganic material in peritubular dentine is composed of crystallites of hydroxyapatite because it takes that form in the other mammalian mineralised tissues. There is evidence, however,

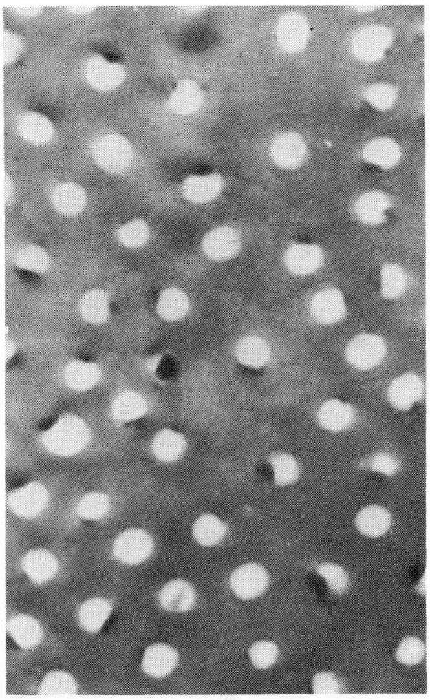

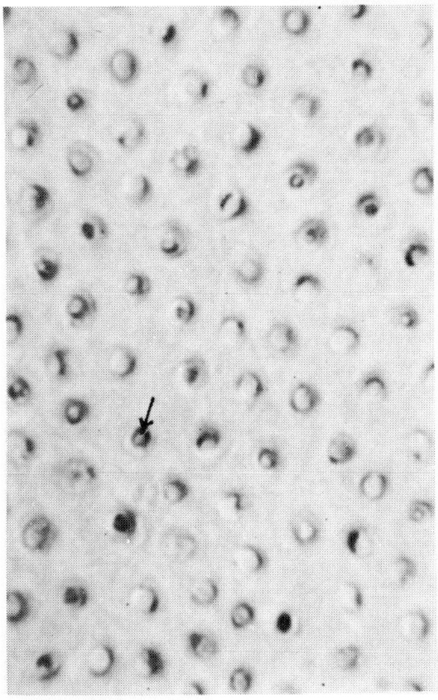

Fig. 194 Transverse section through dentinal tubules. Routinely prepared section. Note the apparently large size of the tubules which are empty apart from an eccentrically placed 'odontoblast process'. Human dentine decalcified in 5 per cent nitric acid, embedded in paraffin wax, and stained with haematoxylin and eosin. × 1200. (*By courtesy of Prof E. W. Bradford.*)

Fig. 195 Transverse section through dentinal tubules. Section prepared by special methods. The odontoblast processes proper are seen as dark rings, each surrounded by a peritubular zone distinct from the rest of the dentine matrix. The arrow indicates an odontoblast process. Human dentine decalcified in the di-sodium salt of ethylene diamine tetracetic acid; embedded in polyethylene glycol and stained with methyl violet. × 1200. (*By courtesy of Prof E. W. Bradford.*)

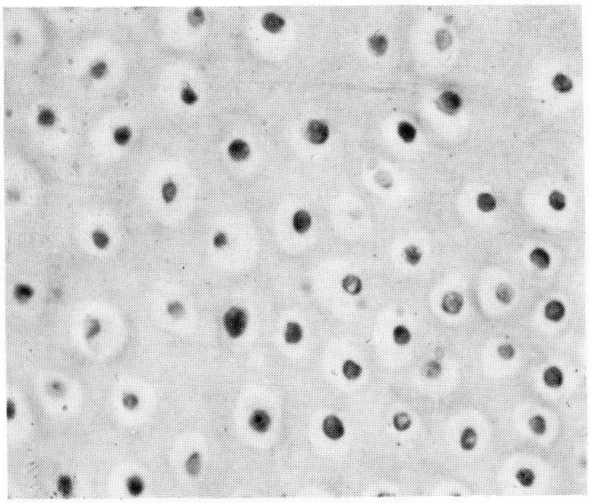

Fig. 196 Ground section of dentine cut transversely to the dentinal tubules and showing the peritubular translucent zones. × 1200. (*By courtesy of the 'Archives of Oral Biology'.*)

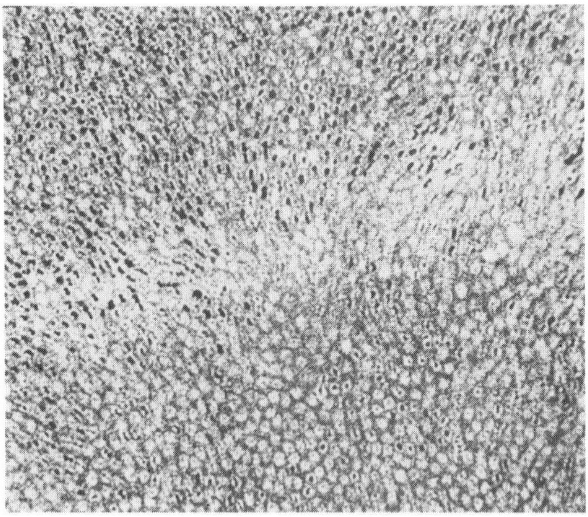

Fig. 197 Microradiograph of a horizontal ground section through an incisor tooth from an elderly subject. A belt of occluded tubules runs across the field. Elsewhere the peritubular dentine shows as radiopaque rings surrounding the radiolucent dentinal tubules. Original magnification ×80.

which suggests that the mineral material in peritubular dentine may well be an amorphous calcium phosphate. This is made up of small globular masses about 250–300Å in diameter (see p. 177).

A peritubular zone is not found along the total length of the dentinal tubule for it is not present in the predentine, and in the crown of a newly completed tooth stops short of the predentine-dentine junction (Fig.

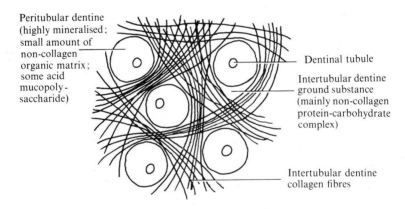

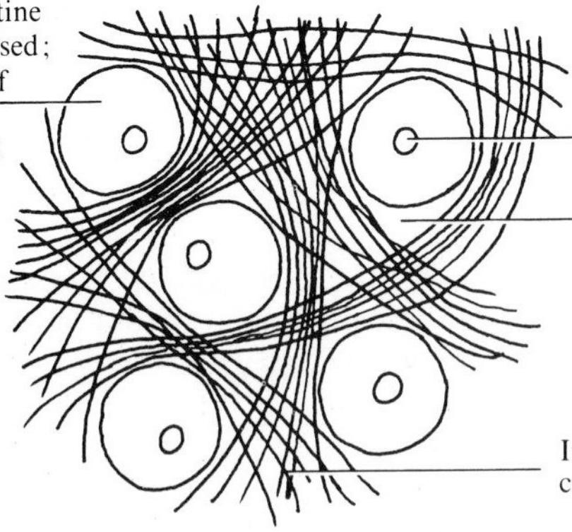

Fig. 198 Diagrammatic representation of a section of fully-formed dentine cut perpendicular to the dentinal tubules. Some details of the structure and composition of the intertubular and peritubular dentine are indicated.

184). As the course of the dentinal tubule is followed towards the outer surface of the dentine the diameter of the odontoblast process becomes narrower and that of the peritubular zone becomes relatively wider. As a result the dentinal tubules are of greater diameter at their pulpal end than towards the outer dentinal surface. It is not uncommon to find, however, individual tubules which show little if any development of a peritubular zone along their course.

Dentinal tubules. The tubules are more closely packed towards the pulp than in the outer part of the dentine; the amount of intertubular matrix, therefore, varies considerably at different levels in the dentine. This is a result of the greater area of the external surface of the dentine compared with its inner or pulpal surface.

The number of tubules is very large for at the pulpal surfaces of the dentine there are 30 000–70 000 tubules per sq mm. It has been calculated that halfway between the pulpal surface and the amelo-dentinal junction the total cross-sectional area of the tubules is equal to a tube of a diameter of 0·3 mm for each square millimetre of dentine. Such a degree of porosity could permit a considerable amount of fluid movement through the dentine. Experimental work carried out both *in vivo* and *in vitro* by the application of various stimuli such as dehydration, cold or heat, to the surface of exposed dentine has demonstrated an outward or an inward movement of fluid in the tubules. Thus the dentinal tubules provide a system in which capillary forces can act for the movement of fluid along their course. The maximum rate of flow can reach as high as 2–4 mm per sec, so that a considerable rate of flow is possible. The movement of fluid in the dentinal tubules may be concerned in the causation of pain through the production of a distorting effect on nerve endings which are present either in the dentinal tubules or close to them in the pulp (see p. 243).

In their course from the pulp to the outer dentine surface the dentinal tubules take a shallow ∽-shaped course, the first curve having its convexity facing rootward. In the crown this double-curved course is arranged so that the dentinal tubules finish considerably farther coronally at the outer dentine surface compared with their commencement at the pulp surface. In the root, however, and also beneath the incisal edge and cusps of the crown, the dentinal tubules take a straighter course (Fig. 188). As well as these primary curves produced by the dentinal tubules, each tubule shows numerous small secondary curves on its course (Figs. 188, 202). These are a result of the spiral track taken by the odontoblast process in its course from the outer dentine surface of the pulp.

At the outer dentine surface the dentinal tubules usually terminate by dividing into two main branches. These or further fine branchings unite with the terminal branches of neighbouring tubules to form a plexus beneath the outer dentine surface (Fig. 199). From a development viewpoint this is, of course, the region where the odontoblast processes and tubules begin. In the root many of the dentinal tubules end in the granular layer of Tomes; some may link up with the canaliculi of the cement. In the crown a few tubules terminate as the enamel spindles.

Interglobular dentine. The calcifying inorganic element of the dentine first appears in the organic matrix as globules, calcospherites, which fuse to form a homogeneous substance. Sometimes, in certain areas of the dentine, these globules remain discrete and unfused, so that areas of the organic matrix remain uncalcified. These areas are bounded by the curved outlines of the adjacent globules and so are known as interglobular dentine (Fig. 200). The dentine tubules may be seen passing through these areas of interglobular dentine, and here a peritubular zone is absent (Fig. 201). These areas have frequently been called interglobular spaces, though in the living tissue no spaces exist. In dried ground sections where the uncalcified organic matrix has shrivelled up and disappeared, the interglobular areas do form actual spaces and appear black when seen by transmitted light (Fig. 204). Interglobular dentine is usually confined to the crown and not far from the amelo-dentinal junction, but in poorly formed teeth may be found in any part of the dentine.

Incremental lines. Formation of the dentine matrix proceeds rhythmically; that is, in alternating phases of activity and quiescence. In sections of the dentine evidence of these phases is provided by the presence of incremental lines (Fig. 185). These lines run at right angles to the dentinal tubules but not parallel to the outer surface of the dentine. They indicate the position of the inner or pulpal surface of the dentine at successive stages in its formation. The lines are known as the contour lines of Owen and, as originally described by him, are produced by the coincidence of small (secondary) curvatures with a similar orientation on neighbouring dentinal tubules (Fig. 202). Very often other lines with a similar relationship to the surface of the dentine are seen. These are due to variations in the degree of calcification of the dentine matrix and so strictly are not incremental lines. Since, however, the advancing front of calcification is always parallel to the surface of the forming matrix they have the same general arrangement (Fig. 168). Sometimes these lines are accentuated by areas of interglobular dentine.

Occasionally evidence of a finer incremental pattern is found in the form of parallel markings which are much closer together than the contour lines of Owen. These are known as the lines of von Ebner.

Neo-natal line. In those teeth in which calcification has commenced before birth, that is, the deciduous teeth and usually the first permanent molar, a particularly accentuated line is found separating the dentine formed before birth and that formed after birth. This line is called the neo-natal line and, as with the similar neo-natal line in the enamel, is produced by the disturbance caused in nutrition and external environment of the child at birth (Fig. 203).

Granular layer of Tomes. Immediately beneath the cement a narrow

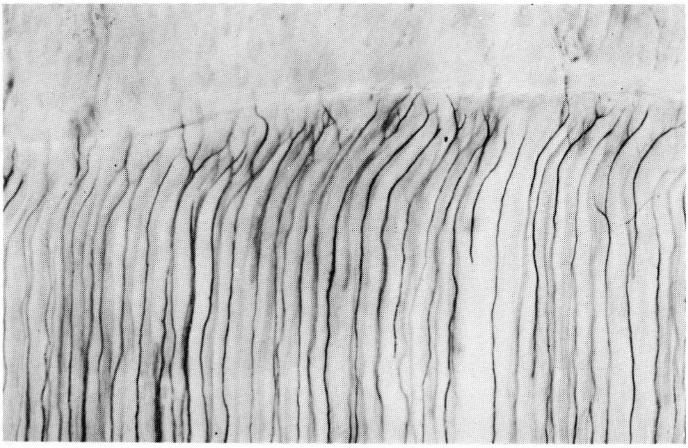

Fig. 199 Ground section showing dentinal tubules and their branching close to the dentine-enamel junction. × 320.

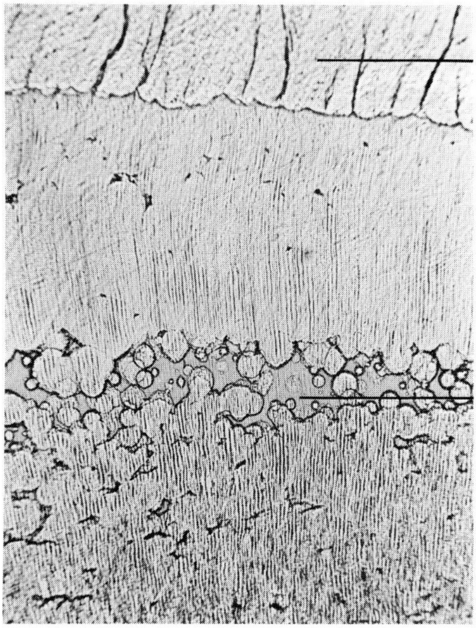

Fig. 200 Interglobular dentine. Ground section. × 80.

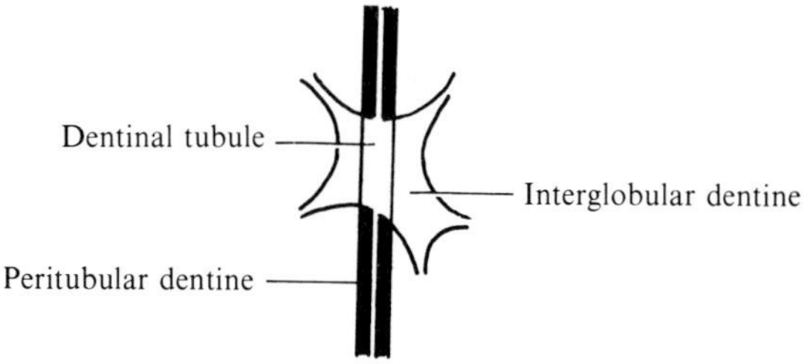

Fig. 201 Diagrammatic representation of a dentinal tubule crossing an area of interglobular dentine; in this area there is an absence of peritubular dentine.

layer of dentine of a granular appearance is always to be seen in ground sections. This layer is a constant feature of the dentine in the root and is known as the granular layer of Tomes (Figs. 204, 224). The granular appearance is produced by what might seem to be minute areas of interglobular dentine. Two suggestions have been made as to its origin. It may be caused by the presence of the coarse fibres found in this zone of the dentine, which could result in certain areas of the zone being less well calcified than the rest of the dentine. Disintegration of the organic material in these areas, during the preparation of ground sec-

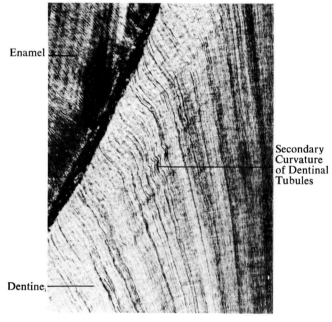

Fig. 202 Contour lines of Owen produced by secondary curvatures of the dentinal tubules. Ground section. × 110.

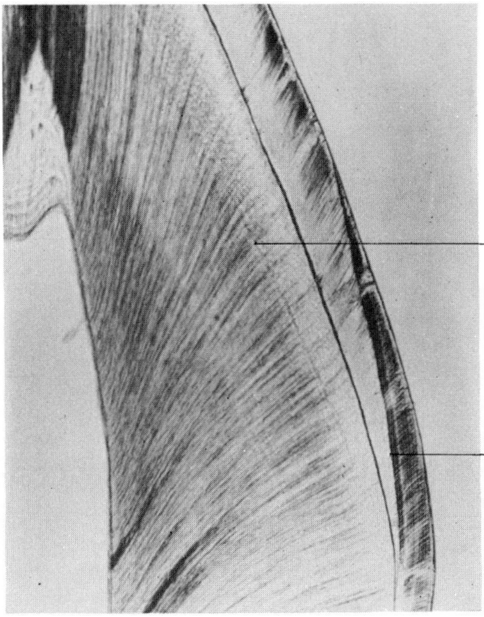

Fig. 203 Neo-natal lines in enamel and dentine. Ground section of deciduous upper central incisor. × 25.

tions, would give the darker appearance of the granular areas. Alternatively it may be due to an interference with the calcification of the surface dentine caused by the inner vascular layer of the dental follicle. This layer is in close relationship to the dentine of the root once the breakdown of the epithelial sheath of Hertwig takes place and before the dentine is again protected by the deposition of cement.

Dentine-cement junction. It is often difficult to determine the boundary between the dentine and the cement, particularly in the region of the acellular cement. External to the granular layer of Tomes there is a narrow zone of a hyaline and amorphous appearance (Fig. 224). This zone appears to belong to the dentine and to separate the granular layer of Tomes from the cement.

It has been shown that there is a delayed mineralisation at the external surface of the dentine, at least cervically, before the deposition of cement occurs and that the mineralisation takes place parallel to the surface of the root. It seems that the narrow zone external to the granular layer of Tomes would correspond to this area of dentine with a different pattern of mineralisation to the bulk of the dentine.

Submicroscopic structure. The collagenous fibrils of the organic basis of the dentine are separated by minute spaces arranged parallel to the direction of the fibrils. It is in these spaces that the submicroscopic crystals of the calcium salts are deposited; the fibrils themselves are not

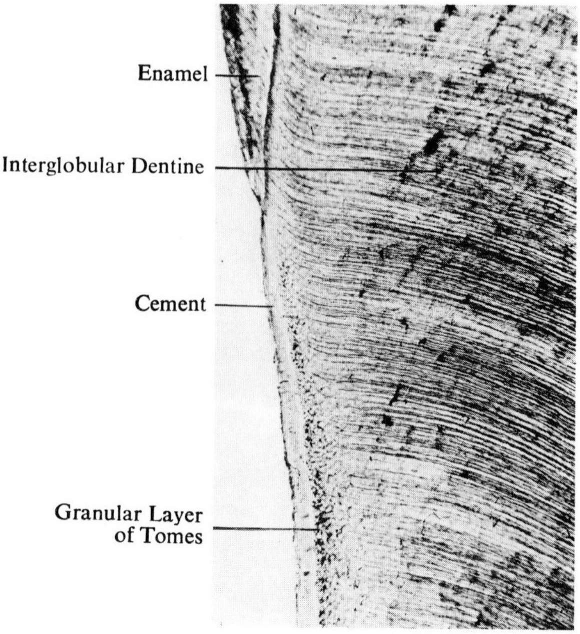

Fig. 204 The granular layer of Tomes at the margin of the root dentine. Note also areas of interglobular dentine which here appear black by transmitted light as this is a dried ground section. × 80.

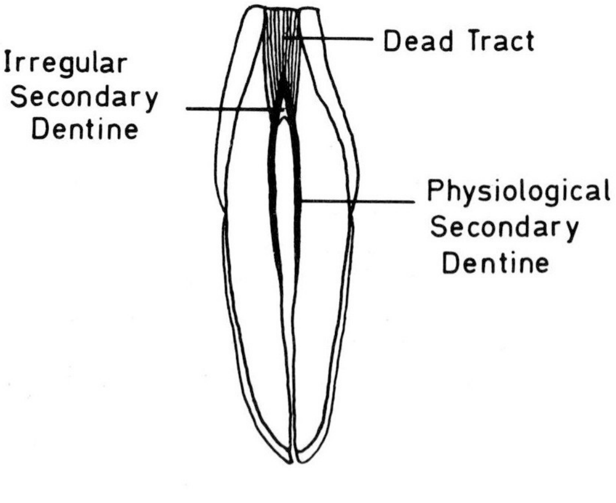

Fig. 205 Diagrammatic representation of a vertical section through a lower permanent incisor with attrition of the incisive edge and the associated dead tract. The distribution of regular and irregular secondary dentine is shown. (*By courtesy of W. Heinemann Medical Books Ltd.*)

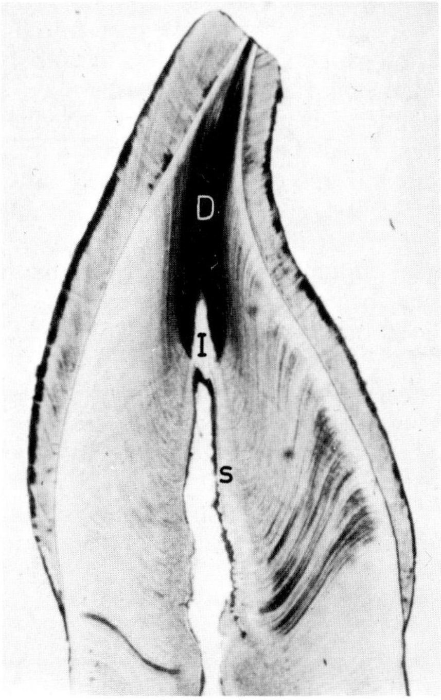

Fig. 206 Vertical section of a permanent incisor showing physiological regular secondary dentine, and an area of irregular secondary dentine in relation to a dead tract. S, physiological secondary dentine; I, irregular secondary dentine, D, dead tract. (*By courtesy of W. Heinemann Medical Books Ltd.*)

calcified but are surrounded by these crystals, the long axes of which are parallel to those of the fibrils. As well as this typical arrangement, it has been found that alternative patterns occur. In some areas of dentine the crystals are arranged radially. In poorly calcified dentine these spherical masses of radially arranged crystals are undisturbed, but in well calcified areas they are deformed by pressure and form semi-lunar areas. Close to the dentinal tubules these crystals form a layer in which their long axes lie parallel to the direction of the tubule.

Innervation of the dentine. The innervation of the dentine is one of the most highly debatable points of dental histology: the staining of nerve fibres, at all times a difficult and uncertain matter, is particularly so in a hard, calcified tissue such as dentine. Due to the nature of the dentine the methylene blue technique cannot easily be employed: on the other hand the silver stains are not sufficiently specific, for connective tissue fibres are sometimes stained as well as nerve fibres. There is general agreement, however, that the myelinated nerve fibres of the pulp, after losing their myelin sheath, pass between the odontoblasts and form a plexus on the surface of the predentine.

From this marginal plexus fibres have been traced into the predentine. Some of the fibres are embedded in the substance of the predentine, others lie in tubules. Some nerve fibres have also been found in tubules in the calcified dentine. The presence of non-myelinated fibres in the tubules of the inner part of the dentine has been confirmed by observation with the electron microscope. The nerve fibres are in close relationship to the odontoblast process (Fig. 192). In some cases at the external limit of the inner third of the dentine complex infoldings of the nerve fibre in the odontoblast process are present. At these situations cellular attachments between the plasma membranes of nerve fibre and odontoblast process occur which appear to be similar to junctional complexes.

Although an innervation of the dentine has been established certain observations on the sensitivity of the dentine are still not explicable on this basis. It has been repeatedly noted that surface anaesthetics, such as cocaine, do not abolish or reduce this sensitivity; moreover pain producing drugs and solutions applied to dentine do not cause discomfort. Attempts have been made to attribute the transmission of stimuli

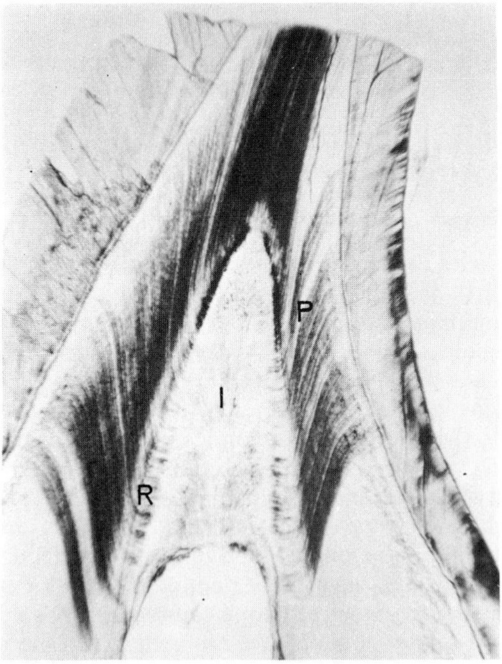

Fig. 207 Primary and secondary dentine. Note the change in direction of the tubules between primary and regular secondary dentine and the irregular arrangement of the tubules in the irregular secondary dentine. Ground section. P, Primary dentine; R, Regular secondary dentine; I, Irregular secondary dentine. ×6.

through the dentine to the agency of the odontoblast processes themselves. Support for such ideas has been adduced on developmental grounds in that the odontoblasts may be derived from neural crest tissue. The evidence in support of the neural crest origins of the odontoblasts is taken, however, from work carried out in amphibians.

Considerable evidence has been derived from *in vitro* and *in vivo* experiments which supports the concept of transmission of pain stimuli, to intradentinal and pulpal nerves by means of a hydrodynamic linkage. Certain agents such as an air blast or dehydrating solutions applied to the exposed surface of dentine produce an outward flow in the dentinal tubules, whereas heat produces an inward flow. An outward or inward flow of only a few micrometres is sufficient to cause pain. Such a movement and distortion of the contents of the tubules could possibly involve the nerve fibres which have been shown to lie in intimate relation to the odontoblast processes in the pulpward part of the dentine.

Regular secondary dentine. It is possible for dentine formation to continue throughout life, though the rate and amount of this formation can vary considerably. During the formation of dentine there is always a border of uncalcified organ matrix between the fully formed dentine and the odontoblasts. This uncalcified zone is known as the predentine or odontogenic zone (Figs. 181, 182).

The dentine which is formed after the dentine (primary dentine) producing the typical form of the tooth has been laid down is known as secondary dentine (Figs. 205, 206).

Physiological secondary dentine is produced without any apparent external stimuli affecting the dentine, and in it the dentinal tubules are comparable to those of the primary dentine both in their regular arrangement and in numbers (Fig. 207). It usually occurs over the whole internal or pulpal surface of the coronal dentine, but can vary considerably in amount in different parts of the same tooth. In multi-root teeth it is much thicker on the floor of the pulp chamber than on the side walls. Between the primary and secondary dentine the dentinal tubules commonly show a considerable change of direction (Fig. 207). The formation of this regular type of secondary dentine is generally believed to be increased by the mild stimuli reaching the pulp as a result of slow attrition of the dentine. It is also found under slowly progressing caries of the occlusal surfaces of molars and in the early stages of cervical cavities.

It is not easy to make a distinction between a primary and a physiological secondary dentine in the root of the tooth. It may be that in the case of the formation of coronal dentine, which takes place before eruption begins, there is sufficient interruption to permit a distinction between a primary dentine (pre-eruptive) and a secondary dentine (post-eruptive). The radicular dentine, on the other hand, is formed either during eruption or immediately afterwards and within a relatively short time.

Irregular secondary dentine. In certain situations such as in abrasion,

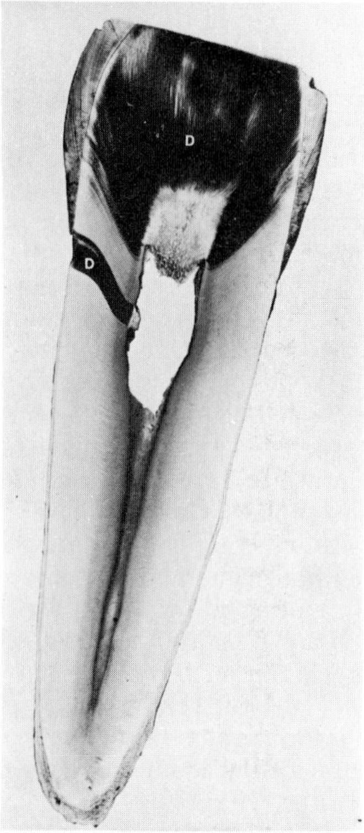

Fig. 208 Ground section of an upper central incisor. Note the dead tracts developed in relation to attrition and to a cervical cavity, and the areas of irregular secondary dentine at the pulpal ends of the affected tubules. D, dead tract.

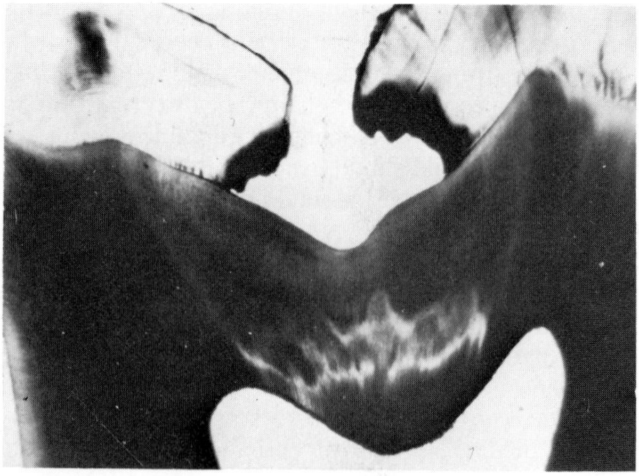

Fig. 209 Ground section of permanent molar with early occlusal caries. Translucent dentine has appeared as a reaction to the caries although no visible destruction of dentine has yet taken place.

or erosion or in any rapid loss of tooth substance, the secondary dentine produced is of a different type and is then best described as irregular secondary dentine. In this form the tubules are much fewer in number and less regular in arrangement than in regular secondary dentine, and frequently there may be a complete absence of tubules. The distinction between the previously formed dentine and this type of secondary dentine is readily made (Fig. 207). At the junction between the two a darkly staining line is often seen in stained sections. Irregular secondary dentine is commonly localised to certain areas of the pulp wall, being found only under those tubules which have been opened up or affected by the causative agent (Figs. 206, 208).

Translucent dentine. As well as the formation of secondary dentine, changes may occur in the dentine itself as a result of loss of tooth substance through physical means or from dental caries. Where the loss of tooth substance is slow and the stimuli transmitted to the pulp are mild, the tooth reacts by production of a narrow zone of sclerosed dentine beneath the surface affected (Fig. 197). In this area the processes of the odontoblasts become progressively reduced in diameter as the tubules are increasingly occluded by a deposition of mineralised material, so that the dentine comes to have a more uniform refractive index. As a result these areas appear translucent when viewed by transmitted light and are known as translucent dentine (Fig. 209). With reflected light these areas appear dark. The light passes through the sclerosed dentine but is reflected from the normal tissue.

In teeth from elderly subjects it is frequently found that much of the dentine, particularly in the roots, has become translucent. This is due to the occluding of the dentinal tubules by calcific deposits over wide areas. It must be considered as an age change.

Dead tracts. It is commonly accepted that where the stimuli to the dentine are stronger, the odontoblast processes in the tubules affected are completely destroyed and the associated odontoblasts destroyed or damaged. These areas of dentine are known as dead tracts and reach from the dentine surface affected to the pulp surface. The tubules are empty and appear black in transmitted light and white in reflected light. They are sealed off at the pulp surface by a deposit of irregular secondary dentine (Figs. 206, 208). Each dead tract is surrounded, and isolated from the rest of the dentine, by a narrow zone of sclerosed dentine.

Dead tracts are commonly found in incisor teeth where attrition has exposed the dentine. It is difficult to believe that the slow progress of attrition produces a more damaging effect on the related odontoblasts than, for example, occlusal caries where translucent dentine is commonly found rather than a dead tract. Moreover the extent of a dead tract usually involves more tubules than those which have been exposed by attrition. It has been shown that dead tracts can occur in incisors which have never erupted and dead tracts are found in some erupted teeth which show little if any attrition (Fig. 210). It would seem therefore

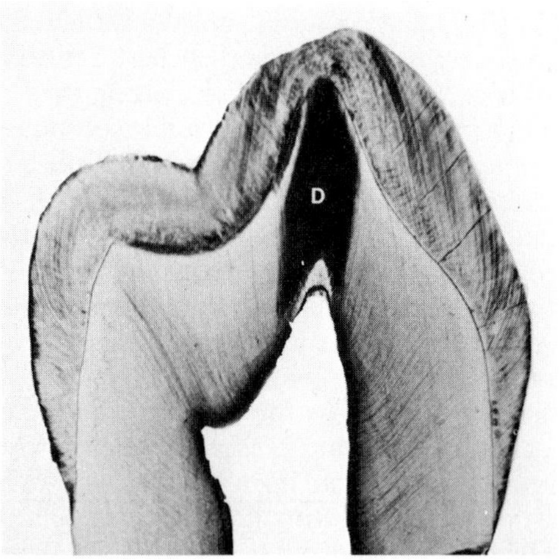

Fig. 210 Ground section of lower premolar showing dead tract, probably due to the degeneration of the odontoblasts in the horn of the pulp. D, dead tract.

that dead tracts are possibly to be considered, in certain situations, as a form of age change and that this may be accelerated by the death of odontoblasts which have been crowded in narrow pulpal horns.

It should be remembered that in dried ground sections of normal teeth the odontoblast processes shrivel up, leaving empty tubules which may be filled with air. These tubules given an appearance similar to that of a dead tract; that is, they appear black in transmitted light and white in reflected light. However, a true dead tract can be distinguished from such tubules by the presence of a deposit of irregular secondary dentine at its pulpal surface (Fig. 210).

Clinical considerations. In cavity preparation it is important to bear in mind the general direction of the dentinal tubules from the pulpal to the external surface of the dentine. Beneath almost all carious areas, with the exception of slowly progressing caries of the occlusal surface of molars a dead tract is to be found. Any cutting of the dentine in this tract does not affect the pulp, as the dentinal tubules forming the tract are sealed at their pulpal end by a calcific deposit. But once the area of the tract is left, the opening up of fresh dentinal tubules may produce a reaction which, if severe, leads to inflammatory changes in the pulp. The direction of the tubules from any part of the crown except the occlusal surface or incisive edge is obliquely downward as well as inward, so that the area of pulp directly involved is considerably more rootward than the position of a carious area involving the tubules (Fig. 188).

The continued formation of regular secondary dentine in the erupted tooth gradually diminishes the size of the pulp cavity and soon obliterates the extremities of the pulpal cornua. This makes exposure of the pulp much less likely to occur in cavity preparation. Regular secondary dentine formation also precludes the eventual exposure of the pulp tissue by heavy attrition, which would otherwise take place.

Both regular and irregular secondary dentine formation increase the time taken by caries to reach the pulp through increasing the width of the barrier to its progress. The extent to which secondary dentine formation occurs, however, varies with different individuals.

The production of an area of translucent or sclerosed dentine constitutes an important barrier to the spread of caries. Bacteria and their toxins are shut off from the pulp tissue, and the carious process spreads laterally rather than pulpally.

BIBLIOGRAPHY

Anderson, D. J. (1976). The nature of pain. In *Scientific Foundations of Dentistry*. Eds. Cohen, B. & Kramer, I. R. H. London: Heinemann.

Anderson, D. J., Hannam, A. G. & Matthews, B. (1970). Sensory mechanisms in mammalian teeth and their supporting tissues. *Physiol. Rev.* **50**, 171.

Bradford, E. W. (1967). Microanatomy and histochemistry of dentine. In *Structural and Chemical Organization of Teeth*. Ed. Miles, A. E. W. New York: Academic Press.

Brännström, M. & Aström, A. (1972). The hydrodynamics of the dentine; its possible relationship to dentinal pain. *Int. dent. J.* **22**, 219.

Eastoe, J. E. (1967). Chemical organization of the organic matrix of dentine. In *Structural and Chemical Organization of Teeth*. Ed. Miles, A. E. W. New York: Academic Press.

Frank, R. M. (1968). Ultrastructural relationship between the odontoblast, its process and the nerve fibre. In *Dentine and Pulp*. Ed. Symons, N. B. B. University of Dundee.

Frank, R. M. (1966). Etude au microscope electronique de l'odontoblaste et du canalicule dentinaire humain. *Arch. oral Biol.* **11**, 179.

Holland, G. R. (1975). The dentinal tubule and odontoblast process in the cat. *J. Anat. Lond.* **120**, 169.

Holland, G. R. (1976). An ultrastructural survey of cat dentinal tubules. *J. Anat. Lond.* **122**, 1.

Johansen, E. (1967). Ultrastructure of dentine. I. *Structural and Chemical Organization of Teeth*. Ed. Miles, A. E. W. New York: Academic Press.

Katchburian, E. (1973). Membrane-bound bodies as initiators of mineralization of dentine. *J. Anat. Lond.* **116**, 285.

Kramer, I. R. H. (1951). The distribution of collagen fibrils in the dentine matrix. *Brit. dent. J.* **91**, 1.

Lehman, M. L. (1967). Tensile strength in human dentin. *J. dent. Res.* **46**, 197.

Lester, K. S. & Boyde, A. (1968). The question of von Korff fibres in mammalian dentine. *Calc. Tiss. Res.* **1**, 273.

Mendis, B. R. R. M. & Darling, A. I. Distribution with age and attrition of peritubular dentine in the crowns of human teeth. *Archs. oral Biol.* **24**, 131.

Mjör, I. A. (1972). Human coronal dentine: Structure and reactions. *Oral Surg.* **33**, 810.

Owens, P. D. A. (1973). Mineralization in the roots of human deciduous teeth demonstrated by tetracycline labelling. *Archs. oral Biol.* **18**, 889.

Symons, N. B. B. (1967). The microanatomy and histochemistry of dentinogenesis. In *Structural and Chemical Organization of Teeth*. Ed. Miles, A. E. W. New York: Academic Press.

Symons, N. B. B. (Editor) (1968). *Dentine and Pulp*. University of Dundee.

Symons, N. B. B. (1976). Dentine and pulp. In *Scientific Foundations of Dentistry*. Eds. Cohen, B. & Kramer, I. R. H. London: Heinemann.

Takuma, S. (1967). Ultrastructure of dentinogenesis. In *Structural and Chemical Organization of Teeth.* Ed. Miles, A. E. W. New York: Academic Press.

Ten Cate, A. R. (1978). A fine structural study of coronal and root dentinogenesis in the mouse: observations on the so-called 'von Korff fibres' and their contribution to mantle dentine. *J. Anat. Lond.* **125,** 183.

13. Pulp

The pulp is composed of loose connective tissue elements on the surface of which is the odontoblast layer consisting of highly differentiated cells. The pulp is a very delicate tissue and is highly vascular. It is derived from the dental papilla, of which it is the part remaining after the formation of the dentine. In virtue of this developmental connection the pulp is involved in the response of the dentine to stimuli, reaching it as a result of loss of or damage to tooth substance. The reaction of the pulp to stimuli of moderate degree is to form secondary dentine; with severe stimuli, the pulp, like other connective tissues, undergoes inflammatory changes. Thus, as well as being concerned in the formation of dentine, the pulp tissue has a defensive function. The pulp is nutritive and sensory to the dentine; these functions are subserved by the blood vessels and nerves contained in it. The young pulp plays a part in the eruption of the teeth to the occlusal plane.

The only form of sensation displayed by the pulp tissue in response to all kinds of stimuli is that of pain. Thus whether the agent be pressure, trauma, heat or cold, or chemical irritant, the same painful sensation is experienced.

Form and relations. The pulp occupies the central cavity, the pulp cavity, of each tooth; that is, the pulp chamber in the coronal and cervical parts of the tooth and the canals in the roots (Fig. 1). At the apex of each root is a foramen or foramina through which pass the blood vessels, nerve fibres, and lymphatics which supply the pulp. The shape of the pulp roughly corresponds with the external shape of the tooth. Under each cusp it is prolonged into a narrow projection, the cornu or horn of the pulp. These are particularly marked in the young tooth (Fig. 211). With increasing age the size of the pulp cavity is diminished by the formation of regular secondary dentine. In multiple-rooted teeth this tends to be deposited to a greater extent on the floor of the pulp chambers than elsewhere, so that the pulp chamber is unequally diminished in size. The space occupied by the pulp may be further restricted by the formation of localised deposits of irregular secondary dentine, which make the form of the pulp cavity irregular.

In erupting and recently erupted teeth the roots and root canals are incomplete, so that between the free margins of Hertwig's sheath the pulp is in wide continuity with the peri-apical tissues (Fig. 92). With the gradual cessation of proliferation of Hertwig's sheath, the root becomes tapered and the root canal and apical foramen narrowed.

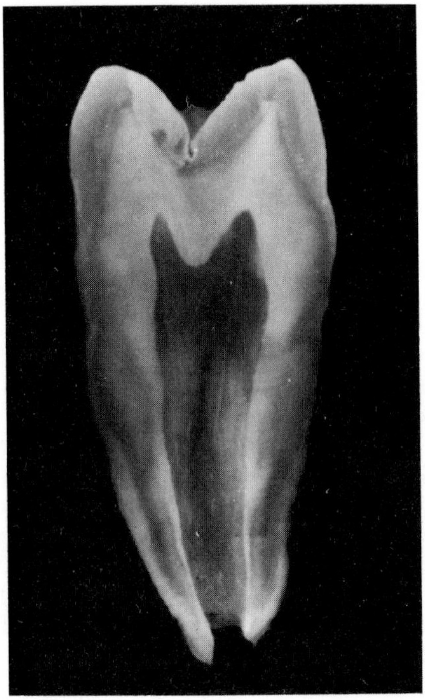

Fig. 211 Upper first premolar, with incomplete root, sectioned vertically showing the pronounced pulpal cornua in the young tooth.

Further narrowing of the apical foramen may be produced by the deposition of cement inside the foramen. Frequently the apical foramen is not single; there may be two or three foramina for each root. This is probably caused by the arrangement of the blood vessels entering the pulp. The apical foramina may sometimes be located to the side of the root apex.

The root canals can vary considerably in shape and in number, showing marked deviation from what might be expected from the external configuration of the root. Irregular curvatures instead of a straight course may be found. Sometimes two separate root canals occur in a single root, or variations between single and multiple canals may be found at different levels in the same root. There may be accessory or lateral canals at any point along the root or neck of a tooth connecting the pulp with the periodontal tissues and quite distinct from the apical connection (Figs. 216, 217). These aberrant openings are presumed to be caused by a localised failure in the formation of Hertwig's sheath, with a consequent lack of odontoblast differentiation and dentine formation at this point, so that the pulp remains in contact with the follicular or periodontal tissues. The gap in Hertwig's sheath is probably produced by the persistence of abnormally placed blood vessels reaching the pulp.

Structure. The pulp is composed of cells and an intercellular substance. The intercellular tissue consists of fibres and an amorphous ground substance of a gelatinous consistency. In addition, there are blood vessels, nerves and lymphatics. In the developing and young pulp the cellular element is very marked, but with increasing age there is an increase in the fibre content and a relative diminution in the number of cells. In the old pulp the number of cells is decreased and the fibre elements are increased.

Cells. The cells of the pulp may be divided into three main types:

1. Odontoblasts.
2. Fibroblasts or fibrocytes.
3. Defence cells.

The odontoblasts are columnar cells on the surface of the pulp (Figs. 177, 178). They have an oval nucleus situated at the end of the cell farthest from the dentine. Each odontoblast has a long protoplasmic process which occupies a dentinal tubule and may traverse the full thickness of the dentine. The appearance of the odontoblasts and the odontoblast layer varies with the stage of tooth development. In the earliest phase of dentine formation the odontoblast layer consists of a single layer of cells regularly arranged and of moderate length. In the later stages of dentine formation and over most of the fully formed tooth the odontoblast layer is much broader, being made up of elongated cells of varying length—the unequal length of the cells makes the odontoblast layer appear as if stratified (Fig. 212). The cells are less columnar and tend to be pyriform, the broadest (basal) part of the cell containing the nucleus, the elongated distal part terminating as the odontoblast process in the dentine.

The length of the odontoblasts also varies in different parts of the adult pulp. The odontoblasts in the coronal part of the pulp are the longest; in the root they become shorter until near the root apex they may be almost flattened.

Immediately beneath the odontoblast layer a cell-free zone can often be demonstrated; this is known as the basal layer of Weil (Fig. 212). It is not seen in the developing tooth. Beneath the odontoblast layer, or beneath the basal layer of Weil if present, there is a narrow zone of pulp tissue in which the cells are more numerous than elsewhere in the general pulp tissue. This subodontoblastic zone of the pulp has a rich capillary network. It is best seen during active formation of dentine.

Apart from the layers mentioned above the pulp tissue has a more or less uniform arrangement of its cell content. The most numerous of the cells are fibroblasts (Fig. 212). They are long flat cells with an oval nucleus; seen from the side they appear to be narrow and spindle-shaped. They have elongated processes which are widely separated and link up with those of other pulpal fibroblasts (Fig. 213). These processes

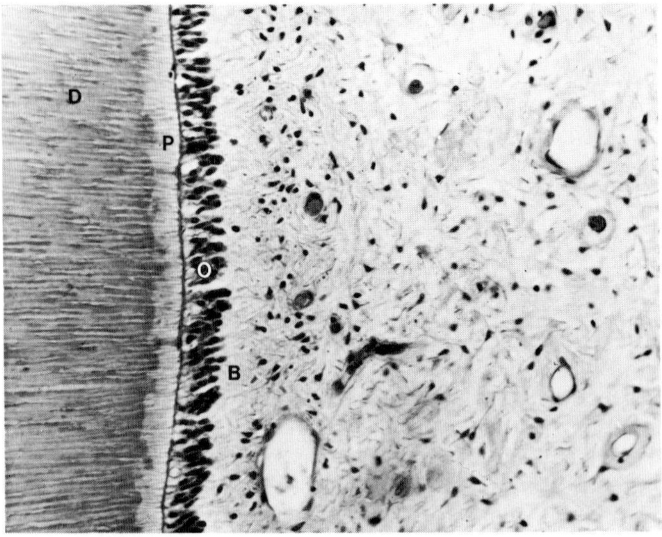

Fig. 212 Odontoblast layer and the adjacent area of pulp tissue. D, dentine; P, predentine; O, odontoblasts; B, basal layer of Weil. Original magnification × 200.

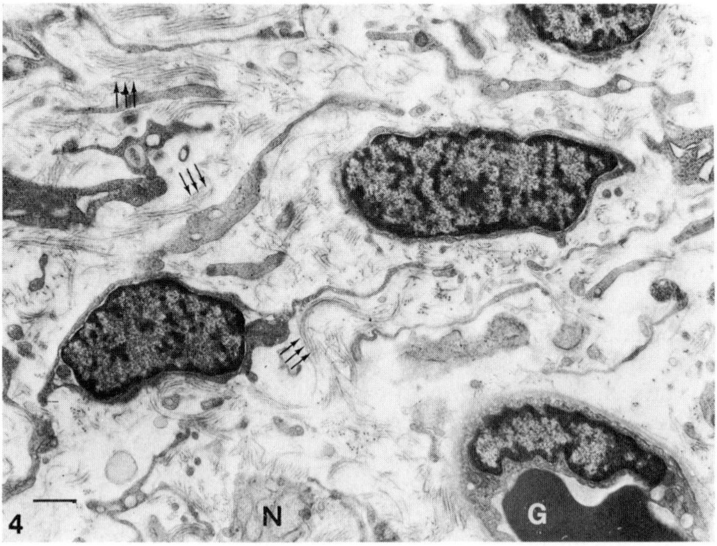

Fig. 213 Central region of the pulp. The bundles of collagen fibres (arrows) and the cellular processes are disposed irregularly. Note the relative poverty of cytoplasmic inclusions in the cells. G, red blood cell in a capillary; N, unmyelinated nerve fibre invaginated in the cytoplasm of a cell. Original magnification × 10 000. (*By courtesy of Dr P.-M. Cahen.*)

give the cells a stellate appearance. The cell outlines are, however, not easily seen in sections stained with haematoxlyin and eosin, and their processes are not readily distinguishable from the fine fibres of the pulp. With the electron microscope the fibroblasts can be seen to be connected together by desmosomal attachments on their processes. The fibroblasts contain a well defined Golgi complex and endoplasmic reticulum with closely associated mitochondria. The fibrocytes show few organelles.

The defence cells forming the third group of pulp cells consist of:

1. Histiocytes (fixed macrophages).
2. Undifferentiated mesenchyme cells.
3. Lymphoid wandering cells.

These cells play an important part in inflammatory reactions of the pulp; under such conditions they have the power of acting as macrophages. In the normal pulp these cells are in a state of rest. They are not easily distinguished from the pulpal fibroblasts with routine histological methods.

The histiocyte is a flat or oval-shaped cell with elongated forms. The nucleus is smaller than that of the fibroblast and is oval or kidney-shaped. The cytoplasm has distinct outlines and stains darkly with a granular appearance. These cells form part of the reticulo-endothelial system and have the power of picking up and storing particles of certain dyes such as trypan blue. In an inflammatory reaction they become freely moving macrophages.

The undifferentiated mesenchyme cells are smaller than the fibroblasts but have a similar appearance. They are usually found lying close to the blood vessels, particularly along the capillaries. These cells have the potentiality of forming other types of connective tissue cells. In inflammation of the pulp tissue they become macrophages.

The lymphoid wandering cells show great variations in size and shape. The smaller ones have a dark-staining round nucleus with little cytoplasm. The larger cells have an eccentric kidney-shaped nucleus. These cells may originate in the blood stream. They can take on the power of acting as macrophages.

Fibres. The bulk of the pulp fibres are very fine, occurring singly or in delicate bundles scattered throughout the pulp tissue (Fig. 213). They are irregularly arranged without any definite pattern. In electron microscope pictures the typical cross-banding of collagen is found. The full abundance and distribution of the fibres cannot be appreciated with ordinary staining methods and silver stains must be used for this purpose. With this method the fibres are shown very clearly as they stain black and are thus known as argyrophil fibres. These include the fibres of von Korff which pass through the odontoblast layer and are very obvious features during the early stages of dentine formation (Fig. 176). There are no elastic fibres in the pulp except for those in the walls of the larger blood vessels.

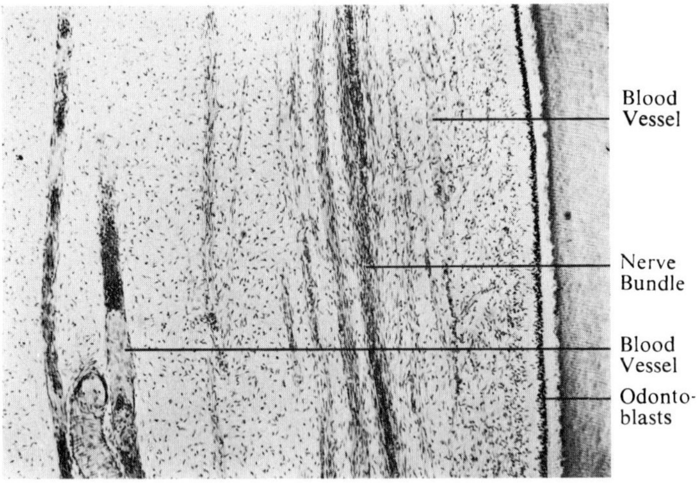

Fig. 214 Blood vessels and nerve fibres of the pulp. Longitudinal decalcified section of pulp. × 70.

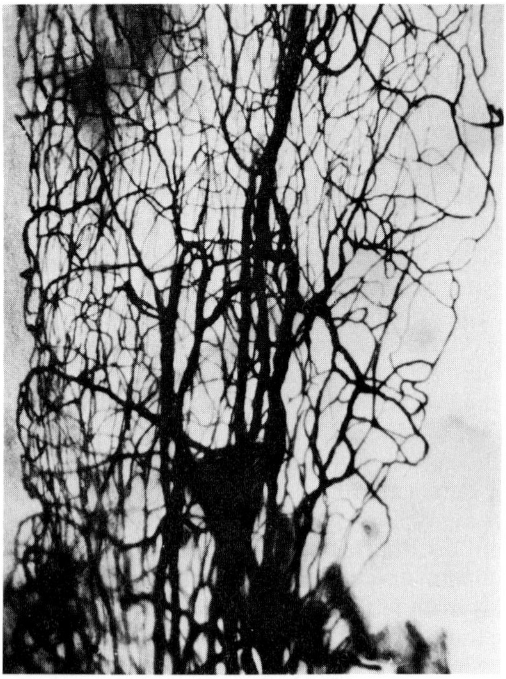

Fig. 215 Blood vessels of the human pulp. The rich vascular supply of the pulp tissue has been demonstrated by injecting the blood vessels with indian ink. (*By courtesy of Prof I. R. H. Kramer.*)

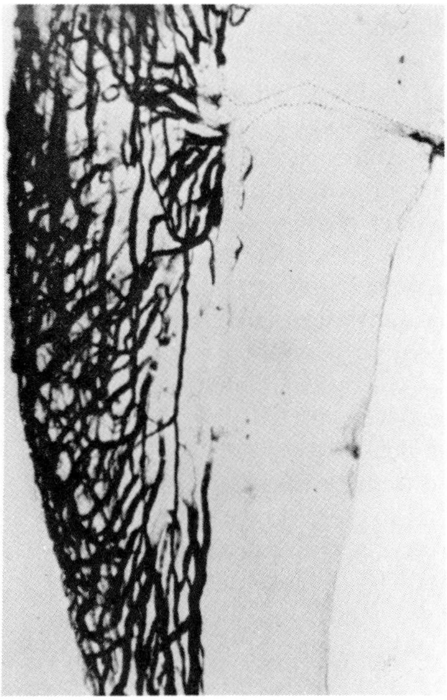

Fig. 216 Part of the root of an upper second deciduous molar. A large vessel passes into the root canal from the bifurcation region, and the venous drainage of this root canal is mainly towards the bifurcation area. × 22·5. (*By courtesy of Prof I. R. H. Kramer and the 'Archives of Oral Biology'.*)

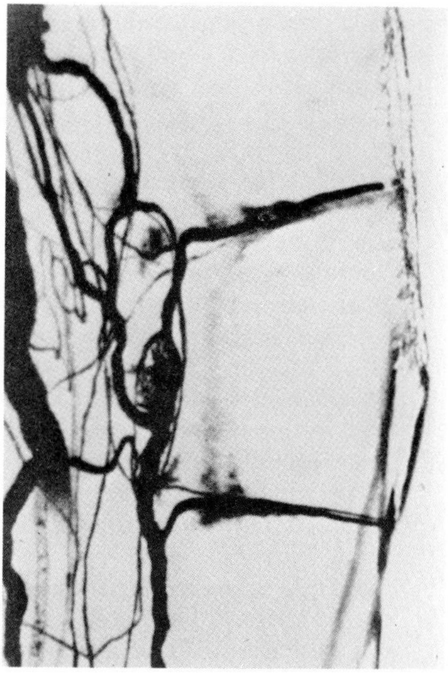

Fig. 217 Root of an upper first permanent molar. Two channels connect the root canal (left) with the periodontal membrane (right). In both cases there is a pair of vessels, a smaller resembling an artery and a larger resembling a vein. × 92. (*By courtesy of Prof I. R. H. Kramer and the 'Archives of Oral Biology'.*)

Blood vessels. The blood supply to the pulp is very rich; it is carried by arterioles which pass through the apical foramina in bundles of three or more. These vessels tend to run in the long axis of the pulp (Figs. 214, 215) giving off branches which anastomose with those of adjacent arterioles and others entering the pulp by separate root canals. The major branching and anastomosis takes place in the pulp chamber. Though the main vascular supply of the pulp is through the apical foramina it is not uncommon, especially in the region of root division in multi-rooted teeth, to find major vessels passing through the dentine to supply one root canal (Fig. 216). Smaller vessels running between root canals and periodontal membrane are fairly common (Fig. 217). At the apical region the arterioles are often embedded in the substance of the nerve bundles; in the pulp generally there is a close relationship between the larger blood vessels and the nerve bundles (Fig. 218). Each arteriole consists of an endothelial lining, a poorly developed tunica media made up of a very few muscle fibres, and a delicate fibrous tunica adventitia. The arterioles of the pulp are notable for the thinness of their walls, and on this account it is very difficult to distinguish the smaller arterioles from capillaries.

The arterioles break up to form a rich subodontoblastic capillary plexus (Fig. 215). From this plexus looping branches pass between the odontoblasts towards the predentine. From the external aspect of many of these loops short thorn-like branches project. It is likely that these represent former capillary loops which have become occluded and lost as a result of the reduction of the pulp which accompanies continued dentine formation. Frequently the peripheral capillary plexus is absent on one aspect of the root canals. Occasionally an isolated capillary loop becomes incorporated in the forming dentine, where it usually becomes cut off from the pulp. The capillary plexus drains into relatively large thin-walled venules, which in turn are gathered together to form several small veins escaping through each apical foramen. As the veins approach the apical foramen they become reduced in number and diameter.

Two kinds of capillaries are found in the pulp. As well as capillaries with a continuous endothelial lining there are also fenestrated capillaries. These have numerous pores about 600 Å in diameter. They are found in areas where important exchanges of fluid take place, and allow a rapid control of fluid and electrolyte interchange between the blood and the interstitial or tissue fluid.

Arterio-venous anastomoses have been demonstrated in the pulp but their importance in the pulpal circulation is not known.

Lymph vessels. Small lymph vessels cannot be distinguished histologically from blood capillaries with the light microscope; therefore before the introduction of the electron microscope the evidence for their existence was largely circumstantial.

In one method the presence of lymphatics may be demonstrated by sealing-in dyes in the pulp, in which case particles of the dye are found in the regional lymph glands. Another method involves the injection or application of lead acetate *intra vitam* and subsequently exposing the white precipitate produced to the action of sulphuretted hydrogen, which produces a black insoluble precipitate of lead sulphide. This is easily distinguished and the course of the lymphatics traced. The lymphatics of the pulp are described as being often perivascular, but larger separate vessels may also be present. Perineural vessels are also described. The lymphatics of the pulp communicate with those of the periodontal membrane.

Nerve supply. Two types of nerve fibres are found in the pulp:

1 Unmedullated fibres of the autonomic nervous system which run along the blood vessels and control the contraction of the smooth muscle in their walls.

2 Medullated fibres which are sensory somatic nerves and carry sensation to the sensory cortex of the brain, where, no matter what the nature of the stimulation may be, the only sensation appreciated is that of pain.

The somatic sensory supply of the pulp is very rich (Fig. 214). Two

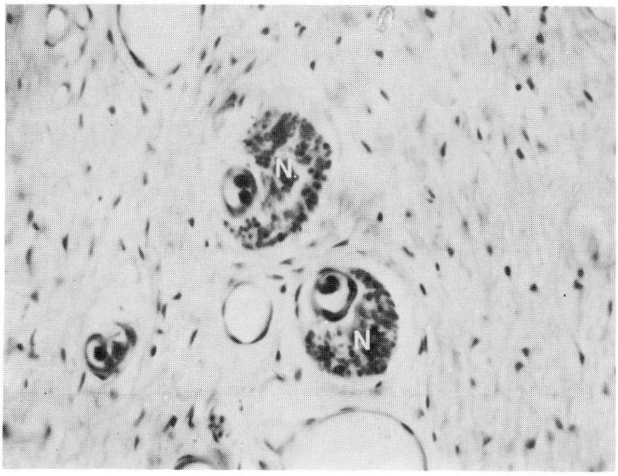

Fig. 218 Section of pulp tissue showing two bundles of nerve fibres, each of which partially surrounds an arteriole. N, nerve fibres. × 250.

or three large trunks enter each root canal, and several small nerve bundles also. Most of the nerves in their course through the root canals are closely associated with the blood vessels. Any branching in the root canal comes almost entirely from the small bundles. The majority of the nerve bundles course direct to the pulp chamber where considerable branching takes place.

Nerve fibres are especially numerous in the pulpal horns, and branches to each horn can always be traced to the same incoming trunks. In incisor and canine pulp chambers the nerve fibres of the main trunks keep a fairly direct course towards the pulpal horns. In other regions of the pulp the majority of the nerve fibres alter their course abruptly on approaching the cell-rich zone below the odontoblasts. The fibres turn off randomly in various directions, and many of them divide, some quite frequently. This results in an interlacing network of fibres below the roof and walls of the pulp chamber, the plexus of Raschkow (Fig. 219). Fibres arising from this plexus cross the cell-free zone of Weil obliquely to reach the odontoblast layer and then turn either abruptly between the odontoblasts towards the dentine or back towards the pulp.

On reaching the predentine most of the fibres turn again, and divide into numerous branches forming a plexus, the marginal plexus, on the surface of the predentine. Branches from this plexus have been traced into the substance of the predentine, others into the dentinal tubules in which they may travel some distance into the calcified dentine (Fig. 220).

The fibres of the marginal plexus are unmyelinated, and in the plexus of Raschkow also most of the fibres have already lost their myelin sheaths (Fig. 221).

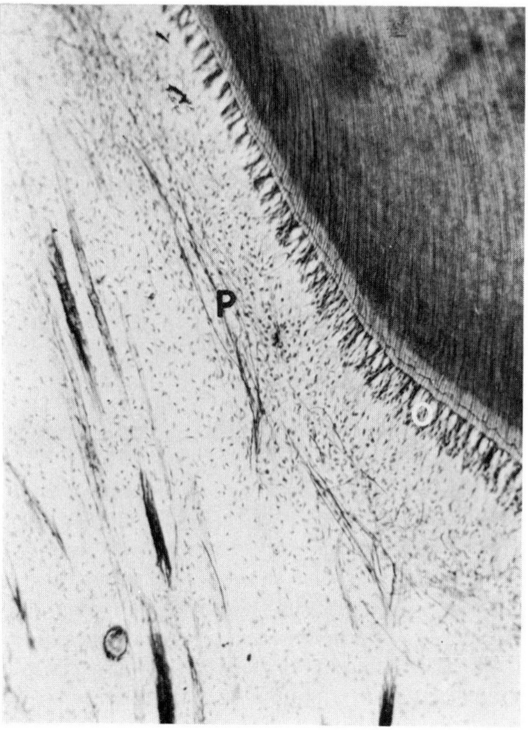

Fig. 219 Section of molar showing the plexus of Raschkow lying below the odontoblasts at the roof of the pulp chamber. At a deeper level in the pulp bundles of thicker fibres are evident. P, plexus of Raschkow. Silver stain. O, odontoblasts. (*By courtesy of Prof R. W. Fearnhead.*)

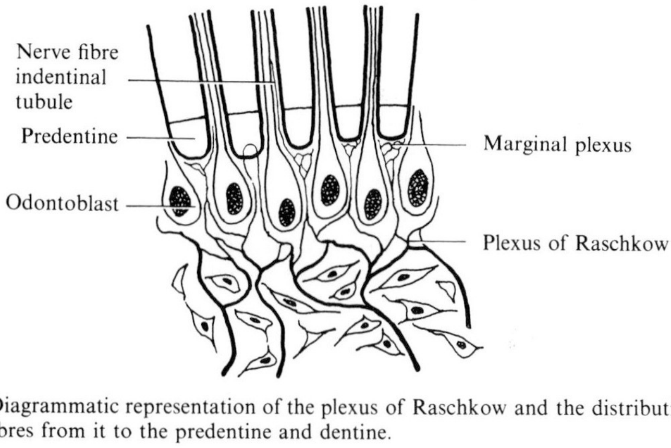

Fig. 220 Diagrammatic representation of the plexus of Raschkow and the distribution of nerve fibres from it to the predentine and dentine.

Age changes. It has previously been pointed out that with increasing age the pulp shows a progressive change in the proportions of cells and fibres, with the result that in the old pulp the cells are few in number and the fibre content is greatly increased. In the old pulp the blood vessels and nerve bundles are also decreased. In these changes the odontoblasts are affected and tend to degenerate; in some areas of the pulp they may have completely disappeared. The total effect is to produce a lessened vitality of the pulp tissue and a lessened response to stimulation.

A further change associated with ageing is the appearance of deposits of calcium in the pulp. These deposits may be in the form of localised masses known as pulp stones (Fig. 222). sometimes large enough to be seen in an X-ray, or alternatively as diffuse calcifications throughout the whole pulp. Since any deposition of calcium in a not normally calcified tissue must be considered as pathological, it is not intended to describe this condition in detail.

Due to the formation of regular secondary dentine, the whole cavity occupied by the pulp becomes progressively narrowed (Fig. 185B). In the young tooth the pulp chamber is larger with pronounced cornua. The cornua become largely obliterated and the pulp chamber very much smaller, especially in multi-rooted teeth through the thick deposits on the floor and roof. The size of the pulp cavity may be further reduced by the formation of irregular secondary dentine, which also gives it an irregular shape.

Clinical considerations. Any agency which opens up the dentinal tubules produces a reaction on the part of the pulp. The type of reaction depends on the nature and severity of the stimulus. Accordingly, whereas the pulp produces secondary dentine in the case of a stimulus of moderate intensity, it responds with an imflammatory reaction where the stimulation is severe. Thus in cavity preparation great care should be taken that the opening up of large numbers of fresh dentinal tubules does not produce a pulpitis. It should be remembered that towards the pulp cavity the cut surface of one square millimetre of dentine contains the openings of at least thirty thousand dentinal tubules. In the actual cutting of the cavity all unnecessary production of heat should be avoided by using sharp burs for limited periods, and if necessary under a stream of water. In the filling of the cavity all irritating filling materials should be avoided. It has been shown that the cements are particularly liable to produce inflammatory changes in the pulp. The pulp should be protected by lining the cavity with a bland non-conducting lining. Zinc oxide and oil of cloves are completely harmless to the pulp. In the preparation of non-carious teeth for crowns or as bridge abutments the possibility of pulp damage is even greater than in cavity preparation, as the pulp has not previously been able to protect itself by secondary dentine formation as would be the case where a carious cavity existed. Moreover, the amount of actual cutting of dentine is over a

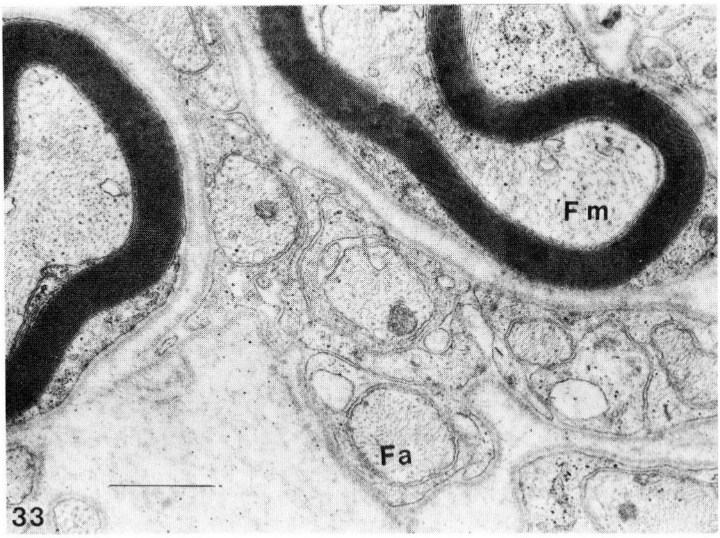

Fig. 221 Transverse section of a group of non-myelinated nerve fibres (Fa) situated between myelinated nerve fibres (Fm). Original magnification ×26000. (*By courtesy of Dr P.-M. Cahen.*)

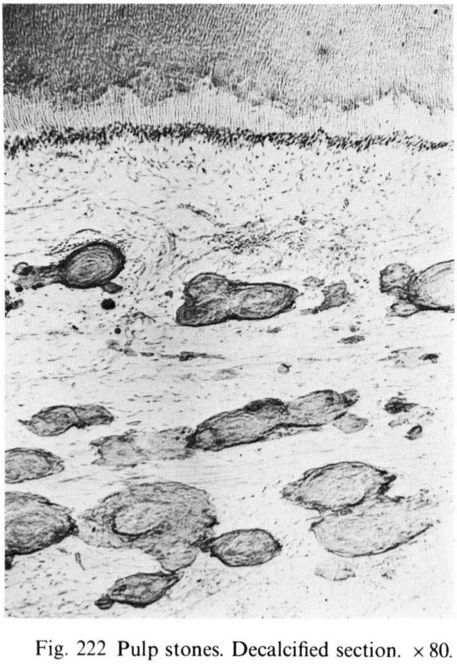

Fig. 222 Pulp stones. Decalcified section. ×80.

much greater area of the tooth, so that many more fresh dentinal tubules are opened up.

Advantage of the protective power of the pulp may be taken in the preparation of deep cavities where discoloured but firm dentine may temporarily be left untouched until secondary dentine formation beneath the cavity has taken place. In the final preparation of the cavity the discoloured dentine may be removed safely, as an exposure of the pulp can be avoided, due to the increased thickness of the dentine.

Since the blood vessels of the pulp are contained by the unyielding walls of the dentine, the hyperaemic and exudative changes accompanying inflammation, which lead to an increase in volume of the tissue, produce in the pulp a great increase in pressure. This compresses the blood vessels and is liable to occlude them, particularly at the apical foramina. The pain experienced with pulpitis is mainly due to the effect of this pressure on the nerve fibres of the pulp. The thin walls of the pulpal blood vessels render .them particularly liable to hyperaemia.

BIBLIOGRAPHY

Brannström, M. (1968). Physio-pathological aspects of dentinal and pulpal response to irritants. In *Dentine and Pulp.* Ed Symons, N. B. B. University of Dundee.

Engström, H. & Öhman, A. (1960). Studies on the innervation of human teeth. *J. dent. Res.* **39**, 799.

Fearnhead, R. W. (1961). The neurohistology of human dentine. *Proc. R. Soc. Med.* **54**, 877.

Frank, R. M. (1975). Reactions of dentine and pulp to drugs and restorative materials. *J. dent. Res.* **54**, B176.

Griffin, C. J. & Harris, R. (1966). Ultrastructure of collagen fibres and fibroblasts of the developing pulp. *Arch. oral Biol.* **11**, 659.

Han, S. S. & Avery, J. K. (1965). The fine structure of intercellular substances and rounded cells in the incisor pulp of the guinea pig. *Anat. Rec.* **151**, 41.

Harris, R. & Griffin, C. J. (1967). Histogenesis of fibroblasts in the human dental pulp. *Arch. oral Biol.* **12**, 459.

Harris, R. & Griffin, C. J. (1968). Fine structure of nerve endings in human dental pulp. *Archs. oral Biol.* **13**, 773.

Kramer, I. R. H. (1960). The vascular architecture of the human dental pulp. *Arch. oral Biol.* **2**, 177.

Marsland, E. A. (1968). The response of the dental pulp to cavity preparation. In *Dentine and Pulp.* Ed. Symons, N. B. B. University of Dundee.

Setzer, S. & Bender, I. B. (1975). *The Dentine and Pulp.* 2nd ed. Philadelphia: Lippincott.

Stanley, H. R. (1962). The cells of the dental pulp. *Oral Surg.* **15**, 849.

Ten Cate, A. R. & Shelton, L. (1966). Cholinesterase activity in human teeth. *Arch. oral Biol.* **11**, 423.

14. Cement

Compared with enamel and dentine little work has as yet been carried out on the cement (cementum) by the use of modern techniques. This is partly due to the difficulty of obtaining enough cement material free from contamination with other tissues.

Development. When the dentine in the root of the tooth begins to form it is at first covered by the epithelial sheath of Hertwig which separates it from the surrounding tissues of the dental follicle. With the disintegration of Hertwig's sheath the inner vascular layer of the mesodermal dental follicle comes into contact with the dentine. Cells of the follicle then differentiate to form cementoblasts. These somewhat cubical cells form a single layer in contact with the dentine. The organic matrix of the cement consisting of fibres and amorphous material is then laid down and is attached to the surface of the dentine. The calcific material forming the inorganic element of the cement is deposited in the amorphous substance in which these fibres are embedded. This deposition is presumed to be under the control of the cementoblasts. These are large cells with vesicular nuclei and prominent nucleoli. They contain basophilic cytoplasm. In appearance they are very similar to osteoblasts. As the cement is formed the principal fibres of the periodontal membrane are attached to it. The embedded parts of the principal fibres are known as Sharpey's fibres.

This process of gradual disintegration of Hertwig's sheath, differentiation of cementoblasts, and laying down of cement continues as the dentine of the root is progressively formed. It is generally accepted that the deposition of the cement begins at the cervical margin of the root; however, recent work suggests that cement deposition does not begin until root formation is well advanced and that from its starting point in the more apical region of the root it spreads towards the crown. During cement formation there is always a thin layer of uncalcified cement matrix on the surface of the already formed cement; it is known as cementoid and is lined by cementoblasts. Cement is formed in unerupted teeth and in teeth developing in dermoid cysts. In some animals it covers the enamel of the crown surface.

Sometimes a localised patch of Hertwig's sheath may show full development of all the parts of the crown portion of the enamel organ, including full differentiation of the inner layer to form a group of ameloblasts. In such areas of the root a circumscribed area of enamel is formed in the midst of the cement; this is known as an enamel pearl. The formation of lateral root canals due to a failure of dentine formation following on a localised failure of development of Hertwig's sheath has already been described (see section on Pulp).

Physical characters and chemical composition. The cement (cementum) covers the whole root of the tooth as a normally thin layer (Figs. 188, 223). Of the calcified dental tissues it most approaches bone in composition, structure, and behaviour. Indeed, from the viewpoint of comparative anatomy it may be considered as a bone of attachment.

Cement is yellowish in colour but rather less so than dentine. It is less hard than dentine. It is composed of an organic matrix and an inorganic element. The organic matrix consists of collagen fibrils embedded in an amorphous cementing substance and as in bone prob-

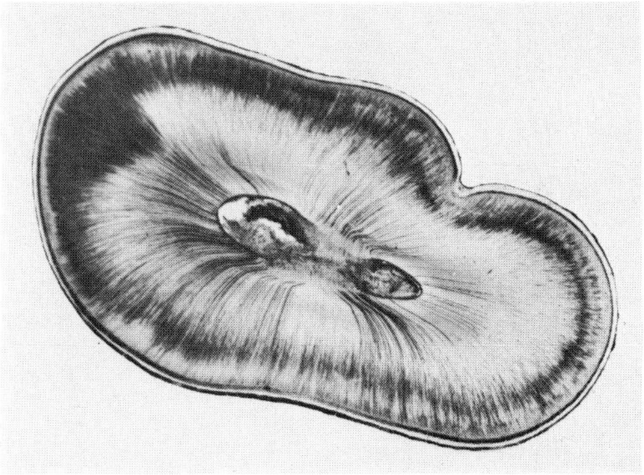

Fig. 223 Transverse section through the root of a tooth in the region of the acellular cement. Note the thinness of the layer of the cement. Ground section. × 6·5.

ably amounts to about 24 to 26 per cent of the total weight. The cementing substance contains acid mucopolysaccharide. The inorganic element is about 70 per cent by weight, with water making up the remainder of the total weight. The calcium salts which largely make up the inorganic element are mainly in the form of apatite molecules. This is deposited as submicroscopic crystallites in the cementing substance between and around the collagen fibrils of the matrix. The *in vitro* exchange of the isotopes of calcium, phosphorous and sulphur is greater in the cement than in the other dental tissues.

Structure and distribution. Two types of cement are recognised depending on the presence or absence of cells, and they are therefore known as acellular (primary) cement and cellular (secondary) cement; both forms are deposited in layers. Deposition of cement probably continues throughout life. A recent study indicates that the thickness of cement increases about three times between 11 and 76 years.

The collagen fibrils of cement are of two kinds. The first group is made up of the embedded parts of the principal fibres of the periodontal membrane, which are known as Sharpey's fibres (Fig. 231). These fibres are formed by the fibroblasts of the periodontal membrane. The other group of collagen fibrils, which constitute the intrinsic group, are formed by the cementoblasts and are found between the Sharpey fibres arranged either randomly or parallel to the surface of the cement. In the acellular cement most of the collagen is provided by Sharpey's fibres whereas in the cellular cement they only constitute a part of the fibre element.

The first formed cement is of the acellular variety, and this usually covers the root from the cement-enamel junction to near the root apex. It appears in ground sections as a thin homogeneous layer (Figs. 223, 224). In the incisors and canines the whole root is frequently covered

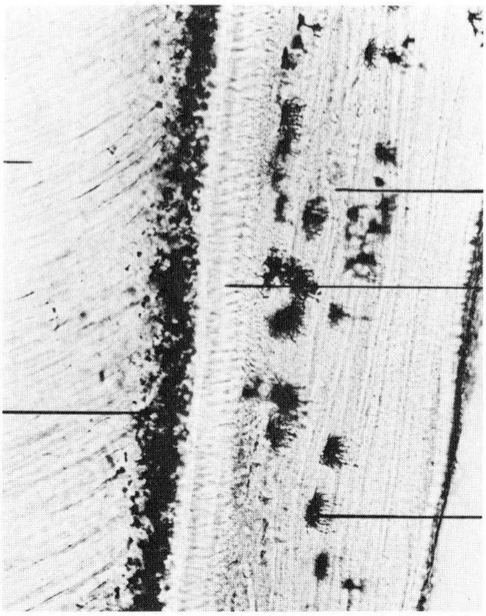

Fig. 224 Ground section showing cellular and acellular cement. Note the incremental lines in the cement. × 135.

by acellular cement alone. Acellular cement consists of layers of collagen fibre containing material which are united by thin fibre-free cementing lines of amorphous substance.

The cellular cement is found in the apical part of the root, gradually increasing in thickness as the apex is approached (Fig. 188). In this region it may considerably add to the length of the tooth. In the anterior teeth the amount of cellular cement is generally very small or it may be entirely absent. In multi-rooted teeth, however, cellular cement extends up to and over the region of the root division, where it may form a thick layer (Fig. 225). The time of appearance of cellular cement is related to the commencement of tooth eruption.

The cement at the apical region is about five times as thick as at the

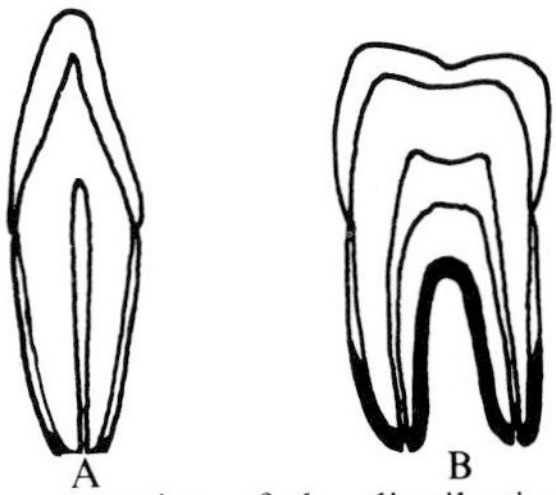

Fig. 225 Diagrammatic representation of the distribution of acellular and cellular cement. Cellular cement shown in solid black. A, incisor; B, molar.

neck of the tooth. Through the apical cement the apical vessels pass to and from the tooth pulp. The apical opening may be single, opening at the apex or to one or other side of it, or multiple. The most constricted parts of the canal or canals are often close to the cement-dentine junction. The most apical part of the earlier formed acellular cement may often be found covered by a later deposition of cellular cement (Fig. 224). Occasionally cellular cement is overlaid by a second layer of acellular cement.

In the cellular cement the cells (cementocytes) are found irregularly distributed, representing cementoblasts which have been left behind and surrounded during cement formation. They are contained in spaces or lacunae like the osteocytes in bone (Fig. 224). Processes of the cells spread out from the lacunae in fine canaliculi through the cement and often anastomose with those of other cells. They do not, however spread out uniformly in all directions round the cell, but are directed towards the periodontal membrane from which the cells obtain their nutrition (Fig. 226). In dried ground sections the lacunae appear as dark spaces (Fig. 224). Immediately around each lacuna the cement is dense and

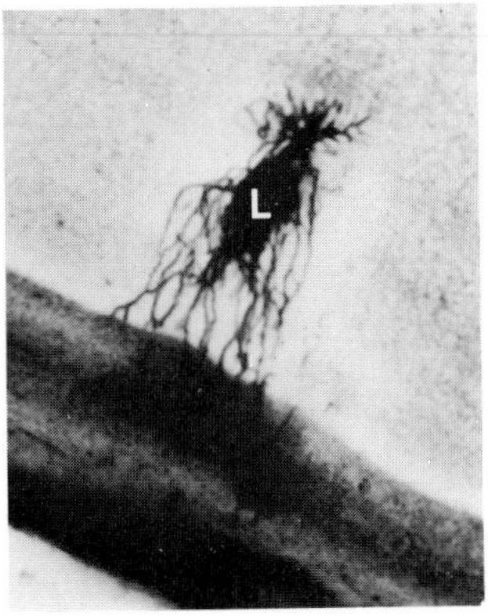

Fig. 226 Lacuna and canaliculi in the cement. The outer layers of the cement are heavily stained with silver. L, lacuna. × 580.

homogeneous and would appear to represent a mineralised ground substance which is deposited by the cementocyte within its lacuna.

In both acellular and cellular cement incremental lines run roughly parallel with the root surface (Fig. 224). These are formed by fibre-free amorphous substance and represent intervals between successive deposition of cement.

Between the dentine and the cellular cement there is often an intermediate layer (intermediate cement) which contains protoplasmic inclusions connecting the dentinal tubules and the cement lacunae. These may be the remains of the sheath of Hertwig which have been trapped between the dentine surface and the rapidly forming cement.

Sharpey's fibres. At the surface of the cement the principal fibres of the periodontal membrane pass into its substance. The fibres, where embedded in the cement, are known as Sharpey's fibres (Figs. 209, 230). In the accelular cement Sharpey's fibres are usually calcified. In the cellular cement each fibre commonly shows an uncalcified core with a calcified periphery. Evidence of such incompletely calcified fibres can be seen in microradiographs. In dried ground sections they appear as dark lines as a result of their disintegration which leaves channels in the cement (Fig. 224).

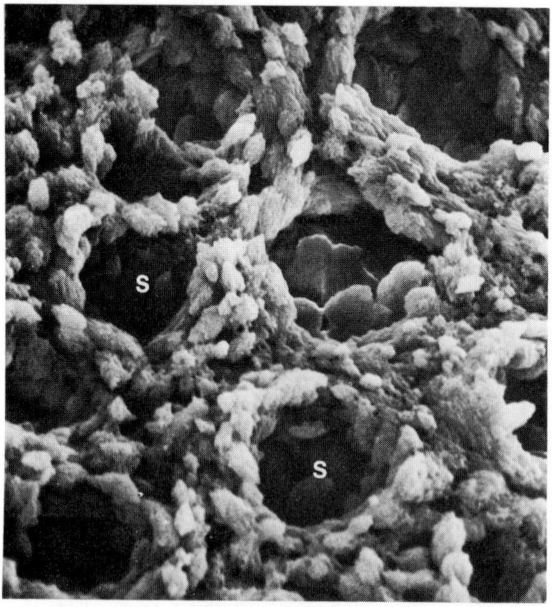

Fig. 227 Forming cement surface from which the organic matrix has been removed. The Sharpey's fibres appear as depressions as they mineralise in such regions after the intrinsic matrix. The nodular pattern of the intrinsic matrix represents the progress of mineralisation within the collagen fibres of the intrinsic matrix. S, Sharpey's fibre. Original magnification × 5000. (*By courtesy of Dr A. Boyde.*)

Sharpey's fibres always emerge from the cement in a straight line and continue across the periodontal interval and into the alveolar bone; stresses are thus always applied in the direction of their long axis. In alternating incremental layers of the cement the direction of Sharpey's fibres varies. This a record of previous movements of the tooth and the deposition of fresh layers of cement to attach the newly orientated fibres.

Permeability. It has been shown that the degree of permeability of the cement varies with age, and that cellular cement is more permeable than acellular cement. In young dogs the acellular cement is at first permeable but soon becomes impermeable; the cellular cement which is at first permeable in both periodontal and dentinal directions becomes impermeable on the dentinal side except in the region of the apex, but remains permeable on the periodontal side. The loss of permeability is attributed to increased calcification with age.

Cement-enamel junction. The relationship of the cement and the enamel is somewhat variable. Most commonly, in about 65 per cent of teeth, the cement slightly overlaps the enamel. In about 25 per cent of teeth the cement and enamel meet, each in a fine edge; and in rather less than 10 per cent the cement and enamel do not meet, leaving an area of exposed dentine. In the latter case gingival recession may lead to the exposure of an area of sensitive dentine in the mouth cavity. In a young fully erupted tooth the epithelial attachment or cuff ends at the cement-enamel junction. With increasing age or with gingivitis the epithelium migrates on to the cement covered root surfaces. This involves a destruction of the periodontal attachment in this area.

Function and functional changes. By the embedding of part of the principal fibres of the periodontal membrane in its substance, the cement provides the means by which these fibres are attached to the tooth and thus the tooth is attached to the alveolar bone.

Since the formation of the cement continues throughout life the attachment of the periodontal fibres can be altered or shifted according to the functional needs of the tooth, and newly formed periodontal fibres can gain attachment to the tooth, replacing fibres which have aged. This necessity for a shifting of periodontal fibres is most obvious in the vertical movement of the teeth during their eruption, but is equally important to allow of the bodily lateral and mesial movement of the teeth in the jaws during their growth and the mesial movements which occur afterwards as a result of approximal wear. Apart from the more obvious movements of the teeth, continual minute adjustments of each tooth occur in response to changing functional stresses.

The loss of tooth substance caused by attrition is partly compensated by the continued addition of cement which occurs at the root apex.

In about 90 per cent of permanent teeth there is evidence of small areas of cement resorption, usually in the apical region. In many cases old areas of resorption show evidence of repair by a later deposition of cement. The demarcation is shown by a deeply staining reversal line.

The cement formed in repair may be cellular, acellular, or both. Sometimes fractured teeth are united by cement deposition.

Clinical considerations. The function of the cement in permitting the alteration of the attachment of the periodontal fibres to the tooth is of prime importance in orthodontic practice. This feature allows of the artifical movement of the teeth as it does their natural movements.

By applying gentle pressure to the crown of a tooth, bone is resorbed adjacent to the root on the opposite side of the tooth and the tooth then can move in that direction. Obviously the cement on the pressure side is under the same pressure as the bone, but cement is much less readily resorbed than bone and so is normally unaffected. This property of the cement is another factor which permits the successful orthodontic movement of the teeth. The pressures employed are low, being ideally not more than 20 g per square centimetre of root surface. If excessive pressures are used, the tissues are damaged and necrosis may occur. Occasionally, even under the range of low pressures used, an extensive resorption of cement may take place and in severe cases this may involve the dentine.

Though the reasons for this resorption of cement are not fully understood, it has been shown that sometimes there is an underlying disturbance in the function of the ductless glands. After the removal of the pressure the resorptions are generally repaired by the deposition of fresh cement which fully restores the contour of the root in all but the very severe cases. Resorption of cement is also produced by occlusal trauma when a single tooth or a group of teeth carry more masticatory stress than normal.

In normal circumstances the cement is always separated from the bone of the tooth socket by the periodontal membrane which is never ossified. Probably the chief factor in preventing ossification spreading from bone to tooth is the continual functional movement between the tooth and its socket. Bone can be deposited in tissue which is continually under tension; it is not deposited in fibres which are continually changing their relationship to one another as are the fibres of the periodontal membrane.

Sometimes, however, and most often in retained deciduous teeth which are protected from the stresses of occlusion and mastication by the adjacent permanent teeth, ossification does take place and the root of the tooth is united over part of its extent with the wall of the socket (anchylosis). As a result of chronic inflammatory conditions anchylosis may take place in relation to permanent teeth.

A more common result of chronic inflammation around the roots of the teeth is to cause a marked deposition of cement, producing an abnormally thickened root (Fig. 228). This thickening may occur over the whole root or may be localised as a mass at the apex. Especially when found as a rounded mass at the root apex, the abnormal formation of cement may make the extraction of the tooth concerned unusually difficult, the diameter of the mass of cement being greater than that of the tooth socket immediately above it. This excessive deposition of cement or hypercementosis may affect one tooth or a number in the same mouth. In a similar way fragments of roots which have been left in the jaws following an extraction frequently become surrounded by a deposition of cement.

When recession of the gingival margin occurs to such an extent that the epithelial attachment and gingival crevice are completely on the root surface an area of cement becomes exposed in the mouth. Such an area of cement loses its vitality as it is cut off from its nutritional supply

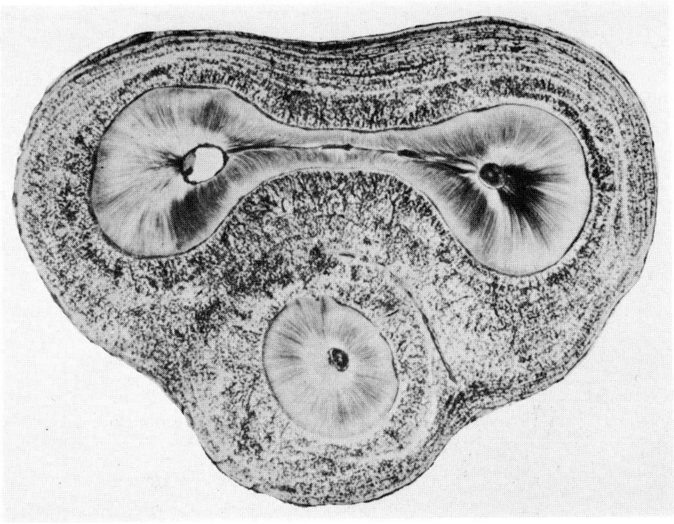

Fig. 228 Hypercementosis of upper molar. Transverse ground section. ×9.

from the gum and periodontal membrane. The exposed cement can easily be removed from the teeth during scaling if great care is not exercised. Furthermore, being thin it can readily be worn away by abrasion. In both instances the underlying dentine is exposed and this is very sensitive. If a lateral root canal should open at such an area of cement which has become exposed through gingival recession, infection of the pulp ensues and an otherwise unexplainable pulpitis results.

Sometimes as a result of trauma part of the cement may break away (cement tear); this usually occurs along the cement-dentine junction. Such fragments may become reattached by the deposition of fresh cement or come to lie in the periodontal membrane with fibres of the membrane attached to both surfaces.

BIBLIOGRAPHY

Bennett, D. T. & Miles, A. E. W. (1955). Observations on the permeability of human calcified dental tissues to penicillin. *J. dent. Res.* **34,** 553.

Blackwood, H. J. J. (1957). Intermediate cementum. *Brit. dent. J.* **102,** 345.

Boyde, A. & Jones, S. T. (1968). Scanning electron microscopy of cementum and Sharpey fibre bone. *Zeitschr. f. Zellforsch.* **92,** 536.

Furseth, R. (1969). The fine structure of the cellular cementum of young human teeth. *Archs. oral Biol.* **14,** 1147.

Henry, J. & Weinmann, J. P. (1951). The pattern of resorption and repair of human cementum. *J. Amer. dent. Ass.* **42,** 270.

Owens, P. D. A. (1976). The root surface in human teeth: a microradiographic study. *J. Anat. Lond.* **122,** 389.

Paynter, K. J. & Pudy, G. (1958). A study of the structure, chemical nature and development of cementum in the rat. *Anat. Rec.* **131,** 233.

Selvig, K. A. (1965). The fine structure of human cementum. *Acta odont. scand.* **23,** 423.

Stones, H. H. (1934). The permeability of cementum. *Brit. dent. J.* **56,** 273.

Zander, H. A. & Hürzeler, B. (1958). Continuous cementum apposition. *J. dent. Res.* **37,** 1035.

15. Periodontal Membrane

Development. Before tooth eruption commences the outer surface of the dental follicle is in contact with, but not attached to, the bone of the alveolus or crypt. As eruption takes place the follicular tissue gradually becomes converted into the periodontal membrane or ligament which attaches the root of the tooth to the bone of the socket (Fig. 229).

After eruption has started the epithelial sheath of Hertwig, separating

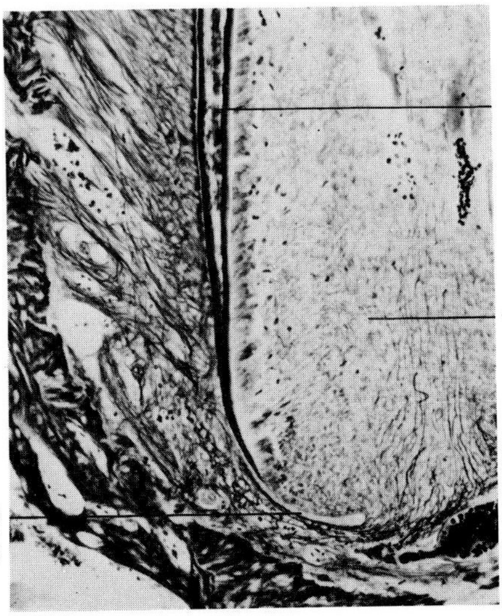

Fig. 229 Section through the developing root of the molar tooth of a rat stained with Wilder's silver stain. Note the obliquely orientated fibres of the developing periodontal membrane attached to the formed part of the root in comparison to the circumferentially arranged fibres of the dental follicle external to the sheath of Hertwig. × 105.

the newly formed dentine from the follicle, begins to disintegrate over the first formed part of the root, forming an epithelial network in place of a continuous epithelial layer. As a result the innermost fibres of the follicle come into direct contact with the dentine of the root and, by the deposition of cement, are attached to the root. At the same time the outermost fibres of the follicle become attached to the developing bony socket.

As the root continues to grow during eruption of the tooth, more and more of the inner fibres of the follicle become attached to the root by cement deposition, and the outer fibres become attached to the wall of the forming socket by a filling in of the alveolus or crypt by bone deposition (Fig. 230).

The first group of fibres to develop are the free gingival attached to the tooth immediately below the cement-enamel junction. The remaining fibres run obliquely from bone to tooth. However, as the tooth erupts the direction of the fibres related to the crest of the alveolar bone

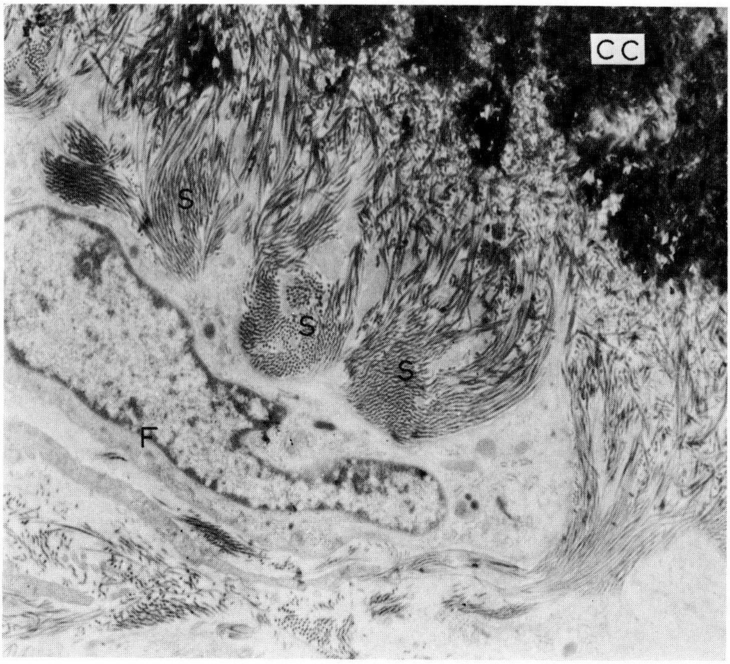

Fig. 230 Developing periodontal membrane with formation of Sharpey's fibres and their attachment to the surface of newly formed cement. S, Sharpey's fibre; F, fibroblast; CC, calcifying cement. Original magnification ×4000.

changes to a horizontal and finally to a position of reverse obliquity to give the alveolar crest fibres. The transeptal fibres between upper central incisors develop only when growth ceases in the overlying suture.

During eruption the fibres attached to the alveolar bone and to the cement intermingle with one another to form an intermediate plexus which persists as a site of fibre adjustment for as long as active eruption continues. After the tooth reaches the occlusal plane the intermediate zone disappears and the periodontal fibres run in a direct course from bone to root of tooth. The intermediate zone is much more readily distinguished in continually growing and erupting teeth, such as the rodent incisor, than in human teeth.

Doubt has been cast on the existence of the intermediate plexus by certain isotope studies. Labelled precursors of collagen, such as tritiated glycine or proline, might be expected to be deposited particularly in the central region of the periodontal membrane where formation of collagen fibres would be required during active eruption. Instead of this a uniform distribution of radioactivity has been found across the width of the periodontal membrane. On the other hand polarised light examination indicates a less well organised central zone in the periodontal membrane during active eruption, that is a region where the collagen is less mature. It is obvious that some mechanism must exist to allow for adjustments in the arrangement of the periodontal fibres as the tooth moves vertically relative to the surrounding bone during active eruption, yet at the same time the attachment between tooth and bone has to be maintained. It is significant that autoradiographic studies have shown a high turnover rate of collagen in the periodontal membrane whereas elsewhere in the body collagen is only very slowly replaced.

Structure. The most important elements of the periodontal membrane are the bundles of collagen fibres which pass from the cement of the tooth to the lamina dura of the tooth socket, to adjacent teeth or into the gingival tissue surrounding the cervical region of the tooth (Fig. 231). These fibres are known as the principal fibres of the periodontal membrane, in distinction to the loosely arranged connective tissue surrounding the blood vessels and nerve fibres of the periodontal membrane. The individual fibres in the bundles are bound together by a cementing substance. The principal fibres can be divided into groups according to the direction in which they run and according to their function (Fig. 232).

1. *Oblique fibres.* By far the greater number of principal fibres run obliquely inward and apically from the alveolar bone to the root of the tooth (Fig. 233). Between the bundles of these fibres there are round or oval intervals where the periodontal tissue is much less dense (Fig. 234). In these areas it forms a reticular framework of loose connective tissue through which the blood vessels, nerves, and lymphatics of the periodontal membrane run in a somewhat spiral course between the bone of the socket and the tooth.

The oblique fibres suspend the tooth in its socket: by their arrangement pressure on a tooth is transformed into tension on the wall of the socket. The relation of the fibres to tooth and socket prevents the apical region of the root being driven down on to the alveolar bone, under normal functional stresses (Fig. 232). In this way the vessels entering and leaving the pulp are not damaged or occluded. Around the apical region of the roots of the teeth the periodontal membrane forms a cushion of looser tissue. The periodontal fibres in this region are sometimes described as a distinct group, the apical fibres. The greater part

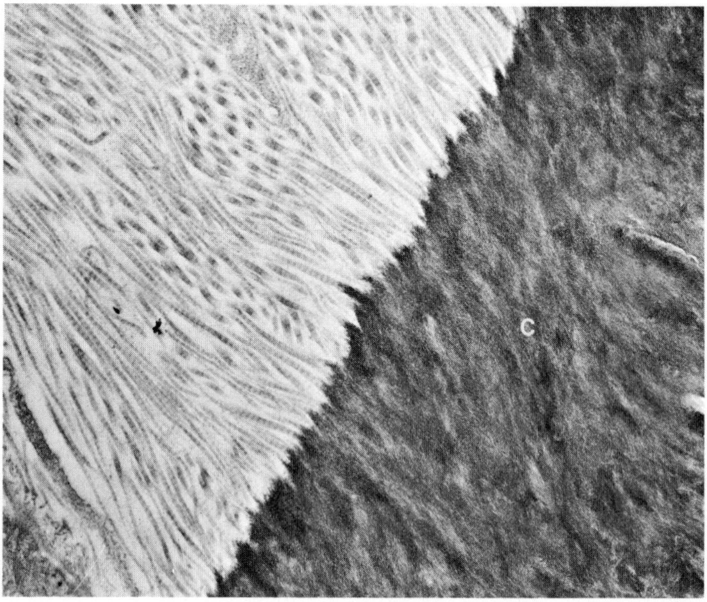

Fig. 231 Electron micrograph showing the densely packed fibrils of the periodontal membrane entering the cement. The typical cross-banding of collagen fibrils is evident. C, cement. Original magnification ×9500 (*By courtesy of Dr K. A. Selvig.*)

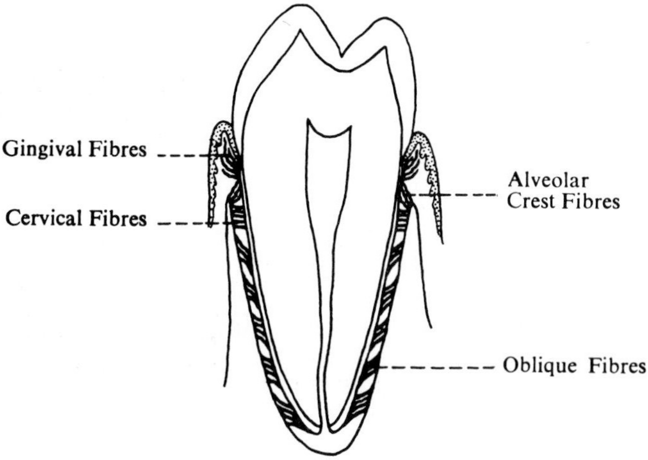

Fig. 232 Diagrammatic illustration of a longitudinal section through a single tooth and its socket to show the arrangement of the oblique principal fibres of the periodontal membrane. The gingival, alveolar crest, and the cervical fibres are also shown.

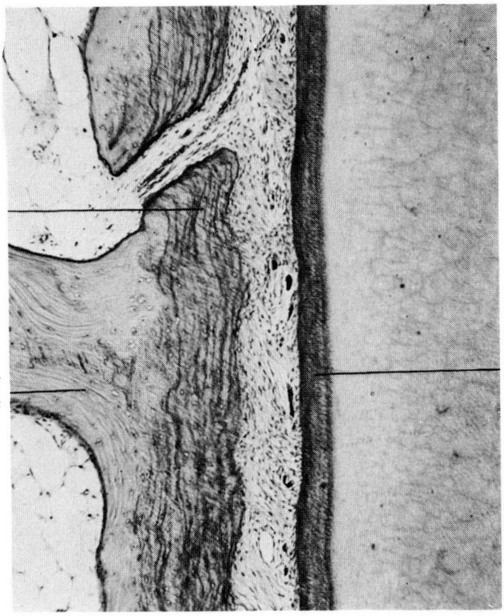

Fig. 233 Vertical section through the periodontal membrane in the region of the oblique principal fibres. A blood vessel may be seen passing through an opening in the lamina dura of the alveolar bone. × 55. (*By courtesy of Prof R. W. Fearnhead.*)

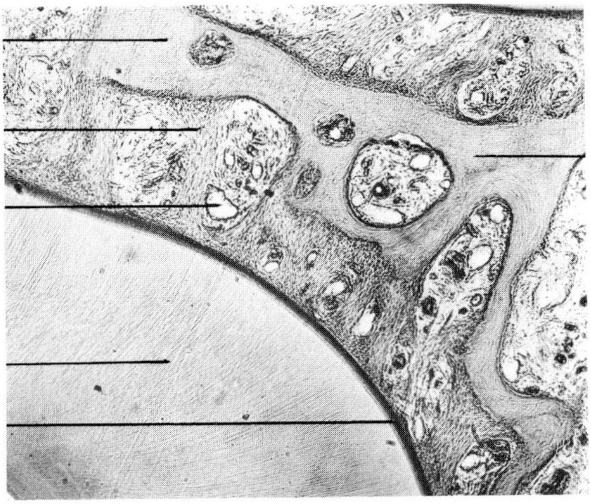

Fig. 234 Periodontal membrane. Note the oval areas filled with loose tissue and containing blood vessels between the bundles of dense fibrous tissue. Transverse decalcified section. × 35.

of the pressure of mastication is transmitted from tooth to socket in the coronal third of the root. In multi-rooted teeth the fibres at the crest of the interradicular septum are somewhat differently arranged from the other oblique fibres as they fan out from this region to the adjacent part of the division of the root. The oblique fibres do not usually run in a strictly radial fashion between points on tooth and socket in the same vertical plane. This arrangement limits the amount of rotatory movement of the tooth.

2. *Horizontal fibres.* In the region of the neck of the tooth a dense group of fibres forms an almost continuous ligament between the root of the tooth and the rim of the alveolar bone at the mouth of the socket. The more superficial fibres form a strong ligament connecting the necks of the adjacent teeth on their mesial and distal surfaces above the level

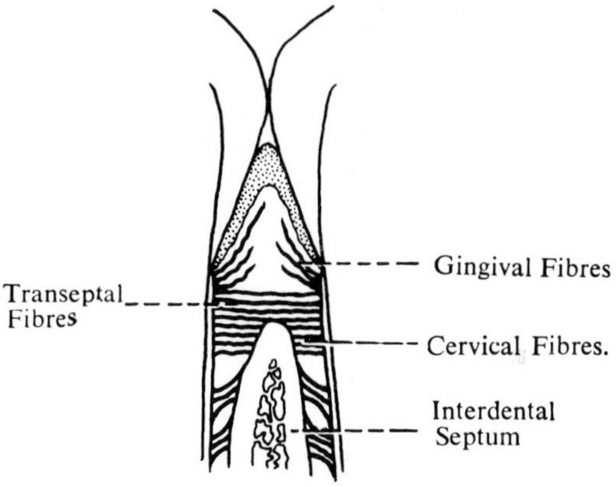

Fig. 235 Diagrammatic illustration of a mesio-distal section through two adjacent teeth and the interdental septum to show the arrangement of the transeptal, cervical and gingival fibres of the periodontal membrane.

of the interdental septum of the alveolar bone and are continuous with the periosteum of the bony septum. These transeptal fibres link the individual units of the dentition together (Figs. 235, 236).

The deeper fibres, usually referred to as a cervical group, pass from the neck region of the root of the tooth to the wall of the socket just within the rim of the socket (Figs. 232, 235). These fibres and the transeptal group have a horizontal course. The cervical group check any tilting movement of the tooth.

After the removal of a single tooth and the repair of its socket the transeptal fibres are reconstructed so as to connect the teeth on either side of the gap. The repair of these fibres, with the subsequent contraction of the fibrous tissue, is one of the factors responsible for the tilting of the teeth on either side of the space left by the lost tooth. The transeptal fibres have been shown to be important in the production of physiological mesial drift of the teeth.

3. *Alveolar crest fibres.* Attached to the cervical part of the cement in relation to the buccal and lingual sides of the teeth, a further group of fibres pass to the alveolar bone. As they are attached to the very rim of the socket they are known as alveolar crest fibres (Fig. 232). These fibres limit tilting and extrusive movements of the tooth and together with the horizontally arranged group are the ones that must first be ruptured in tooth extraction. The deeper horizontal and the alveolar crest fibres are sometimes grouped together as the circular ligament.

4. *Gingival fibres.* From the necks of the teeth fibres pass into the overlying gum, some running vertically into the marginal gingiva close to the epithelial attachment or junctional epithelium, whereas others

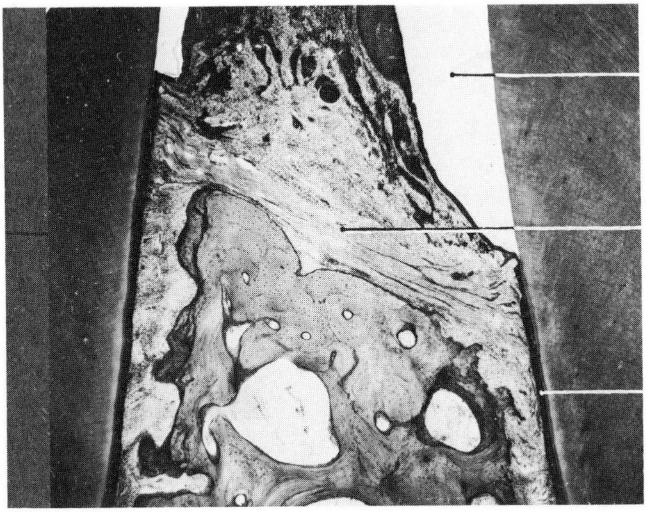

Fig. 236 Mesio-distal section through the two adjacent permanent incisors and the inter-dental bony septum. ×22. (*By courtesy of Prof H. J. J. Blackwood.*)

run in a more horizontal direction (Figs. 232, 235, 236). As well as these fibres which spread radially from the cervical cement into the gingivae there is another group of gingival fibres which are arranged circularly to the teeth (Fig. 258). These fibres lie in the lamina propria of the gingivae above the level of the alveolar bone. The function of both groups of fibres is to hold the gum tightly against the necks of the teeth. The maintenance of these fibres is an important factor in consolidating the epithelial attachment of gum and tooth at the gingival margin and in preventing the formation of pockets between tooth and gum.

The periodontal fibres which have an attachment at one end to cement, are attached at the other end to alveolar bone, gingival tissue, or to the cement of an adjacent tooth. The fibres of the periodontal membrane are not, with the possible exception of the recently described oxytalan fibres, elastic; they are collagen fibres. They do, however, allow a small range of movement to the tooth since at rest they have a wavy course and under tension can straighten out.

Movements of teeth. The forces of mastication produce vertical depressive movements of the teeth, rotatory movements, and tilting movements. These movements are limited mainly by the oblique and horizontal fibres. In depressive movements all the oblique fibres are under tension; in tilting and rotatory movements only part of the oblique or horizontal fibres are under tension, depending on the direction of the thrust on the tooth. In tilting the axis of movement of the tooth is situated a little below the midpoint of the length of the root, therefore the oblique and horizontal

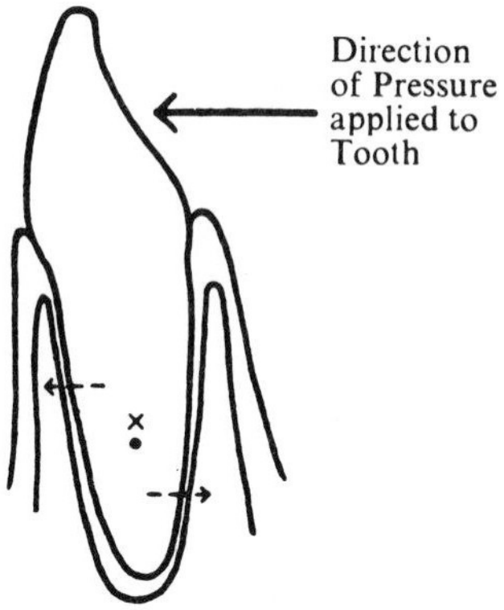

Fig. 237 Diagram to show the tilting produced when pressure is applied to one aspect of the crown of a tooth as in orthodontic treatment. X indicates the axis of movement; the small arrows in broken line indicate the direction of movement of the root around this axis. In these areas the fibres of the periodontal membrane are compressed on one aspect of the root, whereas on the opposite aspect they are under tension.

fibres above this level are under tension on the side of the thrust; below this level the oblique fibres on the side opposite to the thrust are under tension (Fig. 237).

Attention has been directed to the modifying effect on tooth support and tooth movement that is provided by other components of the periodontal membrane apart from the principal fibres. These are the ground substance and tissue fluid of the membrane and the volume of blood contained by its rich vascular supply. These fluid or semi-fluid elements constitute a hydro-dynamic system which is capable of damping down tooth movements and producing recoil effects when a tooth has been subjected to brief intrusive pressures. Where a continuous pressure is applied, as with orthodontic appliances, the tissue fluid is displaced in a gingival or apical direction and gives a squeeze-film effect which damps down the tooth movement. In the sudden but short acting pressures which arise during mastication the blood is displaced into the surrounding alveolar bone through the interconnecting vessels; from there it can return to produce a rebound effect when the pressure is removed.

The combined physical characteristics of the various components of the periodontal membrane are such that when a force is applied to a tooth an initial rapid movement is produced which is followed by a slower movement, when the force is removed there is an initial rapid return movement suceeded by a slower phase.

Thickness of periodontal membrane. At the level where the axis of movement is situated in tilting of the tooth the periodontal membrane is at its narrowest; towards the apex of the root or more cervically it has a greater width. The thickness of the periodontal membrane also varies from tooth to tooth and in different individuals. The normal range of thickness of the periodontal membrane around functional teeth is about 0·1–0·33 mm. The thickness tends to be diminished in non-functional teeth, and around these the bundles of principal fibres lose their definite organisation.

Cells. Throughout the life of each tooth the periodontal membrane is constantly undergoing change brought about by the stress of mastication and by alteration in the position of the teeth. The fibres must be continually repaired, replaced and reattached. The migration of the teeth, which occurs during growth of the jaws and also in adult life as a result of wear at the mesial and distal surfaces, necessitates a considerable amount of periodontal adjustment. The maintenance and replacement of the periodontal fibres is carried out by the fibroblasts which lie on and between the collagen bundles. Attachment of the fibres is produced by the deposition of new bone on the walls of the socket and by the deposition of cement on the surface of the root of the tooth. The fibroblasts are also responsible for the breaking down of the collagen which takes place in the remodelling of the periodontal fibres.

Lying on the surface of the bone of the socket and between the fibres of the periodontal membrane as these pass into the bone are the bone-forming cells, the osteoblasts. These cells are particularly numerous during periods of new bone deposition when they form an almost continuous layer on the surface of the bone. Whenever bone resorption takes place large multinucleated cells, osteoclasts, which have the power of resorbing bone, lie in cut-out spaces, lacunae, on the surface of the bone. During migrational movements of the teeth it is usual to find bone resorption and deposition occurring at the same time; resorption chiefly on the aspect towards which the tooth is moving and deposition chiefly on the opposite side. On the surface of the cement and between the fibres attached to it cement-forming cells, cementoblasts, are to be found.

Defence cells, similar in kind to those occurring in pulp tissue (see p. 253), are to be found in the periodontal membrane; they come into functional activity whenever an inflammatory reaction takes place.

Blood vessels. The main vessels of the periodontal membrane run parallel to the long axis of the tooth and are located close to the wall of the socket. They lie in the loose connective tissue between the bundles of the principal fibres in their course through the periodontal membrane (Fig. 234). Branches are given off towards the tooth and from them capillaries arise which are arranged in a network with a large and irregular mesh(Fig. 238). In the cervical part of the periodontal membrane this pattern is modified so that the capillary vessels form here a denser network. From these vessels single capillary vessels are given off which take a coiled course and then return to the originating network, so that an arrangement resembling that of glomeruli is produced (Figs. 238, 239). More coronally still looped capillaries with coiled arterial parts are found in the region of the epithelial attachment (Figs. 238, 239). Anastomosis between the periodontal vessels and the gingival vessels (see p. 305) takes place in this area.

The blood supply of the periodontal membrane is derived from two sources:

a. From the apical region of the tooth, where, as they traverse the periapical tissue, the vessels to and from the pulp give off and receive

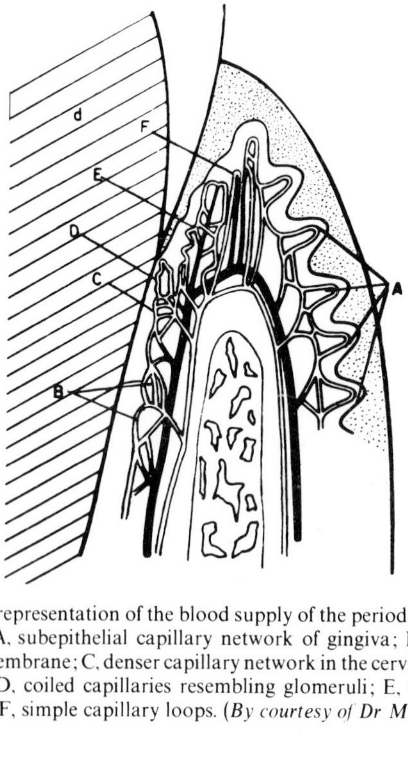

Fig. 238 Schematic representation of the blood supply of the periodontal membrane and the gingival tissue. A, subepithelial capillary network of gingiva; B, capillary network of the periodontal membrane; C, denser capillary network in the cervical part of the periodontal membrane; D, coiled capillaries resembling glomeruli; E, capillary loops with coiled arterial part; F, simple capillary loops. (*By courtesy of Dr M. Kindlová and Arch. oral Biol.*)

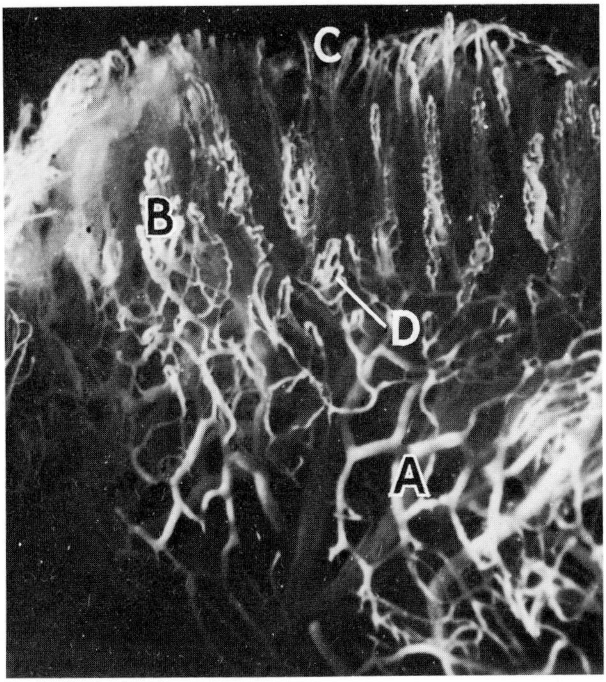

Fig. 239 Latex cast of the blood supply of the periodontal membrane and the adjacent part of the gingival tissue. A, capillary network of the periodontal membrane; B, capillary loops with coiled arterial part; C, simple capillary loops; D, coiled capillaries resembling glomeruli. (*By courtesy of Dr M. Kindlová.*)

vessels passing to and from the periodontal membrane (arterioles and venules).

b. From the gingival tissue. These branches anastomose with the periodontal vessels around the necks of the teeth (Fig. 238).

Blood vessels perforate the lamina dura and form anastomoses between the main periodontal vessels and those of the Haversian systems and cancellous tissue of the alveolar bone (Fig. 233). These vessels probably provide escape routes for blood when the ascending vessels of the periodontal membrane are compressed as a result of the pressure exerted during mastication. The bone-perforating vessels have their origin from branches of either the apical vessels or those of the gingivae. Larger vessels perforate the bone around the margins of the tooth sockets especially in the molar region.

When a tooth is extracted the ruptured vessels pour blood into the socket from below (apical vessels), the sides (alveolar vessels), and from the gums. The blood soon clots and later the clot is invaded by capillaries and fibroblasts and is covered over by proliferation of the oral epithelium. The granulation tissue becomes scar tissue and in this ossification later takes place. The lamina dura usually remains intact for a considerable time, showing in X-rays the outline of the old socket.

Lymphatics. The lymphatics of the periodontal membrane commence in the gums and, after piercing the horizontal group of principal fibres, pass with the vessels and nerves towards the apex of the tooth or of its individual roots where they join those emerging from the pulp. In their further course some follow the blood vessels and nerves towards the front of the face, emerging through the infraorbital and mental foramina, others pass backward towards the infratemporal fossa through the pterygopalatine fossa and the mandibular foramen.

Nerves. The nerves of the periodontal membrane fall into two groups:

1. Non-medullated fibres belonging to the autonomic nervous system which run on the blood vessels and supply the smooth muscle in their walls.

2. Medullated sensory somatic nerves which run in small bundles alongside the blood vessels. They end either in small loops around bundles of periodontal fibres or in small knob-like expansions. Two forms of sensation can be appreciated by the periodontal tissue, pain and pressure. The pressure sense is very delicate so that the slightest contact between the teeth of the two jaws or with substances introduced into the mouth can be appreciated. The nerve fibres from the periodontal membranes of the teeth pass along the mandibular or maxillary divisions of the trigeminal nerve and probably end in the mesencephalic nucleus in the mid-brain. From there secondary neurones pass to the thalamus and thence by tertiary neurones to the sensory cerebral cortex. Reflex arcs, also, are established with the final motor neurons to the muscles of mastication, expression (buccinator and lip muscles), and the tongue muscles, so as to regulate the masticatory apparatus.

Epithelial tissue. Even long after eruption remains of the epithelial sheath of Hertwig are to be found either as isolated columns of epithelial cells or as an incomplete network between the fibres of the periodontal membrane. Such remnants are particularly numerous around the apices of the teeth or at the division of multi-rooted teeth. They are known as the epithelial debris or rests of Malassez (Fig. 240). These epithelial masses are of clinical importance as they may proliferate and form cysts, especially under the stimulus of chronic inflammation of the surrounding tissues. With migration of the teeth and following tooth eruption some of these cell debris may become more widely separated from the teeth and may be found in the alveolar or basal bone of the jaws at some distance from the teeth. They are also frequently found in edentulous jaws.

Clinical considerations. The firm attachment of the periodontal membrane to the cement and to the alveolar bone calls for care in the extraction of teeth. Excessive force used in an uncontrolled manner often leads to portions of the alveolar bone being fractured and, with the adherent gum, coming away with the tooth, leaving an ugly jagged wound.

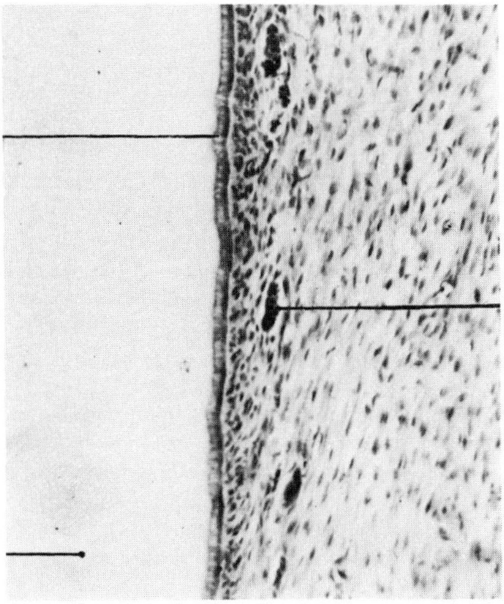

Fig. 240 Epithelial remnants of the sheath of Hertwig in the periodontal membrane of a human tooth. × 110.

Infection of the periodontal membrane may spread from the pulp through the apex or apices of the tooth, giving rise to an abscess or a mass of granulation tissue according to whether the infection is acute or chronic. Apical abscesses often work their way through the adjacent bone and open on the gums or into deeper regions such as the maxillary sinus, the pterygo-palatine fossa, the floor of the nasal cavity, or the floor of the mouth cavity. An abscess may, however, become isolated by a capsule of fibrous tissue so that its migration through the bone becomes very slow or ceases altogether. Such areas of infection are seen in X-rays as dark shadows adjacent to the apices of teeth. Infection may also reach the periodontal membrane from the mouth cavity following infection and destruction of the epithelial attachment of the gum. This type of descending infection (gingivitis) leads to a progressive destruction of the principal fibres of the periodontal membrane, and of the alveolar bone, so that the tooth becomes loosened in its socket. Loose teeth are also sometimes the result of spreading malignant tumours within the jaw, producing a resorption of the internal structure of the aveloar bone. In some adults, and more especially in old people, the bone between the floor of the maxillary sinus and the sockets of the upper molar teeth becomes resorbed so that the periodontal tissue of the apical regions of these teeth becomes continuous with that of the submucosa of the sinus. It is obvious that in such cases infections of the pulps of the teeth spread readily to involve the sinus.

BIBLIOGRAPHY

Bernick, S. (1960). The organization of the periodontal membrane fibres of the developing molars of rats. *Arch. oral Biol.* **2**, 57.

Bevelander, G. & Nakahara, H. (1968). The fine structure of the human peridental ligament. *Anat. Rec.* **162**, 313.

Bien, S. M. (1966). Fluid dynamic mechanisms which regulate tooth movement. In *Advances in Oral Biology*, p. 173. Ed. Staple, P. H. New York: Academic Press.

Cody, F. W. J., Lee, R. W. H. & Taylor, A. (1972). A functional analysis of the components of the mesencephalic nucleus of the fifth nerve in the cat. *J. Physiol.* **226**, 249.

Griffin, C. J. & Harris, R. (1967). The fine structure of the developing human periodontium. *Archs. oral Biol.* **12**, 971.

Griffin, C. J. & Harris, R. (1968). Unmyelinated nerve endings in the periodontal membrane of human teeth. *Archs. oral Biol.* **13**, 1207.

Griffin, C. J. (1972). The fine structure of end-rings in human periodontal ligament. *Archs. oral Biol.* **17**, 785.

Kindlová, M. (1965). The blood supply of the marginal periodontium in *Macacus Rhesus*. *Arch. oral Biol.* **10**, 869.

Kizior, J. E., Cuozzo, J. W. & Bowman, D. C. (1968). Functional and histologic assessment of the sensory innervation of the periodontal ligament of the cat. *J. dent. Res.* **47**, 59.

Levy, B. M. & Bernick, S. (1968). Development and organization of the periodontal ligament of deciduous teeth in marmosets. *J. dent. Res.* **47**, 27.

Melcher, A. H. & Walker, T. W. (1976). The periodontal ligament in attachment and as a shock absorber. In—*The Eruption and Occlusion of the Teeth*. Colston Papers. No. 27. Eds. Poole, D. F. G. & Stack, M. V. London: Butterworth.

Shore, R. C. & Berkowitz, B. K. B. (1979). An ultrastructural study of periodontal ligament fibroblasts in relation to their possible role in tooth eruption and intracellular collagen degradation in the rat. *Arch. oral Biol.* **24**, 155.

Sloan, P., Shellis, R. P. & Berkowitz, B. K. B. (1976). Effect of specimen preparation on the rat periodontal ligament in the scanning electron microscope. *Archs. oral Biol.* **21**, 633.

Smukler, H. & Dreyer, C. J. (1969). Principal fibres of the periodontium. *J. periodont. Res*, **4**, 19.

Ten Cate, A. R. & Deporter, D. A. (1974). The role of the fibroblast in collagen turnover in the functioning periodontal ligament of the mouse. *Archs. oral Biol.* **19**, 339.

Trott, J. R. (1963). The development of the periodontal attachment in the rat. *Acta anat.* **51**, 313.

16. The Alveolar Bone and the Jaws

Alveolar bone, which makes up the alveolar processes and alveolar bulbs of the upper and lower jaws, is that part of the facial skeleton which forms the alveoli and crypts of developing teeth and the sockets of erupted teeth giving protection to the former and providing a means of attachment for the latter. Within the mouth it is covered by mucous membrane. Some authorities limit the use of the term alveolar bone to the lamina dura and call the rest of the bone making up the alveolar process supporting or sustentacular bone. The alveolar bone between the roots of adjacent teeth is known as the interdental septum and it supports the interdental gingival tissue (see p. 305). The bone of the facial skeleton, which supports the alveolar bone, is sometimes referred to as the basal bone. There is, however, no difference in structure between the alveolar and basal bone of the face. If an X-ray of a child of about seven years of age is examined (Fig. 136) it will be seen that the crypts of the successional permanent teeth, and especially the canines, are situated deep in the jaws. The bone in which their crypts are lying is at this stage 'alveolar' bone. In the adult, however, when all the permanent teeth have erupted, the region occupied by these teeth during their pre-eruptive development has become 'basal' bone.

When the teeth have been lost the alveolar bone is gradually resorbed, so that in the upper jaw the floor of the maxillary sinus may be in close proximity to the toothless gums with only a thin layer of bone separating them. The mucous membrane covering the gum is almost on the level of that covering the hard palate. In the lower jaw the mylohyoid and external oblique lines of the mandible lie close to the upper border of the jaw, and in extreme cases the mental foramen may lie close to or at the upper border of the bone. In children in whom there has been complete failure of tooth development (anodontia) the alveolar bone does not develop, but otherwise the growth of the facial skeleton is normal. Teeth implanted in sockets are a characteristic of mammalian dentitions shared only by advanced reptiles such as crocodiles and alligators.

THE STRUCTURE OF ALVEOLAR BONE AND JAWS

When first formed in fetal life the alveolar bone, like the rest of the skeleton, is in the form of an irregular lattice work without any definite structural pattern; there is at this stage no cortical layer (Fig. 113). The developing bone is surrounded by a thick periosteum. This fetal bone is a variety of coarse-fibred bone known frequently as woven bone. During the rapid growth of alveolar bone, which occurs during fetal life, areas of secondary cartilage may appear at the growing alveolar margins.

Compact bone. After eruption of the teeth the alveolar bone gradually takes on its adult form and is made up of a surface cortical layer of dense bone and an interior zone of cancellous bone (Fig. 241). Both compact and cancellous bone are composed of layers of bone arranged in an orderly fashion which are known as lamellae. Lamellar bone unlike woven bone is a fine fibred bone. At the mouths of the tooth sockets the surface cortical bone is continuous with that lining the sockets, the lamina dura or cribriform plate (Fig. 242). There are usually numerous

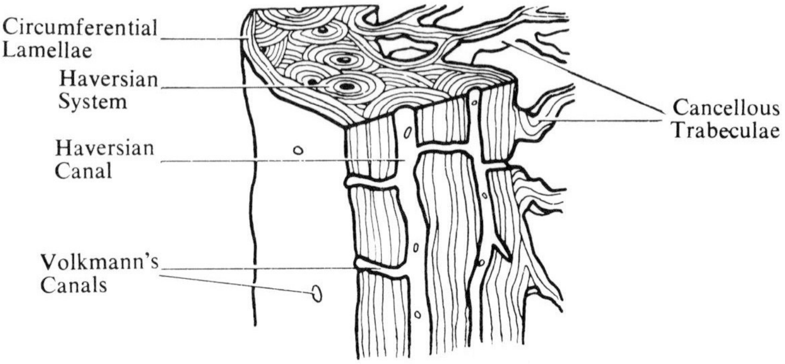

Fig. 241 Diagrammatic representation in three dimensions of a segment of bone illustrating the arrangement of compact and cancellous areas, the lamellar pattern and the vascular channels (Haversian and Volkmann's canals).

openings through which blood vessels reach the adjacent gingival tissue at the mouths of the sockets. The lamina dura is much thinner than the surface layer of cortical bone. The term lamina dura is given to this layer of bone from the dense radiopaque appearance it gives on radiographs (Fig. 243). The deeper portions of the cortical bone of the alveolar surface are made up of Haversian systems (osteones) composed of bone arranged in concentric lamellae around the central blood vessels of each Haversian canal (Fig. 241). Beneath the surface periosteum and where it forms the wall of the tooth sockets the bone is laid down in the form of surface lamellae. In the tooth sockets, however, where the principal fibres of the periodontal membrane are actually attached the lamellar bone is covered by areas of bundle bone. Between the surface lamellae and those forming the osteones there are lacunae which contain osteocytes.

As the replacement of the original woven bone of the jaw takes place two generations of osteones appear. The first or primary osteones are

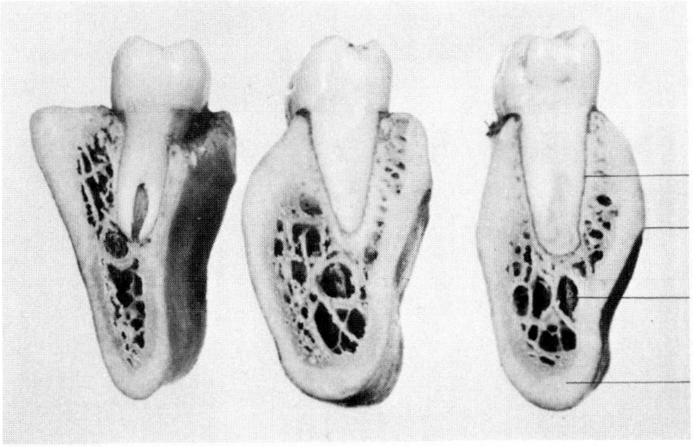

Fig. 242 Sections through the lower jaw to illustrate the distribution of the compact (cortical) and cancellous bone and the formation of the sockets for the teeth. The sections are at the levels of the distal root of the three lower left molars. Note the altering thickness of buccal and lingual alveolar plates from first to third molar. (A) Third molar. (B) Second molar. (C) First molar.

formed within spaces in the structure of the woven bone, the secondary osteones replace areas of woven bone or primary osteones which have been partly or wholly resorbed during the continued process of bone remodelling.

Sharpey's fibres and bundle bone. The fibres of the periodontal membrane pass between the surface layers of the cement and the surface layers of the bone and are inserted into both by bundles of collagen fibres (Sharpey's fibres). Sharpey's fibres occupy definite channels in both bone and cement (Fig. 244). The walls of these channels have a somewhat different composition from the adjacent bone matrix. The bone into which the Sharpey's fibres are attached is a coarse fibred bone and is usually referred to as bundle bone (Fig. 233). Apart from the periodontal fibres it contains fewer collagen fibres than ordinary lamellated bone. Bundle bone is particularly found in those areas of the sockets where recent bone formation has occurred as a result of tooth movement.

The surface of the alveolar bone and the lamina dura is perforated by numerous minute foramina (Volkmann's canals) for blood vessels, and possibly lymphatics, and nerves. These perforations are particularly numerous in the lamina dura and account for its alternative name of cribriform plate. The blood vessels pass from the periosteum and the periodontal membrane into the bone where they anastomose with the vessels of the Haversian canals and with those of the medullary tissue. They are most numerous immediately within the sockets and at the bottom of the sockets.

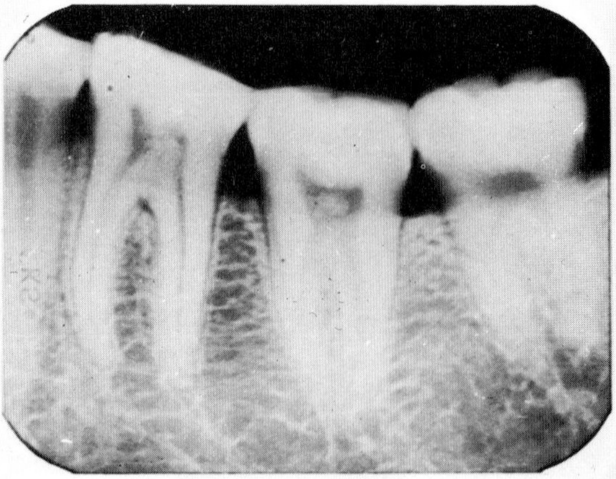

Fig. 243 Radiograph of the lower permanent molars and the surrounding alveolar bone. Especially in relation to the first molar the dense radiopaque line, the lamina dura, can be seen. This is separated from the roots of the teeth by a dark line corresponding to the periodontal membrane.

Cancellous bone. The central cancellous tissue passes between the lamina dura of the sockets and the surface cortical plates of the alveolar bone and between the lamina dura of adjacent sockets (Fig. 245). Its degree of development is related to the forces of mastication. In the incisor-canine region in both jaws the bone forming the outer wall of the tooth sockets is thin and is made up of a union of the surface cortical bone and the lamina dura without any intervening cancellous bone. Cancellous bone is built up of trabeculae which consist of one or more

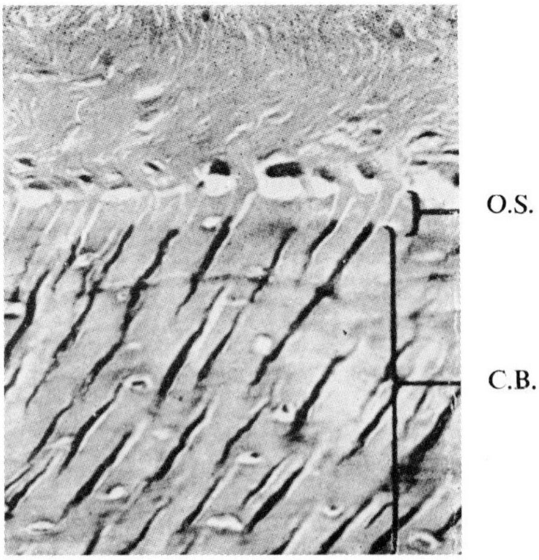

Fig. 244 Sharpey's fibres entering alveolar bone. There is a change in staining as the fibres pass from the uncalcified osteoid layer (O.S.) into the calcified bone (C.B.) ×264. (*By courtesy of Dr J. A. Pedler and the 'Dental Practitioner.'*)

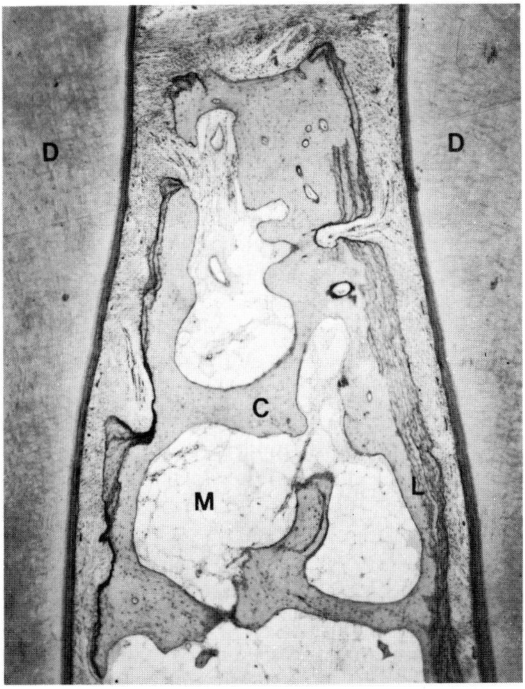

Fig. 245 Vertical section through two adjacent teeth and the interdental bony septum. The interior of the septum is occupied by the trabeculae of the cancellous bone; these surround areas of fatty marrow. In the lamina dura of one socket there are numerous resting lines indicating bone deposition. Adjacent to the other tooth the lamina dura shows resorption areas and reversal lines. These features are present as a result of mesial drift of the teeth. C, cancellous bone; D, dentine; L, lamina dura; M, marrow. × 25. (*By courtesy of Prof R. W. Fearnhead.*)

lamellae surrounding the reticular, vascular tissue of the medullary substance. Between the lamellae are lacunae containing osteocytes.

The trabeculae undergo continual reconstruction through resorption and deposition to meet the changing stresses falling upon them during the development and growth of the dentitions.

Around teeth which have lost their antagonists the cancellous bone of the alveolar process is much reduced although the lamina dura is always intact. Around isolated teeth which have antagonists and those upon which the forces of mastication are excessive the cancellous bone is usually very dense, the trabeculae being numerous and composed of a greater number of lamellae than is normally the case. The cancellous bony tissues enclose irregular marrow spaces which are lined by flattened endosteal cells. During childhood the red marrow is gradually replaced by fatty tissue (yellow marrow) (Fig. 245).

Structure of the mandible. In the lower jaw the alveolar bone is everywhere supported by the body of the mandible (basal bone), the outer and inner alveolar plates of compact bone being continuous with the cortical compact bone of the body of the mandible which forms the outer (buccal) and inner (lingual) surfaces and the lower border. The cortical substance is especially well developed along the lower border, and at the inner and outer surfaces where these are strengthened to form the inner (mylohyoid) and outer (buccinator) oblique ridges (Fig. 242). These ridges bound the retro-molar space behind the last molar tooth and become continuous with the anterior border of the ascending ramus and coronoid process to which the temporal muscle is attached. The thickened lower border of the body of the mandible is continuous with the lower border of the ramus, to which are attached the masseter and medial pterygoid muscles. During the development of the dentition the back part of the alveolar process of the mandible is partly buried in the front of the ascending ramus. This part of the alveolar process, which contains the crypts of the molar teeth prior to their eruption, is the lower alveolar bulb (Fig. 132). After the eruption of the third molar the alveolar bulb becomes filled in with cancellous bone and forms the anterior part of the retro-molar area.

The interior of the body of the mandible is made up of cancellous bone which supports the perforated bony tube of the inferior alveolar canal. Cancellous bone also unites the lamina dura of the tooth sockets to the adjacent cortical bone, forms a thin layer between the cortical bone of the inner and outer surface of the ramus, and supports the cortical bone of the condyle.

Structure of the upper part of the face. In the upper jaw, although the alveolar process is carried by the maxilla in the whole of its extent, the forces of mastication are transmitted to the cranial base along three buttress systems on each side of the face (Fig. 246). At these buttresses the cortical bone is thickened and the cancellous tissue is well developed. Apart from the buttress areas the surface cortical layer of bone in the upper jaw never shows the thickness found in the mandible. In the maxilla the amount of cancellous bone, apart from that found between the tooth sockets, in the hard palate, the maxillary tuberosities, and the facial buttresses, depends upon the size of the maxillary sinus which excavates a large area which would otherwise contain bony trabeculae. Over a great part of the facial, infratemporal, and orbital surfaces of the maxilla only a thin plate of cortical bone separates the mucous membrane of the sinus from adjacent structures.

The anterior buttress of the upper facial skeleton is the frontal process of the maxilla which lies in front of the sinus and forms the lateral boundary of the nasal cavity on each side. Through the anterior buttress the forces of mastication are transmitted from the incisor and canine teeth to the frontal bone.

The middle buttress is formed by the zygomatic process of the maxilla (the key ridge) and the zygomatic bone. Through the zygomatic bone

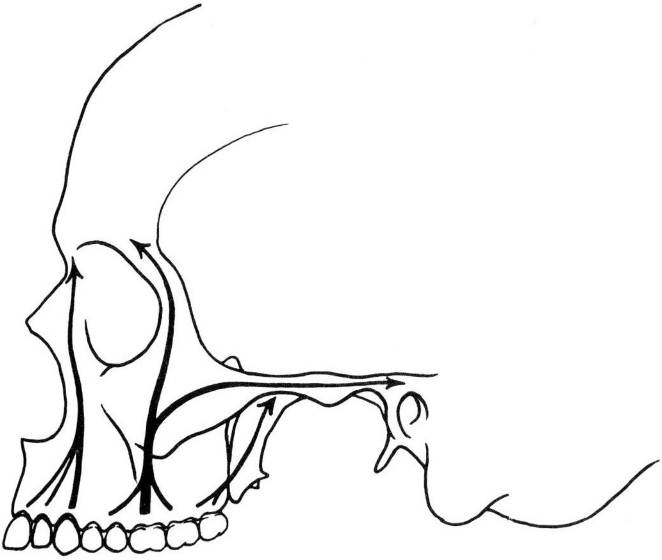

Fig. 246 Diagram showing the facial buttresses. The direction of the thrust from the teeth along the buttresses to the cranial base is shown by arrows. (*After Sicher and Tandler.*)

the forces of mastication, acting on the molar teeth, are transmitted to the frontal bone around the outer surface of the orbital cavity and to the base of the skull along the zygomatic arch.

Behind the maxilla is supported by the pterygoid plates of the sphenoid and the tuberosity of the palatine bone, together making up the posterior buttress.

The arch of the hard palate also greatly strengthens the upper alveolar process. The upper teeth, therefore, are implanted in a body basis formed by the alveolar process and hard palate and this in its turn is attached to the skull base by strong buttresses of bone. This arrangement allows for the large excavations necessary for the nasal cavities, sinuses, and orbital cavities in the upper part of the face, while at the same time establishing a firm base against which the lower jaw can act in the process of mastication.

In the upper jaw the alveolar bulb, which contains one after another the crypts of the developing permanent molars, faces into the pterygopalatine fossa (Fig. 133) but is quite free of any contact with the pterygoid plates. After the eruption of the third molars the remains of the alveolar bulb become filled in with cancellous bone forming the maxillary tuberosity. In old age the tuberosity may become partly invaded by the maxillary sinus.

CHANGES IN THE ALVEOLAR BONE DURING TOOTH ERUPTION AND MIGRATION

As the teeth erupt and their roots develop the alveolar cavities and crypts in which they lie are replaced by sockets. At the same time the dental follicles are reorganised to form the periodontal membranes (see p. 272). These processes involve a reconstruction of the bony tissue adjacent to the teeth, which is especially marked in the case of multi-rooted teeth.

Superficially to the developing and erupting permanent teeth, the bone between the roof of each crypt and the alveolar margin is resorbed along the line of the gubernacular canal. Meanwhile the floor of the crypt is filled in from below as the newly deposited bone adapts itself to developing roots of the erupting teeth. A breakdown in the proper balance between bone resorption and deposition results in the growing teeth becoming trapped and distorted in their cryps. Such a condition occurs in cleidocranial dysostosis in which the teeth are delayed in their eruption and their roots are bent and often stunted.

Throughout childhood the alveolar bone (alveolar processes) of both jaws grows in vertical height so as to 'fill in' the space created by the downward growth of the mandible relative to the cranial base and the upper facial skeleton. In this way the functional teeth are maintained in occlusion. The alveolar processes also grow forward and outward during childhood as a result of bone deposition on their facial surfaces. During adult life in fully functional dentitions in which there is attrition of the occlusal surfaces and incisive edges of the teeth, growth at the alveolar margins assists in maintaining the normal height of the masticatory region of the face.

During the period of facial growth there is a reconstruction of the socket and crypts in relation to the forward and outward migration of the teeth, which involves a resorption of the lamina dura adjacent to their mesio-buccal surfaces. The process of resorption is, however, not continuous, and during the rest periods the normal thickness of the lamina dura is regained. On the other surfaces of the tooth sockets and crypts, including the floors of these cavities, bone deposition maintains the normal thickness of the periodontal or perifollicular space. The new bone is laid down in lamellae which run parallel to the surfaces of the crypts and sockets, or as bundle bone where periodontal fibres are actually attached. These parallel lamellae are replaced at a deeper level by Haversian systems (Fig. 247) but remains of the parallel lamellae, or of bundle bone, are often found among the Haversian systems and indicate the former position of crypt and socket surfaces. At a deeper level still the Haversian systems are replaced by cancellous bone. Bone deposition and internal reconstruction, like bone resorption, are intermittent processes so that throughout the period of facial growth the teeth move, the periodontal attachment is maintained, the

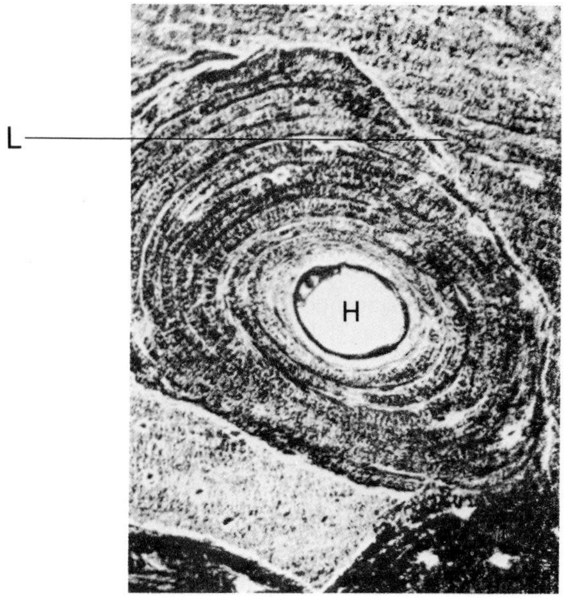

Fig. 247 Haversian system showing the constituent circular lamellae. In the upper right-hand quadrant of the system resorption has taken place and here a reversal line appears. The section is stained with silver to show the fibres in the lamellae. The cement-lines are unstained. H. Haversian canal; L. circular lamellae. ×264. (*By courtesy of Dr J. A. Pedler and the 'Dental Practitioner.'*)

sockets and crypts are reconstructed, and the lamina dura remains intact.

Evidence of these alternating phases of bone deposition, quiescence, and resorption may be seen histologically in both lamina dura and the individual trabeculae of the cancellous bone. The periods of quiescence are represented by cement lines which stain differently from the surrounding bone (Fig. 245). Successive increments of bone are separated by regular cement lines which are usually parallel to each other; these are referred to as resting lines. In distinction to these, other lines of irregular outline made up of a series of concavities, Howship's lacunae, are to be found. These are known as reversal lines as they represent the limit of a phase of bone resorption on which fresh bone deposition has occurred (Fig. 247).

Clinical considerations. In fractures of the jaws the alveolar bone is usually involved with tearing of the attached gum. Functional teeth may be loosened or lost when fracture lines involve the tooth sockets, and teeth developing in their crypts may be damaged. Abscesses commencing from teeth with infected pulps develop in the alveolar bone (see p. 283), and may form extensive sinus tracks within the bone. Neoplasms (epitheliomas and sarcomas) may develop from parts of the oral epithelium, from remains of the dental epithelium, from remains of primary or secondary cartilages, or from the mucous membrane of the nasal cavity or maxillary sinuses and invade the jaws, including the alveolar bone. Areas of necrosis involving alveolar bone may develop in poorly nourished children following sepsis resulting from oral infections, and in operations or compound and multiple fractures. The alveolar bone is early involved in periodontal disease with destruction of the tooth sockets beneath the infected gums.

The alvolar bone, gum (gingiva), epithelial attachment, periodontal membrane, and cement together make up the supporting structures of the teeth which are sometimes grouped together as a functional and clinical unit—the periodontium (p. 43)—and it is these tissues which are involved in parodontal disease.

BIBLIOGRAPHY

Bourne, G. H. (1972). *The Biochemistry and Physiology of Bone*. 2nd ed. New York: Academic Press.

Boyde, A. & Hobdell, M. H. (1969). Scanning electron microscopy of lamellar bone. *Z. Zelforsch.* **93**, 213.

Manson, J. D. (1963). The lamina dura. *Oral Surg.* **16**, 432.

Moore, W. J. (1975). Bone growth and remodelling. In—*Applied Physiology of the Mouth*. Ed. Lavelle, C. L. B. Bristol: Wright.

Parfitt, G. J. (1962). An investigation of the normal variations in alveolar bone trabeculation. *Oral Surg.* **15**, 1453.

Ritchey, B. & Orban, B. (1953). The crests of the interdental alveolar septa. *J. Periodont.* **24**, 75.

Scott, J. H. (1955). Basal and alveolar bone. *Dent. Practit.* **5**, 381.

Scott, J. H. (1968). The development, structure and functions of alveolar bone. *Dent. Practit.* **19**, 19.

Simpson, H. E. (1969). The healing of extraction wounds. *Brit. dent. J.* **127**, 550.

17. The Mucous Membrane of the Mouth and Related Structures

Over the margin of the lips the oral mucous membrane is connected to the skin covering the outer surface of the lips by a transitional zone, the red or vermilion border of the lips. The lamina propria of this zone shows prominent dermal papillae which penetrate well into the covering epithelium so that the blood in the papillary vessels gives the red colour to the area. Unlike the mucous membrane of the inner aspect of the lips the transitional zone shows some degree of keratinisation. As there is a virtual absence of glands related to the epithelium of the transitional zone the surface tends to become dry unless moistened by saliva.

Within the mouth the oral mucous membrane surrounds the necks of the teeth and provides the covering for both the vestibule and the mouth cavity proper. At the bottom of the vestibular sulcus the mucosa is reflected from the alveolar processes of the upper and lower jaws to the lips and cheeks. In the mid line of the upper and lower jaws is a fold of mucous membrane, the frenum or frenulum, which connects the lip to the gum. On the cheek opposite the upper second permanent molar is a papilla which marks the opening of the duct of the parotid gland.

Inside the mouth cavity proper the mucous membrane covering the alveolar process of the lower jaw is reflected to form the covering of the floor of the mouth and then covers the inferior surface and the dorsum of the tongue. In the median plane a fold of mucosa, the frenulum of the tongue connects the anterior part of the inferior surface of the tongue to the floor of the mouth. On either side of the frenulum is a small papillary elevation, the sublingual papilla, which shows the opening of the duct of the submandibular salivary gland on its summit. Stretching in a backward direction from the sublingual papilla between the tongue and gums is a ridge of mucous membrane, the sublingual fold. This is produced by the underlying sublingual salivary gland and it carries the numerous minute openings of the ducts of the gland. The mucous membrane of the lingual gingivae in the upper jaw is continuous with that covering the hard and soft palate, which form the roof of the mouth cavity.

The oral mucous membrane, like the skin, is composed of a surface epithelium and a deeper connective tissue layer, the lamina propria or corium (Fig. 248). The epithelial layer is of either ectodermal or endodermal origin, depending on its relation to the oral membrane in embryonic life. The lamina propria is of mesodermal origin. The

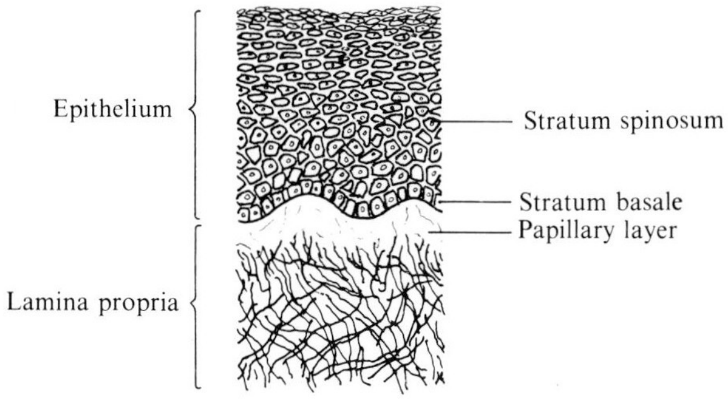

Fig. 248 Diagrammatic representation of a section through an area of oral mucous membrane showing its basic layers.

epithelium of the oral mucosa, however, is lubricated and protected by the secretion of mucus and it is this feature which gives rise to the term mucous membrane. In the case of oral mucosa the mucus is produced either by small glands which lie immediately deep to the mucous membrane in the submucosa or by the large submandibular and sublingual glands which are placed some distance from the mucosa. Mucus is a combination of the glycoprotein, mucin, and water.

There are two major functions which are common to all parts of the oral mucosa. These are the protection of the underlying tissues from harmful environmental agents and the reception and passage of various kinds of sensory information.

Though the oral mucous membrane has this basic structure and functions in all parts of the mouth cavity, yet it is modified in certain regions

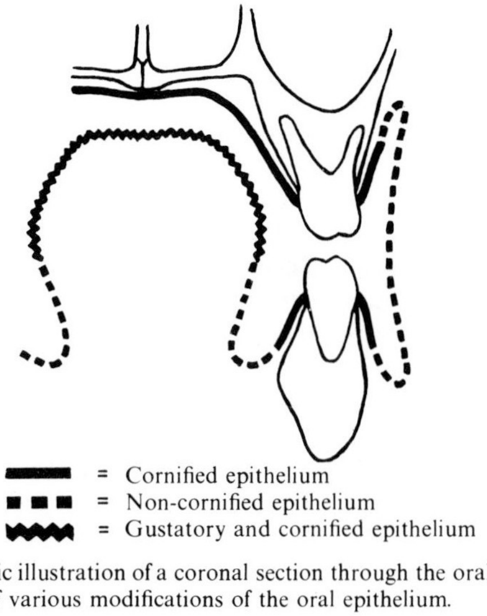

Fig. 249 Diagrammatic illustration of a coronal section through the oral cavity to show the respective areas of various modifications of the oral epithelium.

in accordance with a more localised function. (Fig. 249). Thus, in the region of the gums and hard palate, it may be described as a masticatory or cornified mucosa since it is adapted to meet the friction produced in mastication (Fig. 250). Over the cheeks, lips, soft palate, floor of the mouth, and under-surface of the tongue, where the mucous membrane is less exposed to mastication, it is a more simple lining mucosa. The mucous membrane on the dorsum of the body of the tongue shares the characteristics of a gustatory and a masticatory mucosa. The oral mucosa may be further modified by the presence or absence of a submucous layer; this largely determines the firmness or looseness of its attachment to the underlying bone or muscles.

The oral epithelium. The epithelium is of the stratified squamous variety and is separated by a basal lamina from the underlying lamina

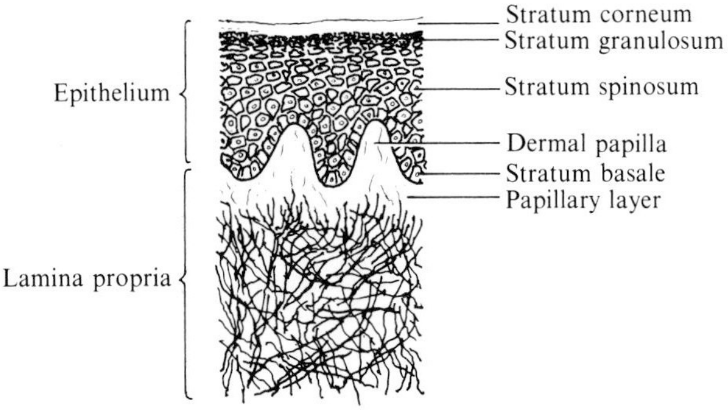

Fig. 250 Diagrammatic representation of a section through an area of cornified (keratinised) oral mucous membrane, and showing its constituent layers.

propria (Fig. 251). In electron micrographs the basal lamina consists of an amorphous moderately dense layer, about 330–600 Å thick, the lamina densa, and separated from the cell membranes of the epithelium by an interval of 400–450 Å, the lamina lucida (Fig. 252). As in the skin, several distinct layers may be distinguished in the epithelium. The cells lying directly upon the basal lamina are cuboidal or low columnar and are known as the stratum basale; since much of the cell division responsible for the more superficial cells takes place in this layer they are often described as the stratum germinativum. Immediately above this single layer of cells there are several layers of somewhat larger polyhedral cells; some cell division takes place in these layers. The cells are separated from each other by an intercellular space but are connected across this by intercellular bridges or processes (Fig. 253). The presence of an acid mucopolysaccharide, possibly chondroitin sulphate B, has been demonstrated in the intercellular spaces, and this substance acts as an intercellular cement. The processes, which are readily seen, give these cells a characteristic 'prickly' or 'spiny' appearance, and this is expressed in the name given to the layer, the stratum spinosum (Fig. 253). With the

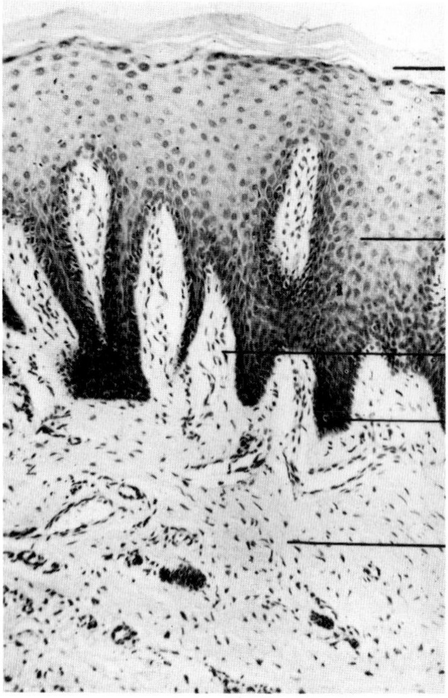

Fig. 251 Oral mucous membrane. Two of the dermal papillae in this section have been cut tangentially so that they appear surrounded by the epithelial layer. × 110.

electron microscope each intercellular process is seen to be composed of narrow cytoplasmic extensions which arise from adjacent cells and are closely applied to each other. These cytoplasmic extensions are well supplied with desmosomes, to which thick bundles of tonofilaments are attached (Fig. 254).

Overlying the stratum spinosum the epithelial cells may be arranged in two further layers, the stratum granulosum and the stratum lucidum. The stratum lucidum is, however, absent or poorly developed in the mouth cavity. The stratum granulosum is composed of flattened cells, two or three thick; these contain the granules of kerato-hyaline which give this layer its name. On the gums, hard palate, and dorsal surface of the body of the tongue an additional layer, the stratum corneum, is found superficially. This layer is structureless, the individual cell outlines and the nuclei having disappeared. Keratinisation, the formation of a stratum corneum, commences before birth on the vestibular and lingual aspects of the alveolar ridges. As these are not regions of masticatory stress it would appear that the process is genetically determined.

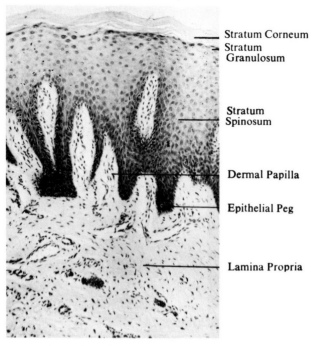

As the cells of the oral epithelium age and pass more superficially, so they become flattened and show considerable changes in organisation which in areas where a stratum corneum is produced lead to a

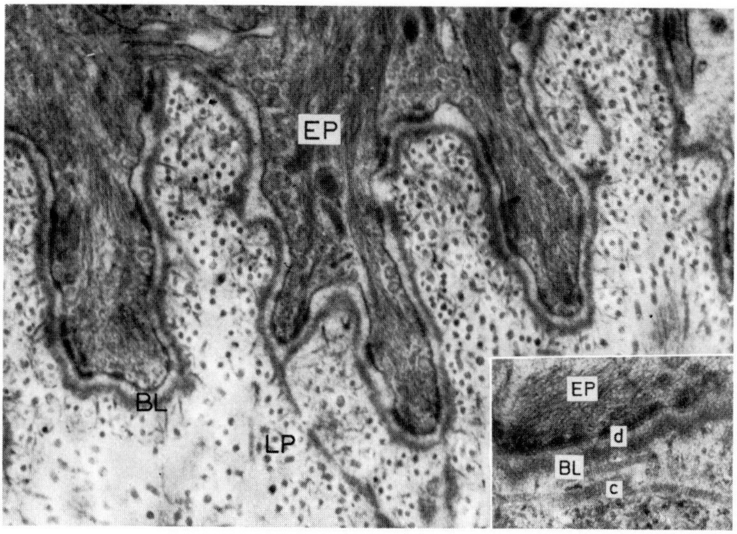

Fig. 252 Epithelium-connective tissue junction. Note amorphous basal lamina (BL) separating oral epithelial cells (EP) from the underlying lamina propria (LP). Original magnification ×35000. *Insert.*—Higher magnification of basal lamina area. EP, Epithelial cell; d, modified desmosome, or hemidesmosome; BL, basal lamina; C, collagen fibrils. Original magnification ×60000. (*By courtesy of Dr M. A. Listgarten and Amer. J. Anat.*)

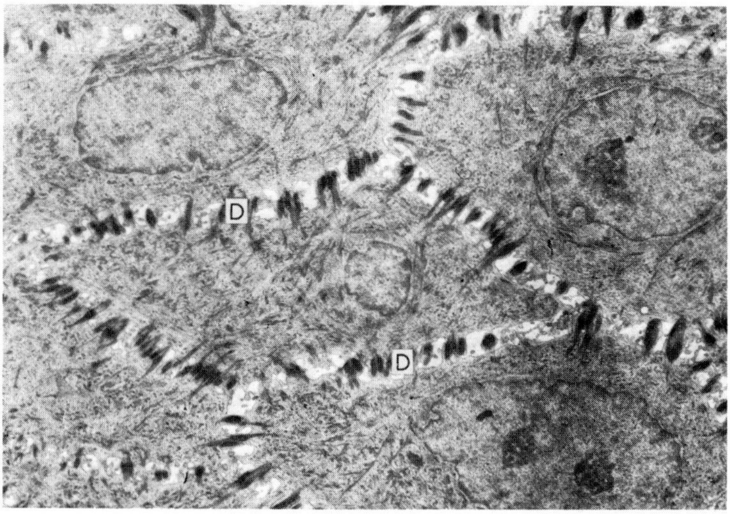

Fig. 253 Cells of stratum spinosum. Note the large number of desmosomes (D). Original magnification ×5800. (*By courtesy of Dr M. A. Listgarten and Amer. J. Anat.*)

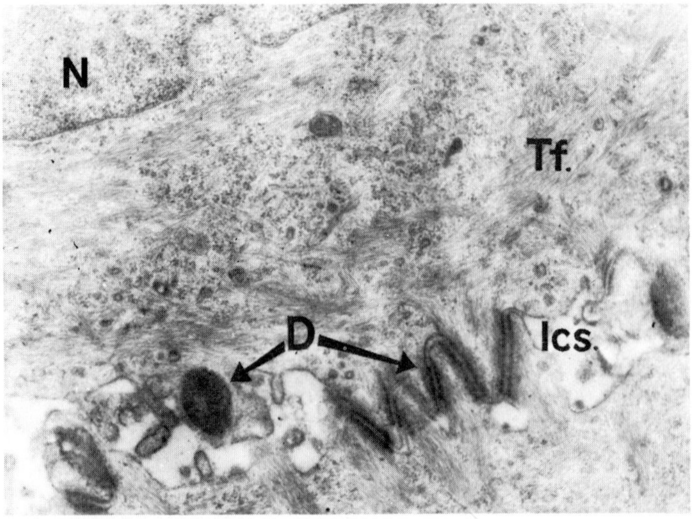

Fig. 254 Detail of cell in the stratum spinosum. Note the fibrillar nature of the cytoplasm. N. nucleus; Tf. tonofilaments; D. desmosomes cut in different planes; Ics. intercellular space. Original magnification ×26000. (*By courtesy of Dr M. A. Listgarten and Amer. J. Anat.*)

complete loss of cellular structure (see p. 170). The most superficial cells of the stratum spinosum show flattening, as do the cells of the stratum granulosum; and the surface cells of this layer have pyknotic nuclei. The surface cells are shed into the mouth cavity or form the stratum corneum where this exists. The desquamation of the surface cells may be related to alterations in the structure of the desmosomal attachments which occur in the more superficial layers of cells. The degenerated cells are normally washed away by the secretions of the salivary and mucous glands. In conditions of ill health where the glandular secretions are reduced the dead cells form part of the white 'coat' found on the tongue and around the necks of the teeth.

Keratinisation, the development of a surface horny layer (the stratum corneum), occurs on the surface of the gums and over the hard palate in healthy mouths in which the function of mastication is well developed. The absence or poor development of a stratum corneum, especially in the epithelium of the lips, cheeks, and floor of the mouth, gives the red colour to the oral mucous membrane as the deeper epithelial layers are more transparent and the vascular tissue of the lamina propria shows through them. The intercellular spaces which exist in the stratum spinosum and the deeper layers of the stratum granulosum allow a circulation of tissue fluid. The more superficial cells of the latter layer are closely arranged so that no tissue fluid can pass through this layer to the surface or to an overlying stratum corneum.

There is considerable variation in the rate of shedding of cells from the surface of the oral epithelium in different parts of the mouth cavity and a corresponding variation in the rate of replacement of the cells in the germinative layers. The replacement rate in non-keratinised areas is much quicker than in keratinised regions. The oral epithelium shows a faster turnover than the epidermis of the skin and a slower rate than the epithelium of the intestinal tract.

In addition to the ordinary cells a distinct cell form is found in the oral epithelium apart from that of the tongue. These cells are concerned in pigment production and are chiefly found in the more basal layers of the epithelium. They are generally larger than the ordinary epithelial cells, but can only be seen, however, with special staining methods. Long, slender branching processes pass out from them and ramify in the intercellular spaces amongst the other epithelial cells. These branching cells have been given a variety of names, but melanocyte and dendritic cell are most commonly used. The term melanocyte refers to the pigment, melanin, which is produced by these cells and is subsequently passed on to the other epithelial cells in which it is stored. The oral melanocytes are exactly similar to the melanocytes which occur in the epidermis of the skin. It has been shown that these latter cells are of neural crest origin.

In the more superficial parts of the oral epithelium dendritic cells are present which do not have the ability to form melanin and these are often called Langerhans cells. The so-called 'clear' cells that are to be seen in the oral epithelium have been identified with these non-melanin producing dendritic cells. The relationship between the basal melanocytes and the high-level non-melanin producing cells is not clear.

In the basal parts of the oral epithelium other 'clear' cells are found. These are not dendritic and are known as Merkel cells. A nerve fibre is often found close to the Merkel cell and this association supports the concept that these cells act as touch receptors.

The lamina propria. The lamina propria, corium, or 'dermis' is a layer of dense connective tissue made up largely of bundles of collagen fibres and the fibroblasts and fibrocytes related to them. It is everywhere permeated by an amorphous ground substance which also contains some elastic fibres, blood vessels, lymphatics, and sensory nerve fibres and their endings. In addition there are various kinds of defence cells, such as histiocytes, undifferentiated mesenchyme cells, mast cells, and cells derived from some form of leucocyte and associated with inflammatory reaction.

The connective tissue of the lamina propria provides most of the mechanical properties of the oral mucosa. The number and arrangement of the collagen fibres determines the resistance of the mucosa to deformation and the degree to which it is extensible. The elastic fibres bring about the return of the mucosa to normal after the collagen fibres have been extended.

Immediately below the oral epithelium is a layer of fine fibres which constitutes the papillary layer (Figs. 248, 250). Elsewhere in the corium the fibres are much coarser.

The lamina propria of the mucosa lining the inner surfaces of the lips and cheeks, the soft palate, the floor of the mouth, and the inferior surface of the tongue is thin. In most areas of the mouth the junction between the epithelium and the lamina propria is not smooth and regular, but is thrown up into folds so that in most sections numerous finger-like processes of the lamina propria, the dermal papillae, interdigitate with what would appear to be similar processes of the epithelium, the epithelial pegs (Figs. 251, 252). Actually the epithelial pegs are not finger-like processes but form a series of interconnecting ridges. In this manner the surface of contact between lamina propria and epithelium is increased, allowing a greater opportunity for the passage of nutritive material from the blood vessels of the lamina propria to the non-vascular epithelium. The numbers and height of the epithelial ridges and the dermal papillae are greater in areas of masticatory mucosa compared with lining mucosa. The dermal papillae contain a subepithelial capillary network, and the terminations of the nerve fibres of the lamina propria.

The sensory nerve endings found in the oral mucosa may be either free nerve terminations or may have a coiled form, varying in degree of complexity(Fig. 255). The latter have been classified as simple, complex, and compound forms. Most of the various endings lie beneath and close to the epithelium of the mucosa, but some free nerve terminations penetrate between the basal epithelial cells, and a few pass more superficially. The anterior part of the oral cavity is most plentifully supplied with nerve endings of all kinds. Nerve fibres frequently converge towards groups of endings from several directions; this arrangement may serve as the structural basis for accurate sensory discriminations.

The submucous layer. A submucous layer is present in certain regions of the mouth cavity (Fig. 256). It is a fat containing connective tissue layer of varying thickness, but much more loosely constructed than the lamina propria. It contains the larger arteries from which arise the smaller branches which run in the lamina propria, and the larger veins into which the venules drain. The larger nerve fibres for the mucous membrane run in the submucosa. Mucous glands are present whose ducts penetrate the overlying mucous membrane to open in the mouth cavity. There is a well-marked submucous layer present in the floor of the mouth and at the fornices of the vestibule; and beneath the mucosa covering the alveolar bone between the fornices of the vestibule and the gum tissue (gingivae) there is also a definite though thinner submucosa. Here the mucosa is loosely attached to the underlying tissues. Elsewhere the lamina propria of the oral mucous membrane is bound down to the underlying bone (gums and hard palate) or to adjacent muscles (lips, cheeks, soft palate, and tongue).

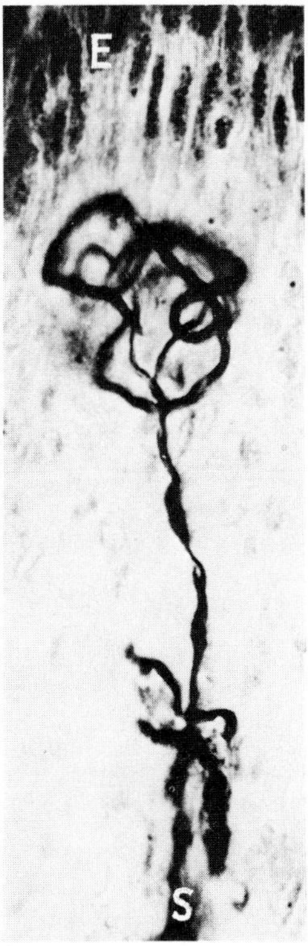

Fig. 255 Coiled nerve ending in the human palate. S. stem axon; E. epithelial cells. Silver impregnation method. ×430. (*By courtesy of Prof A. D. Dixon and the 'Archives of Oral Biology'.*)

The gingivae and the alveolar mucosa. The mucous membrane related to the teeth and the alveolar bone is divided into the gingival and the alveolar mucosa. The gingivae or gums surround the necks of the teeth and cover the adjacent part of the alveolar bone; the alveolar mucosa covers the rest of the alveolar bone beyond the gingivae (Fig. 257). The two parts are separated by a scalloped line called the muco-gingival, or alveolo-gingival junction, except on the palate where the gingival mucosa merges imperceptibly with the rest of the mucous membrane.

In a general way the gingival margin follows the contour of the cervical margins of the teeth, though at a different level. The level depends on the age of the individual; in the young adult it is placed coronally. Apart from its marginal area, the gingival mucous membrane is firmly and directly attached to the underlying bone and necks of the teeth (Fig. 258). The distance from the base of the epithelial attachment to the crest of the alveolar bone remains fairly constant during life. The length of the epithelial attachment is much less constant than this region

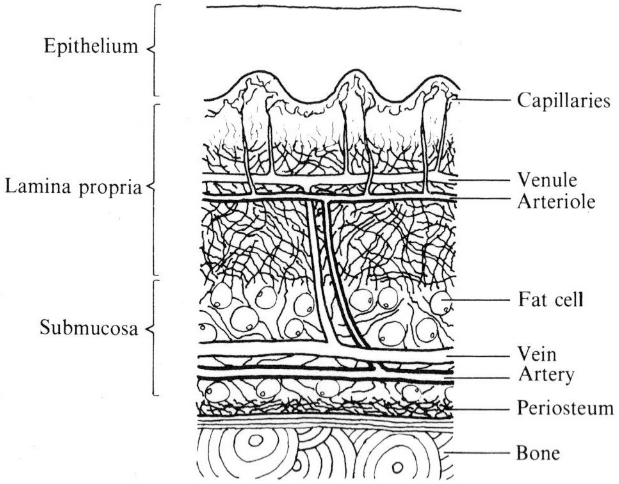

Fig. 256 Diagrammatic representation of a section through an area of oral mucous membrane where there is an underlying submucosa. The vascular supply for the mucous membrane is shown.

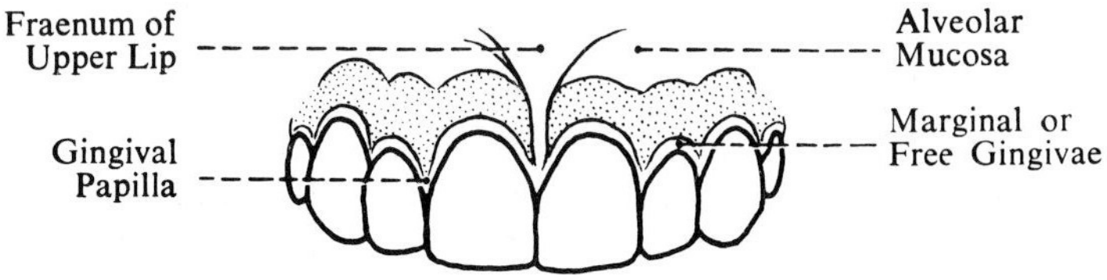

Fig. 257 Diagram to show the arrangement of the gingival mucosa. The attached area of the gingival mucosa is shown stippled.

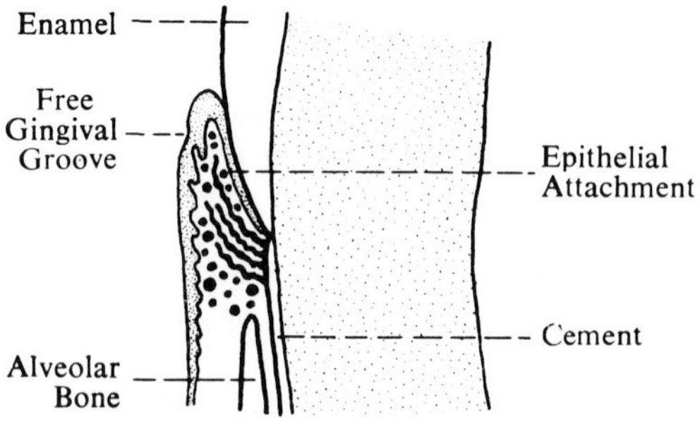

Fig. 258 Diagram to show the arrangement of the parodontal tissues at the cervical region of a tooth. Only the radial and circular gingival fibres of the periodontal membrane are indicated.

which may be described as the connective tissue attachment. The marginal or free gingiva is marked off from the attached gingivae by a shallow groove, the free gingival groove (Fig. 258). This groove is about 1 to 1·5 mm from the actual gingival margin and follows its contour both labially and lingually. Sometimes the free gingival groove is imperceptible. The actual margin of the gingivae is known as the gingival crest and here the gingival epithelium forms the outer boundary of the gingival crevice or sulcus. The surface of the marginal gingiva is smooth. At the bottom of the gingival crevice the gingival epithelium becomes continuous with that of the epithelial attachment or junctional epithelium (Fig. 258). The latter shows only shallow epithelial ridges; the junction with the underlying lamina propria, as seen in section, is smooth and regular.

Anastomosis between the periodontal blood vessels and those of the gingivae takes place in the tissue coronal to the alveolar crest. From this region looped capillaries with coiled arterial parts arise and are situated close to the epithelial attachment. These are of greater calibre than those found more apically in the periodontal membrane. The coiled arterial part of the capillaries encircles a thick venous limb and finally drains into it. It is probable that these vessels are related to the nutritive requirements of the tissues at the dento-gingival junction. The capillary loops related to the epithelium covering the external surface of the gingival tissue consist of straight slender loops with arterial and venous limbs of equal length (Fig. 238).

Between the adjacent, approximal surfaces of the teeth the interdental gingival tissue connects the lingual with the labial or buccal gingivae, and here the marginal gingiva takes the form of a wedge-shaped process, usually known as the interdental papilla. The height of the interdental tissue depends on that of the particular interdental space. Deep to the interdental gingival tissue are the transeptal fibres of the periodontal membrane and then the crest of the interdental septum of bone (Fig. 235). Groups of fibres, the alveolo-gingival fibres, arise from the crest of the interdental septum and radiate into the adjacent connective tissue of the free and attached gingivae. Immediately beneath the contact area the height of the so-called interdental papilla is less than that found lingually and labially or bucally (Fig. 259). There is thus a central depression between two peaks, one lingual and the other labial or buccal; because of this the interdental gingival tissue has been compared to the mountainous feature known as a col.

Unlike the marginal gingiva the rest of the gingival mucosa has a stippled surface. The stippled appearance is due to the attachment of collagen fibres to the basement membrane between the epithelial ridges. The disappearance of this characteristic is often the first indication of the presence of gingivitis. The lamina propria of the attached or stippled gingiva merges into the periosteum of the alveolar bone; the mucous membrane here forms a mucoperiosteum. The lamina propria gains its attachments to the teeth through the gingival fibres of the periodontal membrane. In addition to the radially arranged fibres there are others in the lamina propria which run circularly to each tooth (Fig. 258). Both groups of fibres assist in maintaining the gingivae in close relationship to the teeth and in supporting the epithelial attachment.

The gingival mucosa is firm and dense, and in it the epithelial ridges and dermal papillae are pronounced. It is commonly stated that the gingivae are keratinised and this is probably the ideal condition. Actually, however, in a large number of individuals the gingival epithelium

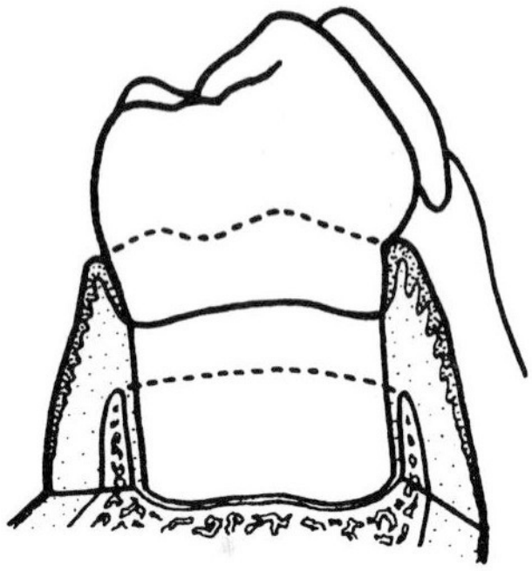

Fig. 259 Diagrammatic illustration of a lower tooth with the parodontal tissues cut away to show the relationship of the alveolar bone and the interdental gingival tissue. The margins of the interdental bony septum and the interdental gingival tissue are indicated in broken line. Note that the interdental gingiva shows a buccal and a lingual papilla and dips beneath the contact area.

show no keratinisation or an incomplete keratinisation. In the latter case though the cells of the surface layer have lost their boundaries their nuclei remain and are very flattened and pyknotic; the condition is known as parakeratosis.

The alveolar mucous membrane is different in structure and attachment from the gingivae and may easily be distinguished in the living subject from the gingivae by the difference in colour; the normal gingivae are pink, whereas the alveolar mucosa is red. The alveolar mucous membrane is thin, has no stratum corneum, the epithelial pegs and dermal papillae are absent or poorly developed. Due to the presence of a submucous layer the alveolar mucosa is not so firmly attached to the underlying bone.

The epithelial attachment. The adherence of the gingival tissue to the teeth is provided not only by the attachment of its connective tissue to the cervical part of the roots of the teeth but also by a layer of cells which is known as the epithelial attachment or junctional epithelium. This layer, together with the gingival epithelium, serves to cover and protect the underlying gingival connective tissue, the periodontal membrane, the root of the tooth and the crest of the alveolar bone. In providing the actual seal for the union between the teeth and the gingivae the epithelial attachment has a key role to play. This is a unique situation in the body in that hard, mineralised structures, the teeth, protrude through the surface integument of the body.

Since the epithelial attachment or junctional epithelium is derived from the reduced enamel epithelium which covers the crown of the erupting teeth it differs in its origin and constitution from the rest of the epithelial layer covering the gingival tissue, which is a part of the oral epithelium (Fig. 100).

Unlike the latter it does not keratinise, and as it has certain mechanical weaknesses it represents a region where pathological changes may be initiated due to the penetration of foreign elements. This is particularly the case in the interdental regions where the epithelial covering of the interdental gingival tissue is produced by the meeting and fusion of the reduced enamel epithelium related to the approximal surfaces of two adjacent teeth. In a well formed and regular dental arch the junctional epithelium is protected by the convexities of the crowns of the teeth and on their labial, buccal and lingual aspects by the adjacent keratinised or parakeratinised epithelium of the gingival margin.

The junctional epithelium is a layer of stratified epithelium of about 12 to 18 cells thick, though at its apical or cervical margin it may be only two or three cells thick. In the young healthy adult it extends from the enamel-cement junction some distance, usually about 2–3 mm, coronally over the enamel surface and meets and fuses with the gingival epithelium at the base of the gingival sulcus (Fig. 258). In cases of gingival recession its cervical margin proliferates rootward and the junctional epithelium becomes related to the cement in part, or wholly in extreme cases (Fig. 102).

Some authorities distinguish the zone of epithelium lining the gingival sulcus as the sulcular epithelium, intervening between junctional epithelium and the oral epithelium at the gingival crest.

The junctional epithelium is composed of two layers, a basal layer adjacent to the gingival connective tissue and a supra-basal layer nearer the tooth. The single row of cells of the basal layer are cuboidal or slightly flattened. The cells of the supra-basal layer are flattened and are arranged parallel to the enamel surface. Compared with the oral epithelium there are few desmosomal interconnections between the cells of the junctional epithelium.

The junctional epithelium is connected to the underlying connective tissue of the gingiva by a basal lamina and hemidesmosomes similar to the arrangement found in the oral mucosa between the epithelial layer and the lamina propria. On the enamel surface the plasma membranes of the epithelial cells show hemidesmosomes and a layer similar to a basal lamina is present between the cells and the enamel. Sometimes the basal lamina is related to cuticular structures interposed between it and the surface of the enamel. At present there is doubt as to the origin of these cuticles. The alternative suggestions have been: either they are produced by the cells of the epithelial attachment, or are derived from organic constituents of the saliva or tissue fluid, or may represent denatured haemoglobin derived from compressed and degenerated erythrocytes which have resulted from local haemorrhage.

The cells of the junctional epithelium show many of the characteristics of actively protein and polysaccharide secreting cells in their large cisternae of endoplasmic reticulum and prominent Golgi complexes. Especially below the gingival crevice the cells of the junctional epithelium show a considerable concentration of lysosomal elements. They possess only a few bundles of cytoplasmic filaments compared with keratinising cells such as those of the oral epithelium.

The abundant content of organelles shown by the cells of the junctional epithelium is concerned with the constant reformation of the hemidesmosomes and basal laminae on its enamel and connective tissue aspects. The small amount of cytoplasmic filaments results in a lack of rigidity of the cells. The junctional epithelium proliferates rapidly and has a rapid turnover rate. The desquamating cells that result are shed at its coronal end into the gingival sulcus. The cells of the junctional epithelium approach the gingival sulcus in a vertical arrangement and so, together with their lack of rigidity, form a mechanically weak zone in the gingival tissues where foreign bodies may be intruded (Fig. 104). Leucocyte emigration around the teeth takes place preferentially through the junctional epithelium. As a result of the combination of these features the junctional epithelium or epithelial attachment constitutes a rather weak zone of rapidly permeable epithelium which allows the movement of molecular or cellular bodies from either oral cavity into the parodontal tissues or in the reverse direction; yet due to its proliferative activity this epithelium possesses considerable powers of repair and renewal.

The hard palate. The mucous membrane covering the hard palate has everywhere a stratum corneum. Peripherally the gingival part of the mucosa is in the form of a mucoperiosteum. Along the midline of the palate also there is no submucous layer, for here the lamina propria is directly attached to the bone, forming the so called palatal raphe, which runs posteriorly from the incisive papilla (Fig. 260). Immediately behind the incisor and canine teeth the mucous membrane has a thick lamina propria and is firmly attached to the underlying bone. In the region of the molar teeth on each side there is an area between the papatal raphe and the gingival mucosa where a submucous layer is present (Fig. 261). Here the greater palatal vessels and nerves run forward from the greater palatine foramen, and numerous mucous glands are to be found. Though a submucosa is present in this part of the hard palate, the mucous membrane is not loose as elsewhere in the mouth cavity where a submucosa exists, for here the lamina propria is attached

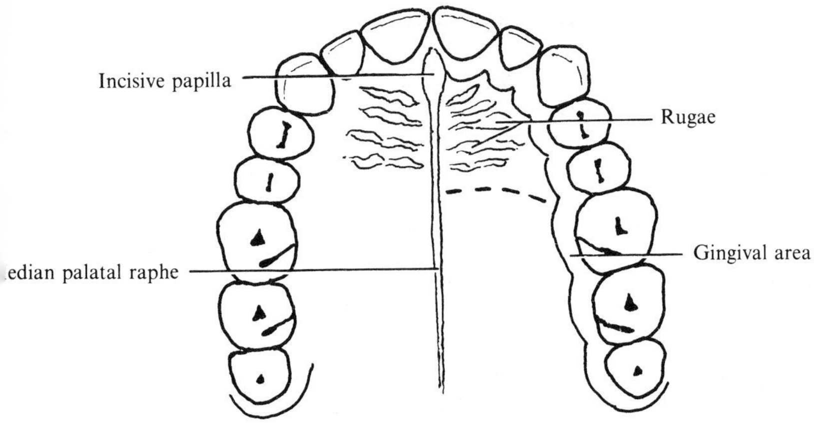

Fig. 260 Diagrammatic illustration of the hard palate. On one side of the palate a scalloped line indicates the limits of the gingivae. On the same side a broken line shows the posterior limit of the anterior area where the mucous membrane of the hard palate is in the form of a mucoperiosteum.

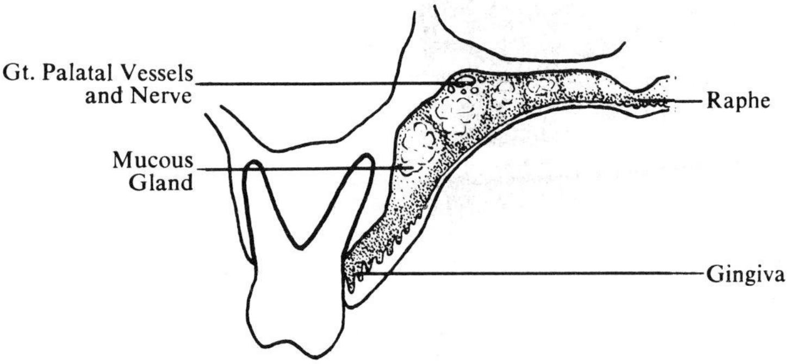

Fig. 261 Diagrammatic illustration of the structure of the hard palate in the region of the first upper molar. The fibrous strands which pass through the submucosa and connect the lamina propria to the underlying bone are shown.

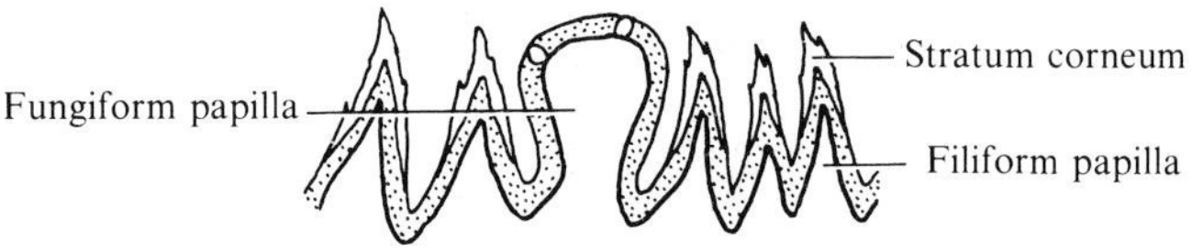

Fig. 262 Diagrammatic representation of a section through the epithelium of the anterior two-thirds of the tongue showing filiform and fungiform papillae. Two taste buds are shown in the epithelium of the fungiform papilla.

to the periosteum of the bone by fibrous strands which pass through the submucous layer.

The palatine ridges or rugae form transverse elevations on the anterior part of the hard palate (Fig. 260), and consist of a core of connective tissue covered by epithelium. In man they vary greatly in number (two to eight on each side), in form, and in size. They appear early in fetal life (about 20–30 mm C.R. stage) and apart from growth in size and in the spacing between them do not alter during life (Fig. 90). Their relation to the teeth varies, the last ridge is usually related to the first or second molar in the permanent dentition. They are much better developed in some other mammals, especially in the ungulates, and in the whalebone whales they give origin to the characteristic baleen plates. When well developed they assist in grasping the nipple during suckling and in the adult assist in mastication. It has been shown that some of the ridges found on the palate of the rat contain numerous touch corpuscles and also taste corpuscles, so that tongue and palate together can act as 'oral fingers' in tactile analysis of the food and other objects brought into the mouth cavity.

The soft palate. The epithelium covering the lower or oral surface of the soft palate is continuous with that of the hard palate and is of the stratified squamous type; that covering the upper or nasal surface is a ciliated columnar epithelium. The lamina propria on both surfaces is attached to the adjacent musculature except in the region of the palatal mucous glands which lie in a submucosa between the mucous membrane and the more deeply placed muscle tissue. The junction between the hard and soft palate is often indicated by a slight transverse crease, and by a change in colour from the paler mucosa of the hard palate to the deeper colour of the soft palate.

The tongue. The dorsal surface of the tongue is divided into a large anterior part and a much smaller posterior part by a v-shaped groove, the sulcus terminalis, the opening of which is directed forward. The mucous membrane covering the anterior part is different in appearance from that covering the posterior part.

The mucous membrane of the anterior part of the dorsal surface is studded with a great number of closely set projections which are called papillae (Figs. 262, 263). These are of three kinds in man; filiform, fungiform, and vallate. The filiform are by far the most numerous and are arranged roughly in rows which run parallel to the v-shaped groove. Each filiform papilla is conical in shape and consists of a central core of connective tissue covered by epithelium. The surface of the papilla is cornified, especially towards its tip. Small secondary papillae may project from the filiform papillae. The filiform papillae provide the masticatory element to the mucosa of the dorsum of the tongue. Between the papillae are areas of non-specialised mucous membrane which permit the marked changes that occur in the shape of the tongue.

The fungiform papillae are found scattered over the mucous mem-

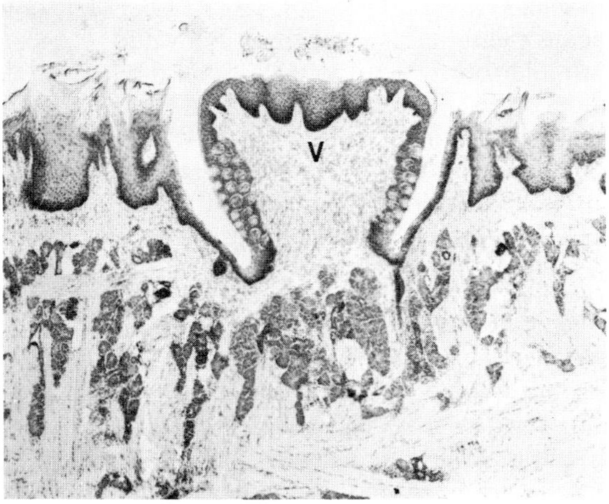

Fig. 263 Section of vallate papilla showing numerous taste buds in the epithelium forming the inner wall of the surrounding groove. On either side of the vallate papilla there are a number of filiform papillae. V, vallate papilla. ×40.

brane, but chiefly towards the tip of the tongue. They are roundish elevations projecting above the general level of the surface. In life they can be readily distinguished as small red spots since the rich blood supply of the connective tissue core shines through the thin non-cornified epithelium. A few taste buds are present in the epithelium of the fungiform papillae.

The vallate papillae are eight to twelve in number and are arranged along but anterior to the v-shaped groove. They are considerably larger than either the filiform or the fungiform papillae, but unlike these do not project above the general level of the mucosa. Each vallate papilla is marked out by a deep circular groove, and in a vertical section has an inverted cone shape (Fig. 263). The epithelium covering the connective tissue core is smooth, and the part which forms the inner wall of the circular groove contains a large number of taste buds; the outer wall may contain a few. Into the bottom of the circular groove open the ducts of small serous glands, the glands of von Ebner, whose secretion washes the groove clear of debris.

Over the posterior part of the tongue the mucous membrane is more smooth and regular. It is, however, slightly raised by a number of round or oval swellings each of which is produced by a mass of lymphoid tissue, known as a lingual follicle. On the surface of each swelling there is a minute opening which leads into a deep epithelial lined pit, the crypt. These masses of lymphoid tissue constitute the lingual tonsil, which forms part of the lymphatic zone between the mouth and nose on the one hand and the pharynx on the other. The lymphatic zone is completed by the tonsils and the pharyngeal lymph tissue (adenoids).

The Retro-molar regions. Behind the last member of the lower dental arch the mucous membrane is firmly bound down to the most posterior part of the alveolar process and to the base of the ramus (retro-molar triangle). In the upper jaw the mucosa is firmly attached to the surface of the alveolar bulb or the maxillary tuberosity extending upwards to a variable extent on their posterior surface. Here the mucosa is in close relationship to the pterygoid hamulus and the tendon of the tensor palati as this enters the soft palate. There may be a few mucous glands in the retro-molar region of each jaw.

Nerve supply and blood supply

The palate area. The sensory nerve supply to the mucous membrane of the hard and soft palate is through branches of the palatine nerves and the nasopalatine nerve. The palatine nerves are branches of the maxillary divisions of the trigeminal nerve given off in the pterygo-palatine fossa and enter the mouth through the greater and lesser palatine foramina at the back of the hard palate. The nasopalatine nerve is also a branch of the maxillary division of the trigeminal nerve and reaches the palate, with its accompany artery, through the incisive foramen. The palatine nerves are accompanied by the palatine arteries which are given off from the third part of the maxillary artery in the pterygoid-palatine fossa. The mucous membrane of the hard palate is neither very sensitive nor very vascular but, as in the scalp, bleeding may be slow to cease as the blood-vessel walls are kept from contracting by the collagenous fibres of the muco-periosteum.

The vestibular area. The blood and nerve supply of the vestibular surface of the upper gums in the region of the premolars and molars is from branches of the superior alveolar (dental) vessels and nerves which pass from the maxillary division of the trigeminal nerve and its infrarobital branch in small canals in the outer wall of the maxillary sinus. They also supply the upper teeth and the mucous membrane of the sinus. The nerves of the vestibular surface of the lower gum are branches of the inferior alveolar (dental) nerve and of the buccal nerve which are given off from the mandibular division of the trigeminal nerve; the vessels for this area are branches of the inferior alveolar (dental) vessels which arise from the first part of the maxillary artery in the pterygoid fossa at the inner surface of the ramus of the mandible. The inferior alveolar (dental) vessels and nerve run within the mandible in the mandibular canal and supply the lower teeth. The nerve supply to the mucous membrane of the upper lip and to the upper gum in the incisor and canine region is from the descending (labial) branches of the infrarorbital nerve through the infraorbital foramen. The blood supply of the upper lip and front part of the gum is from the superior labial branches of the facial artery and the labial branches of the infraorbital artery, which is one of the terminal branches of the maxillary artery. The nerve supply of the lower lip and incisor gum region is from the mental branch of the inferior alveolar (dental) nerve; the blood supply is from the inferior labial branch of the facial artery and from the mental artery, the latter a terminal branch of the inferior alveolar (dental) artery. The sensory nerve supply to the mucous membrane of the cheek is from the buccal branch of the mandibular division of the trigeminal nerve; the blood supply is from branches of the buccal artery, the facial artery, and the posterior superior alveolar (dental) artery.

The sublingual area. The sensory nerve supply to the mucous membrane of the floor of the mouth is through branches of the lingual nerve and its sublingual branch; branches of these nerves also supply the lingual surface of the gum of the lower jaw. The blood supply of the floor of the mouth is from branches of the lingual artery (a branch of the external carotid artery) and from branches of the submental artery, a branch of the facial artery.

The tongue. The sensory nerve supply of the anterior two-thirds of the dorsum of the tongue is through branches of the lingual nerve, a branch of the mandibular division of the trigeminal (fifth cranial) nerve. The nerve supply of the posterior one-third of the dorsum of the tongue is through branches of the glossopharyngeal (ninth cranial) nerve. The nerve fibres from the taste buds of the anterior two-thirds of the tongue pass for part of their course towards the brain in the lingual nerve which they leave in the pterygoid fossa to join the facial (seventh cranial) nerve via the chorda tympani nerve. As part of the seventh cranial nerve these taste fibres enter the midbrain. The nerve fibres from the taste buds on the posterior third of the tongue and on the pillars of the fauces pass to the brain stem along the glossopharyngeal (ninth cranial) nerve. The blood supply of the tongue is from branches of the lingual artery. The vertical fibrous septum in the centre of the tongue prevents any extensive anastomosis between the vessels of the two sides.

Lymph drainage

The palatal area. The chief drainage is backward and then outward at the side of the soft palate to pierce the superior constrictor muscles to enter the upper deep cervical glands. Some lymphatics pass first to the retropharyngeal group of glands.

The vestibular area. In the region of the lips and the anterior part of the cheeks the drainage is downward to the submental and submandibular glands. Posterior to this the lymphatics pierce the buccinator or superior constrictor to reach the upper deep cervical glands.

The sublingual area. Lymphatics pierce the mylohyoid diaphragm to enter the submental glands or run backward to the submandibular group.

The tongue. From the tip of the tongue lymphatics run to the submental glands; from the sides and dorsum to the submandibular group; and from the posterior surface they pierce the superior constrictor to join the upper and deep cervical glands. Some lymphatics from the tip and dorsum may bypass the submental and submandibular glands to run directly to the deep cervical chain.

THE SALIVARY GLANDS

The glands which secrete saliva are numerous and most of them are found in close relationship to the oral cavity. However, the largest of the salivary glands, sometimes known as the salivary glands proper, are three paired glands, the parotid, the submandibular and the sublingual which lie some distance from the oral cavity. The smaller glands are situated below the oral mucosa in the lips, cheeks, tongue and palate.

There are two varieties of saliva secreted, serous and mucous. The word serous implies a thin, watery secretion whereas a mucous secretion is a more viscid one. This characteristic is produced by the presence of a glycoprotein, mucin, which when mixed with water forms mucus. The glands themselves are classified as serous, mucous or mixed depending on the nature of the saliva produced. The parotid is a serous gland whereas the submandibular and sublingual are mixed glands. Although mixed the secretory cells in the submandibular gland are mostly serous and in the sublingual gland most of the cells are mucous. The salivary glands are compound tubulo-alveolar glands; this means that the terminal ramifications of a branching duct system end as clusters of secretory cells which are known as alveoli or acini.

Partitions of connective tissue, known as septa run into the substance of the glands dividing them into lobules. The lobules are made up of groups of alveoli. The larger branches of the duct system run in connective tissue septa between the lobules and so are known as interlobular ducts. Smaller branches which enter the substance of the lobules are described as intralobular ducts (Fig. 264). The part of the duct system interposed between the alveoli and the rest of the collecting and excretory channels is known as the intercalated duct. This has a narrow diameter and is constituted of low cuboidal cells. The intercalated ducts are long in the parotid but are short or absent in the sublingual gland. Striated ducts are found between the intercalated ducts and the larger excretory channels, and are mainly intralobular in position. The cells of the striated ducts form a single layer and are columnar and regularly arranged. The perpendicular striations which give these ducts their name are found in the basal zone of the cytoplasm. The striations are produced by numerous infoldings of the basal part of the cell membrane associated with mitochondria arranged parallel to the infoldings. The striated ducts modify the saliva produced by the alveoli by secreting water and inorganic salts. The larger excretory ducts have an epithelium which is columnar and towards their opening into the oral cavity this becomes pseudo-stratified. As there are a number of variations in the arrangement of the duct system in various animals the above description of the arrangement in man may not apply in detail to other mammals.

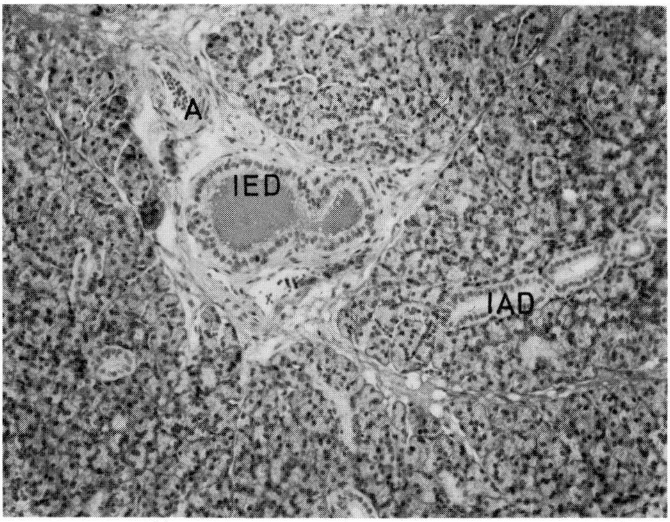

Fig. 264 Serous salivary gland. The cells of the secretory alveoli are more densely stained than those of mucous acini. The nuclei are centrally placed in the cells. Both interlobular (IED) and intralobular (IAD) ducts are to be seen. A, interlobular artery. Original magnification ×25.

The secretory cells of the alveoli show differences depending on whether they are serous or mucous. The cytoplasm of the serous cells has a granular appearance, this is produced by zymogen granules which are intracellular concentrations of the enzyme, ptyalin, found in the secretion of the serous cells (Fig. 264). The nucleus is rounded and is situated towards but not at the basal end of the cell. In the basal zone of the cell the cytoplasm is strongly basophilic due to a high content of RNA. This is particularly associated with the ribosomes of the well-formed endoplasmic reticulum which produces the protein of the zymogen granules. The lumen of the serous alveoli is very small and barely perceptible.

The cytoplasm of the mucous secreting cells generally gives a lightly stained, rather 'empty' appearance (Fig. 265). This is due to the content of mucinogen, the precursor of mucin. In most ordinary preparations, the mucinogen is either lost in preparation of the section or is not stained and so the lightly stained cytoplasm which contains it has a vacuolated appearance. In suitably fixed sections the mucinogen, due to its content of carbohydrate, gives a strong positive coloration with the PAS method. The nucleus is flattened and is placed close to the base of the cell. The mixed glands may be composed of varying combinations of mucous and serous alveoli but more commonly the serous elements are found as crescentic shaped groups of serous cells, the so-called demilunes, which cap the mucous alveoli.

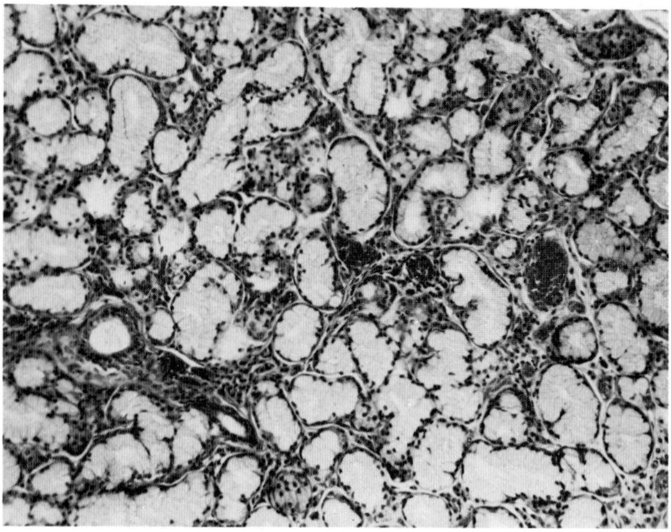

Fig. 265 Mucous salivary gland. The cells of the secretory alveoli show an 'empty' appearance and the nuclei are arranged close to the base of the cells. Original magnification ×25.

The serous and mucous alveoli can vary in appearance depending on the secretory activity of the gland. If the gland is in a resting condition the cells are large and are full of granules or droplets, whereas if the gland has recently been active the cells are shrunken and there are few granules or droplets.

The secretory alveoli are surrounded by a loose basket-like network formed by the processes of special cells that lie against the bases of the secretory cells. These are the myoepithelial cells which are believed to help in the expulsion of the secretion from the secretory cells into the duct system, by virtue of the contractile nature of their long cytoplasmic processes.

The salivary glands have a rich blood supply (Fig. 266). The larger vessels run in the interlobular septa. Around the secretory alveoli there is a capillary plexus.

The salivary glands have both a sympathetic and a parasympathetic nerve supply. Much controversy has occurred about the significance of this double nerve supply. It would appear that either sympathetic or parasympathetic stimulation can produce a secretion even though the sympathetic supply contains vasoconstrictor fibres. The sympathetic fibres are derived from the superior cervical ganglion and reach the glands along the course of branches of the external carotid artery. The parasympathetic fibres arise from either the facial or the glossopharyngeal nerves. The submandibular gland, the sublingual gland, anterior lingual glands, the palatal glands and those of the upper lip

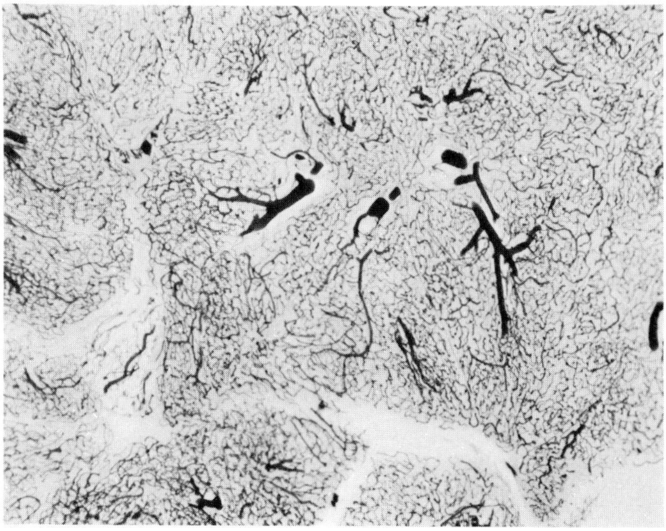

Fig. 266 Salivary gland. Section of an injected preparation showing the rich vascular supply throughout the lobules. Original magnification × 20.

and upper part of the vestibule are supplied by the facial nerve, whereas the parotid gland and those of the lower lip and lower part of the vestibule are supplied by the glossopharyngeal. The parasympathetic fibres reach the submandibular, sublingual and anterior lingual glands via the chorda tympani branch of the facial nerve, the lingual nerve and the submandibular ganglion. The terminal (postganglionic) neurones arising in the ganglion pass to the glands along branches of the submental and lingual arteries and the lingual nerve. The palatal glands and those of the upper lip and upper part of the vestibule are innervated via the greater petrosal nerve, the nerve of the pterygoid canal and the pterygopalatine (sphenopalatine) ganglion. The terminal neurones from the ganglion pass to the glands along the palatine vessels. The parasympathetic fibres reach the parotid gland via the lesser petrosal nerve and the otic ganglion. The terminal neurones from the otic ganglion reach the parotid gland with the auriculo-temporal nerve. In the case of the glands of the lower lip and lower part of the vestibule the postganglionic neurones from the otic gland are supplied along branches of the inferior alveolar (dental) and buccal nerves.

The glands opening into the vestibule of the mouth are the parotid gland, the duct of which opens opposite the second upper molar tooth in the adult, and the small labial and buccal glands. The majority of these lie between the lip and cheek muscles and the mucous membrane, but some larger glands in the cheek lie outside the buccinator muscle which is pierced by their ducts. The parotid gland is a serous gland, the labial and buccal glands are mixed, producing both mucous and serous secretions.

The glands opening into the floor of the mouth are the submandibular and sublingual glands and the anterior lingual glands. Some of the elements making up the sublingual glands open into the duct of the submandibular gland, whereas others open directly into the floor of the mouth cavity. The submandibular and sublingual glands are mixed.

The glands of the palate lie between the oral mucous membrane and the muscles of the soft palate and extend forward into the hard palate, and into the anterior pillar of the fauces (palato-glossal arch). Together with the glands at the back of the tongue they form a mucous secreting gland field surrounding the oropharyngeal opening.

The glands of the tongue are both mucous and serous. In the posterior third of the tongue there are numerous mucous glands, but some are also present at the tip and margins. The anterior lingual glands are mixed though mainly mucous, and lie beneath the under surface of the tongue near the tip forming a group on each side of the frenulum. The serous glands of the tongue mostly lie close to the vallate papillae and their ducts open into the sulci of these papillae.

The serous secretion help to remove epithelial debris and food particles from the surface of the gums, cheek, and dorsum of the tongue, whereas the mucous secretions help to bind together the masticated food to form a bolus and protect the oral epithelium from the abrasive action of food particles (see also p. 335).

Clinical considerations. A knowledge of the structure of the oral mucous membrane is necessary in planning the extent and form of artificial dentures. Whenever possible the denture base should rest upon the mucous membrane where it is closely related to underlying bone, and avoid excessively heavy contact with the mucous membrane where it is not so supported, *i.e.*, the soft palate, floor of the mouth, and sites of reflection from alveolar bone to the lips and cheeks in the vestibule.

In giving injections of local anaesthetic solution the injection should be made when possible into those regions where there is a submucosa. If an injection must be given into a mucoperiosteum, *e.g.*, over much of the hard palate, it must be given very slowly so as to avoid tearing the collagen bundles and producing after-pain.

The normal appearance of the mucous membrane covering the dorsal surface of the body of the tongue should be fully appreciated since many diseases, systemic as well as local, can alter this appearance considerably. The changes so produced are of value in the diagnosis of such conditions. Ulceration from various causes is frequent, and the possibility of carcinoma must always be borne in mind.

BIBLIOGRAPHY

Arnim, S. S. & Hagerman, D. A. (1953). The connective tissue fibres of the marginal gingiva. *J. Amer. dent. Ass.* **47**, 271.

Barker, D. S. (1967). The dendritic cell system in human gingival epithelium. *Archs. oral Biol.* **12**, 203.

Bowman, A. J. & Latham, R. A. (1968). Differential development and structure of keratinizing mucosa of the upper denture bearing area. *Dent. Practit.* **18**, 349.

Cohen, B. (1959). Morphological factors in the pathogenesis of periodontal disease. *Brit. dent. J.* **107**, 31.

——— (1962). A study of the periodontal epithelium. *Brit. dent. J.* **112**, 55.

Dixon, A. D. (1963). Nerve plexuses in the oral mucosa. *Arch. oral Biol.* **8**, 435.

Garrett, J. R. (1976). Structure and innervation of salivary glands. In *Scientific Foundations of Dentistry*. Eds. Cohen, B. & Kramer, I. R. H. London: Heinemann.

Jones, J. H. (1973). The oral mucous membrane markers of internal disease. *Brit. dent. J.* **134**, 81.

Landay, M. A. & Schroeder, H. E. (1979). Differentiation in normal human buccal mucosa epithelium. *J. Anat. Lond.* **128**, 31.

Listgarten, M. A. (1964). The ultrastructure of human gingival epithelium. *Amer. J. Anat.* **114**, 49.

——— (1966). Electron microscopic study of the gingivo-dental junction of man. *Amer. J. Anat.* **119**, 147.

Meyer, J., Alvares, O. F. & Gerson, S. (1976). Structure and function of the oral mucosa. In *Scientific Foundations of Dentistry*. Eds. Cohen, B. & Kramer, I. R. H. London: Heinemann.

Schroeder, H. E. (1969). Melanin containing organelles in cells of the human gingiva. *J. Periodont. Res.* **4**, 1.

——— (1969). Ultrastructure of the junctional epithelium of the human gingiva. *Helv. odont. Acta.* **13**, 65.

——— (1976). Gingival tissue. In *Scientific Foundations of Dentistry*. Eds. Cohen, B. & Kramer, I. R. H. London: Heinemann.

Squier, C. A. & Meyer, J. (1971). *Current Concepts of the Histology of Oral Mucosa*. Eds. Springfield: Thomas.

Squier, C. A., Johnson, N. W. & Hopps, A. M. (1976). *Human Oral Mucosa*. Oxford: Blackwell.

Tolman, D. E., Winkelmann, R. K. & Gibilisco, J. A. (1965). Nerve endings in gingival tissue. *J. dent. Res.* **44**, 657.

Waterhouse, J. P. & Squier, C. A. (1967). The Langerhans cell in human gingival epithelium. *Archs. oral Biol.* **12**, 341.

SECTION IV

The functional anatomy of the oral cavity

18. The Relation of Structure and Function in the Mouth Cavity

When the mouth and the related structures are at rest the teeth are slightly separated and the lips are in contact forming an anterior oral seal. The tip of the tongue lies against the mucous membrane of the hard palate immediately above and behind the upper incisors. The margin of the tongue rests lightly against the lingual surfaces of the teeth, and there is usually a slight space between the dorsum of the tongue and the palate. The soft palate rests against the pharyngeal surface of the tongue forming a posterior oral seal so that the mouth cavity is cut off from the pharynx.

The upper lip is normally in light contact with the labial surfaces of the upper incisors. The cheeks are in contact with the buccal surfaces of the premolar and molar teeth and adjacent gums. In some children the lower lip may be trapped between the upper and lower incisors which tends to produce protrusion of the upper teeth and backward inclination of the lower teeth. In mouth breathing both the anterior and posterior oral seals are broken and air is drawn through the oral cavity.

The teeth are implanted in their sockets so as to resist the pressures tending to dislodge them (see p. 34). The arrangement of the periodontal fibres permits a certain amount of buffering movement. It is this movement which produces the wear at the contact areas of the mesial and distal surfaces.

In dentitions in which the occlusal relationships are normal the pressures are evenly spread over the teeth. If, however, a malocclusion exists then excessive pressures tend to fall upon individual teeth.

In the resting mouth there is very little space between the various parts. Space is provided for food by lowering the mandible, depressing and retracting the tongue and opening up the vestibular region. Once food is introduced mastication takes place in a closed cavity, the lips being in contact and the soft palate resting against the back of the tongue.

The rest position of the mandible. When at rest the lower jaw occupies a position which is determined by the state of tonic contraction of the muscles of mastication. In this activity the muscles counteract the action of gravity through the proprioceptive reflex mechanism which is maintained by the stimulation of sensory endings in the disc and capsular tissue of the jaw joints and in the muscles. The resting position varies in different individuals and with the state of tonic contraction of the muscles. These relax, for example, during sleep. In the normal resting position of the mandible the occlusal surfaces of the teeth are separated. The amount of separation may be judged by the distance the lower incisors move in relation to the incisive edges of the upper teeth as the jaw moves from the occlusal to the resting position. This distance is usually 2–5 mm. From the rest position the lower teeth are carried into occlusion with the upper teeth (centric occlusion) as the elevating muscles contract.

The mouth cavity, containing the teeth and the tongue and into which open the salivary glands, is constructed to receive food and, by the complex mechanism of mastication, to prepare it for the process of swallowing, which terminates the act of mastication. The movements of mastication take place at the temporo-mandibular joints.

THE TEMPORO-MANDIBULAR JOINT

The temporo-mandibular joint is a highly specialised synovial joint which shows a number of unusual features. The articulating mandibular and temporal surfaces are formed, not by articular cartilage, but by a thick layer of fibrous tissue. The joint shows an articular disc which divides it into two joint cavities, a superior and an inferior, in which very different kinds of movement are produced, sliding or translatory in the superior compartment and rotatory in the inferior compartment. The right and left mandibular condyles are carried by a single bone, the mandible, so that every movement of the lower jaw involves both temporo-mandibular joints. One feature of the temporo-mandibular joint is unique, in that closing (elevating) movements of the jaw are finally stopped by the meeting together of the teeth in occlusion.

Apart from the production of movement at a joint the muscles are concerned in the stability of the joint; this is particularly the case with the temporo-mandibular joint where there is little congruence between the articulating surfaces and there is only one ligament, the lateral temporo-mandibular ligament, of any functional significance.

At the temporo-mandibular joints the mandibular condyles articulate with the glenoid fossae and articular eminences of the temporal bones (Fig. 28). The long axis of the head of each condyle, between the lateral and medial poles, is about 15–20 mm. The extended axis of each condyle meet at an angle of 140°–160° at about the level of the anterior border of the foramen magnum. The glenoid fossa is separated from the tympanic plate behind by the squamo-tympanic fissure. The postero-lateral lip of the fossa forms the variable post-glenoid tubercle. The roof of the glenoid fossa is a thin plate of bone separating the upper joint cavity from the dura mater associated with the temporal lobe of the brain. The glenoid fossa is continuous in front with the convex articular eminence. It has no anterior margin or lip so that anterior dislocation of the head of the condyle into the temporal fossa is a common consequence of excessive forward movement of the condylar head. The articular surfaces are covered by a layer of dense fibrous tissue, and are separated by a complete articular disc so that two cavities are present in each joint (Fig. 267). The joint capsule is attached below to the articular margin of the head of the condyle, and above to the

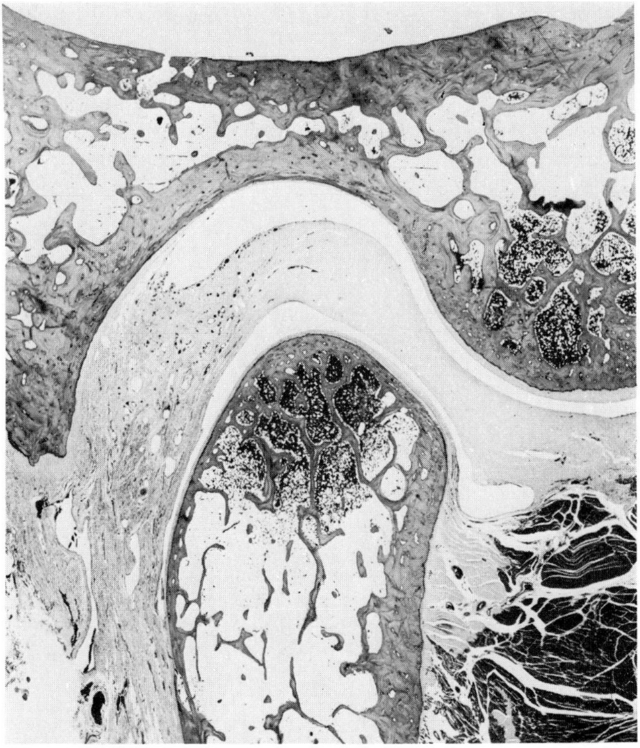

Fig. 267 Sagittal section through the mandibular joint of a human subject of 35 years of age. The central part of the articular disc is avascular compared with the posterior part which shows numerous blood vessels. Note also the layer of fibrous tissue which forms the articular surfaces on both mandibular and temporal aspect of the joint. × 4·5. (*By courtesy of Prof H. J. J. Blackwood.*)

margins of the glenoid fossa and articular eminence. At the sides the capsule is strengthened by collateral ligaments of which the lateral one, the temporo-mandibular ligament, is the strongest (Fig. 268). This ligament limits the range of movement of the condyle, preventing it coming in contact with the tympanic plate behind and passing beyond the articular eminence in front. Behind the capsule is intimately united with the upper and lower attachments of the articular disc; in front the capsule is poorly developed. The accessory ligaments of the joint (spheno-mandibular and stylo-mandibular) have little if any effect in regulating mandibular movements.

The articular disc, composed of densely packed collagen fibres, is firmly attached to the mandible at the outer and inner poles of the head of the condyle, which it fits closely like a cap so that only rotary movements can occur between the condyle and the disc. Behind the disc becomes looser in texture and divides into an ascending limb and a descending limb. The former is attached with the capsule to the anterior margin of the squamo-tympanic fissure, the latter to the posterior surface of the head and to the neck of the condyle. Unlike the rest of the disc the looser posterior part is vascularised and is not normally subjected to any pressure from the condyle. This part of the articular disc

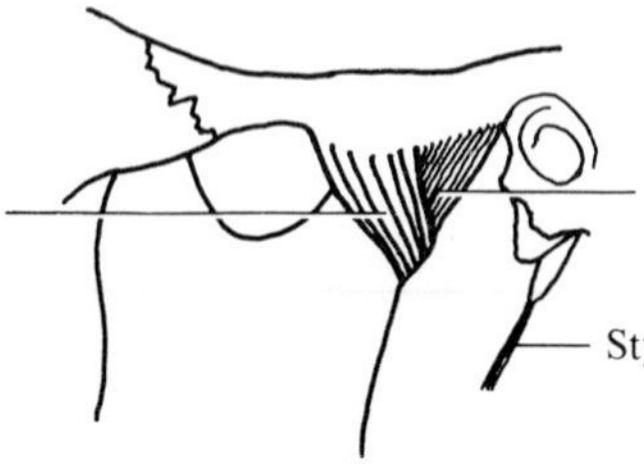

Fig. 268 Diagrammatic representation of the temporo-mandibular joint showing the capsule and the lateral temporo-mandibular ligament.

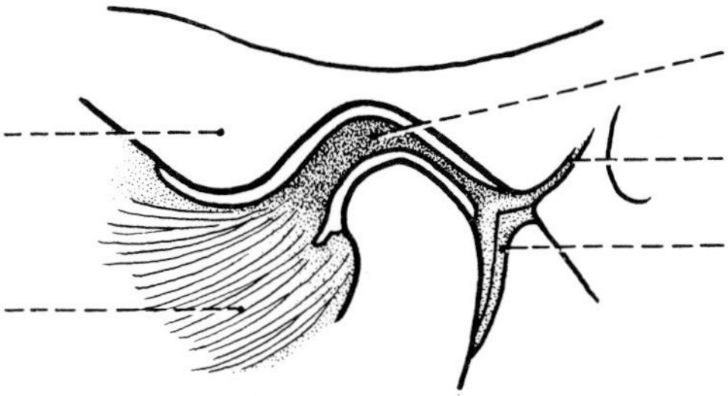

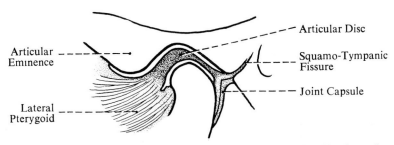

Fig. 269 Diagram of a sagittal section through the mandibular joint. The sharp distinction between the joint capsule and the tissue of the articular disc is purely diagrammatic.

is covered by a vascular synovial membrane. The synovial membrane is absent over the articular areas of the condyle, glenoid fossa and articular eminence, and also the dense articulating region of the disc. In front the disc has no direct attachment to the mandible but passes forward to the anterior edge of the articular eminence (Fig. 269). The upper joint cavity between the disc and the articular fossa is much more extensive than the lower compartment. As the result of the elasticity of the back part of the disc and capsule, the disc can pass forward with the head of the condyle from the glenoid fossa to the articular eminence.

The space vacated by the condyle during its forward excursion is filled in by the posterior part of the disc, the capsule, and extracapsular tissues. Forward movement of the condyle and articular disc is produced by the contraction of the lateral pterygoid muscle which is inserted into the antero-medial aspect of both structures.

Until adult life is reached the articular surface of the condylar head is separated from the underlying bone by the following layers (Figs. 81, 270):

1. A superficial fibrous perichondrium continuous with the periosteum covering the neck of the condyle, and forming the articular surface of the condyle.
2. A deep cellular layer of the perichondrium, which by the proliferation of its cells regulates the growth of the cartilage of the condyle.

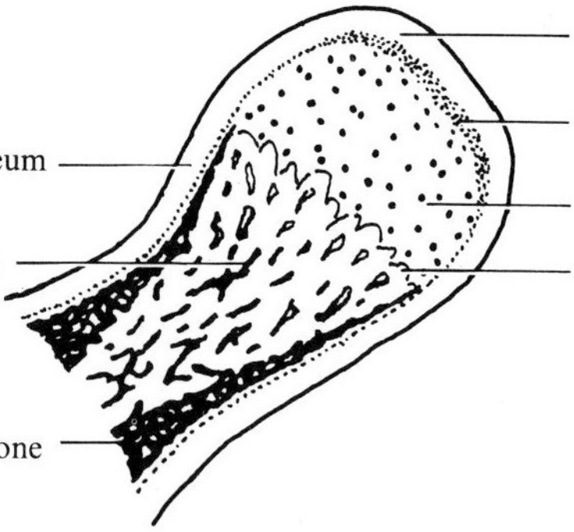

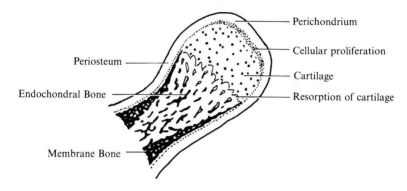

Fig. 270 Diagrammatic representation of a section through the head of the mandibular condyle where a zone of secondary cartilage is present.

3. The secondary growth cartilage of the condyle, which at its lower surface is replaced by bone throughout the period of facial growth. This cartilage is a growth cartilage and not an articular cartilage. It corresponds rather to the epiphyseal plate of a long bone.

When growth of the mandible ceases the zone of secondary cartilage is much reduced in thickness and becomes separated from the marrow cavity beneath by a layer of bone which is continuous with the cortical bone over the other surfaces of the condyle. Throughout the whole period of skeletal growth the condylar cartilage serves to maintain the proper relationship of the condyle to the temporal surface of the joint as well as acting as a growth centre for the mandible. After the cessation of growth the persistent layer of cartilage at the condyle probably continues to be responsible for articular adjustments.

The structure of the tissues at the articular surface of the condyle indicates that the temporo-mandibular joint is not a weight-bearing joint.

Mandibular movements. The movements of the mandible are produced by the bilateral muscles of mastication acting on both the temporomandibular joints, and to a lesser extent by the supra-hyoid muscles. The degree of their action and the extent of the movements produced are controlled by sensory proprioceptive impulses from the mucous membrane of the mouth, the periodontal membranes of the teeth, the articular capsule and disc, and from the muscles themselves. In each joint the basic movements are rotation of the condyle beneath the disc (lower joint compartment) and sliding movement of condyle and disc together in relation to the glenoid fossa and articular eminence (upper joint compartment). The actual movements taking place at the temporo-mandibular joints are combinations of the following:

1. Protrusion.
2. Retrusion.
3. Opening movement, which is in part a protrusion of the lower jaw and in part a rotation around a horizontal axis.
4. Closing movement, the mouth can be closed in any position between extreme protrusion and retrusion.
5. Rotation, in which one condyle is held in its glenoid fossa and the other rotates around it as around a vertical axis.

Protrusion and retrusion can be bilateral or unilateral; when unilateral they involve rotation towards the opposite side. The lower jaw can be moved backwards and forwards either with the teeth in sliding contact or in various degrees of separation.

The process of mastication or breaking up of portions of food introduced into the mouth cavity can be divided into three basic activities: chopping and slicing, carried out chiefly by the incisors and canines; munching or crushing, a simple vertical action of the cheek teeth; and chewing, a combination of vertical, antero-posterior and side-to-side movements involving the whole dentition.

Except in the case of closing movements, which are limited by the occlusion of the teeth, the range of each movement is determined chiefly by the pattern of muscle activity and to a lesser degree by the capsule and its collateral ligaments. The most frequent type of dislocation, as already indicated, is forwards so that the heads of the condyles come to lie beyond the limit of the articular eminence in the temporal fossae. This may follow excessive opening movements.

The lateral pterygoids, assisted by the medial pterygoids, are the prime movers in forward protrusion; the posterior, horizontal fibres of the temporal muscles are the antagonists and relax as the lateral pterygoids contract. The masseters, medial pterygoids, and anterior, vertical fibres of the temporals (synergists), remain in tonic contraction and prevent separation of the teeth by preventing any rotation of the mandible. In protrusion the condyles of the mandible with the articular discs are drawn downward and forward onto the articular eminences by the contraction of the lateral pterygoid muscles. The extent of this movement is limited by the attachment of the discs and the posterior fibres of the joint capsules to the back of the glenoid fossae.

During retrusion the head of the condyles with the articular discs are carried back into the glenoid fossae as a result of the contraction of the posterior fibres of the temporal muscles, the lateral pterygoids relaxing (antagonists) and the remaining muscles of mastication keeping the teeth in contact.

In opening the mouth the lateral pterygoids carry the heads of the condyles and with them the articular discs forward and downward on to the articular eminences as in protrusion; at the same time the posterior fibres of the temporal muscles relax. The masseters, anterior fibres of the temporals, and the medial pterygoids also relax and this permits the mandible to rotate around a horizontal axis. The opening movement is at first a rotation of the heads of the condyles beneath the articular discs, and later a forward movement of the condyles and discs on to the articular eminences. As a result the angle of the mandible moves backwards as the head of the condyle moves forward. This rotatory movement is assisted by the digastric muscles acting on the body of the mandible from a fixed hyoid bone. The axis around which the mandible rotates does not remain fixed during the opening movement but probably moves downward and forward along a line passing from the head of each condyle to the opening of the mandibular canal.

In closing the mouth the masseters, temporals, and medial pterygoids are the prime movers. In closure with protrusion the lateral pterygoids contract and are assisted by the medial pterygoids. As a result the heads of the condyles remain in a forward position on the articular eminences. In closure with retrusion the posterior fibres of the temporal muscles act with the masseters and the pterygoids relax, allowing the condyles to return to the glenoid fossae.

In swinging the jaw from one side to the other (rotatory movements) the condyle of the side towards which the jaw is moving is carried back into the glenoid fossa by the posterior fibres of the temporal of that side and held there by the tonic contraction of all the muscles of that side. On the other side the lateral pterygoid pulls the condyle and articular disc forward and inward on to the articular eminence so that the jaw rotates around the fixed condyle.

Relations of the teeth during mastication. In the movements of protrusion, retrusion, and rotation the teeth can be kept in contact with one another and the food is ground between the premolars and molars. As the food is crushed and ground between the teeth it passes over their buccal and lingual surfaces into either the vestibule or the mouth cavity proper. Contraction of the buccinators, the mylohyoids, and tongue muscles returns the food to the grinding surfaces of the teeth for further mastication. The direct attachment of the mucous membrane of the cheek to the buccinator muscle prevents the appearance of loose folds which might otherwise be damaged by the teeth during mastication.

The curvatures of the buccal and lingual surfaces of the teeth protect the epithelial attachment of the gingival mucosa from injury, and the cornification of the epithelium of the gums and hard palate renders these parts better adapted for wear and tear.

When the incisor teeth are used in biting, the lower jaw is protruded, opened and then closed in the protruded position so that at the end of the movement the teeth meet edge to edge. From this position the incisive edges of the lower incisors slide upwards and backwards in contact with the lingual surfaces of the upper incisors. Meanwhile the cheek teeth come into contact at their buccal cusps, and from this position the lower teeth slide backward into normal (centric) occlusion in which the mesiolingual cusps of the upper molars are at rest in the central fossae of the lower molars (p. 38).

At the commencement of side-to-side movement of the lower jaw the buccal cusps of the lower cheek teeth are between the buccal and lingual cusps of the upper teeth (centric relationship) (Fig. 271). On moving to the right (right lateral occlusal relation) the buccal cusps of the right lower molars come into contact with the buccal cusps of the upper teeth, and the lingual cusps of the lower molars with the lingual cusps of the upper teeth. On the left side the lower buccal cusps come into contact with the upper lingual cusps. In moving to the left (left lateral occlusal relation) a reverse relationship is established. In this way the teeth are maintained in occlusal balance on both sides of the face. In these movements the mandible tilts downwards slightly on the opposite side to the direction of its movement. The lower molars pass over the upper molars in a path which is approximately parallel to the oblique ridges of the upper molars.

These dental movements are of course correlated with the movements of the mandibular condyles in relation to the glenoid fossae and the articular eminences.

Mastication in man can either occur as a chopping or crushing action or as a chewing action. In the former, the mandible opens and closes

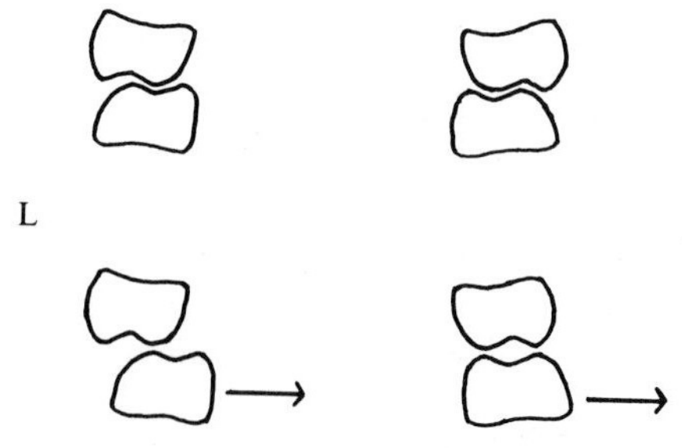

Fig. 271 Diagrammatic representation of the occlusal relationships of the upper and lower molars. In the upper part of the diagram the cheek teeth are in centric relationship. In the lower part of the diagram the altered cuspal relationships brought about by movement of the lower jaw to the right are shown. L, left side; R, right side.

with the minimum of protrusive and side-to-side movement; the teeth returning directly to the position of normal (centric) occlusion. In the latter, protrusive and side-to-side movements play an important role as described above and the teeth only return to the position of centric occlusion at the end of each chewing act.

Individuals with a considerable degree of overbite in their occlusion tend to use a chopping action during mastication as this type of occlusal relationship presents free side to side and protrusive movements, whereas in persons with little overbite a proper chewing action can readily take place.

During mastication the contacts between the teeth stimulate the proprioceptive nerve endings of the periodontal membranes and so regulate, co-ordinate and modify the action patterns of the muscles of mastication. The muscles themselves, and especially the elevating muscles, contain muscle spindles which are concerned in regulating their action. The information which is passed back to centres in the central nervous system from the periodontal membranes and the muscles is supplemented by messages from other nerve endings in the capsule and disc of the temporo-mandibular joint and in the oral mucous membrane (see p. 332).

In the act of closing the mouth great pressures can be exerted upon the teeth and considerable pressure would tend to fall upon the condyles in the glenoid cavities. The pressure on the condyles, which might damage the adjacent growth cartilage, is, however, relieved by a special muscle mechanism whereby during clenching of the jaws the condyle is held away from the glenoid fossa by a synergic contraction of the posterior fibres of the temporal muscles and the lower head of the lateral pterygoid. As a result the condyle is pulled downward by the latter as the coronoid process is elevated by the former in a rotary movement which is the reverse of that which acts in opening the jaws.

Chewing is usually carried out at one side of the mouth at a time. Some people commence chewing on one side and then transfer the food to the other. Most of the work takes place between the premolars and the first permanent molars. The normal pattern of masticatory activity is readily upset by painful teeth or conditions such as ulceration of the mouth cavity. The extent to which food is chewed before swallowing varies to a considerable extent in different individuals. The fundamental action is to break the food into particles of a size to permit easy swallowing. When the jaws are closed and the teeth clenched, the cheek teeth tend to migrate mesially and, providing approximal contact between the teeth is maintained, this mesial movement is transmitted to the anterior teeth.

Movement of the teeth in mastication. During mastication the teeth move in their sockets, and these slight movements help to prevent damage to the teeth, which would more readily occur if the teeth were rigidly attached to the jaw bone.

It has been shown that as a result of forces applied to them in a lateral or a vertical direction the teeth move in two phases. The teeth move rapidly at first when the forces are low and more slowly when the forces are increased; finally a level is reached where pain occurs and no further movement takes place. The point at which the teeth stop moving rapidly has been recorded at somewhat different levels for lateral and vertical movement; these range from 50–100 gm to 300–600 gm respectively.

The strength of the bite. Studies with the dynamometer which have been carried out on the forces which can be exerted between the teeth show that in the molar region a bite of about 50 kg can be produced in young adults with good dentitions. In the Eskimo a figure as high as 150 kg has been recorded. The biting force diminishes towards the front of the mouth and in the incisor region a biting force of only about a third or less of that in the molars can be produced. The level of the biting force can be raised in the individual by practice.

The limits to the biting force between the teeth are determined by the power of the masticatory muscles and by the sensitivity of the periodontal membranes to pain. The different forces found between different teeth are probably due to such factors as the relative position of the teeth (and the dynamometer) to the insertions of the elevating muscles of the jaw, the greater root area available for attachment in the molars as compared with the incisors and by a greater sensitivity of the incisors. The last two factors may well be inter-related in that the same force falling on teeth with different attachment areas would produce different degrees of displacement, and therefore more pain in the teeth with smaller roots.

In normal mastication very much smaller forces are produced than in the static experiments with the dynamometer, for the forces are only as high as 6 kg.

The neural control of mastication. In mastication the lower jaw is moved so that the dental arches are properly aligned and the requisite forces can be transmitted through the teeth in occlusion. During the process of mastication there is a constant flow of information from the structures involved in the process back to the central nervous system. This information is derived from four main sources:

a. the masticatory muscles themselves
b. the temporo-mandibular joint
c. the periodontal membranes
d. the oral mucous membrane.

In this way a great variety of information is made available on various aspects of mastication such as the actions of the masticatory muscles, the movement or position in space of the lower jaw, the force applied to the teeth by the contraction of the masticatory muscles and the position and nature of the food present in the oral cavity. Information from these four sources is carried along branches of the trigeminal nerve to its sensory nuclei. There are three such nuclei situated along the length of the brain stem from the mid-brain to the cervical spinal cord. The main sensory nucleus of the trigeminal nerve is situated in the pons on the lateral side of the trigeminal motor nucleus and is associated with touch and deep pressure sensation. The descending or spinal nucleus of the trigeminal nerve is found in the medulla oblongata and extends from there into the upper part of the cervical spinal cord. It is related to pain and temperature sensation. The sensory fibres reaching these two nuclei have their cell bodies in the semilunar ganglion. The third sensory nucleus of the trigeminal nerve is that situated in the mid-brain, the mesencephalic nucleus. The incoming fibres to it carry proprioceptive information from the muscles of mastication and probably also from the periodontal membranes. These sensory fibres are unique in having their cell bodies in the mesencephalic neucleus and not in a ganglion outside the central nervous system, like the other sensory fibres of the trigeminal nerve or the incoming sensory fibres of the spinal cord which have their cell bodies in the spinal ganglia.

Fibres from all three trigeminal sensory nuclei synapse directly with the cells of the motor nucleus of the fifth nerve. Those from the mesencephalic nucleus form the monosynaptic reflex arcs for the proprioceptive control of the masticatory muscles. The motor nucleus also receives connections which derive from the cerebral cortex, the cerebellum, the reticular formation, the hypothalamic-amygdaloid areas, the caudate nucleus, and the nuclei of other cranial nerves especially the seventh and twelfth cranial nerves. The control of the motor neurones on the masticatory muscles is thus employed on a very wide basis of relevant information.

Impulses from higher centres in the cerebral cortex can pass down large motor neurones of the pyramidal tract, the so-called alpha (α) route, to stimulate directly the lower motor neurones leading to the masticatory muscles; the cell bodies of the latter neurones are the large motor cells of the trigeminal motor nucleus of the pons. However it is generally accepted that the more usual pathway involves the gamma (γ) route, the monosynaptic reflex arc from the masticatory muscles. Efferent fibres from smaller motor cells of the fifth nerve motor nucleus pass to the highly specialised end organs in the muscles, the neuromuscular spindles, to activate the modified muscle fibres of the spindle. The central 'nuclear bag' region of the spindle contains numerous nuclei and the parts of the muscle fibres found there are non-contractile. From this region large fast firing proprioceptive fibres run up to their cell bodies in the mesencephalic nucleus. The axons of these unipolar cells travel to the trigeminal motor nucleus to synapse there with the large motor cells. In this way a 'feed-back' system is incorporated in the activation of the masticatory muscles and as required by the situation a reflex stimulation or inhibition of these muscles can readily occur. (Fig. 272).

Mastication is neither a wholly voluntary or a wholly involuntary activity. It can be initiated by impulses reaching the motor cells of the trigeminal motor nucleus from the cerebral cortex, but following on this initiation the act of mastication can continue by purely involuntary control. In this sense there is a similarity between the actions of walking and mastication. When the jaws are brought into occlusion and a certain level of force is exerted on the teeth a reflex inhibition of the jaw elevating (closing) muscles is brought about by impulses from the nerve endings in the periodontal membranes so that excessive pressures do not fall on the teeth. At the same time a reflex stimulation of the jaw opening muscles occurs and this in turn produces a stretching of the jaw closing muscles with consequent involvement of the muscles spindles in these muscles. The jaw closing reflex is produced, the mandible closes and the activity of the jaw opening muscles is inhibited. Again on closure of the jaws impulses from the periodontal membranes and possibly also from parts of the oral mucous membrane inhibit the action of the jaw closing muscles and stimulate the jaw opening muscles. In this way the alternating cycle of opening and closing movements of the jaws which occurs during mastication is maintained.

The masticatory cycle can be divided into three phases; (a) opening, (b) closing and (c) an occlusal phase. In the opening and closing phases

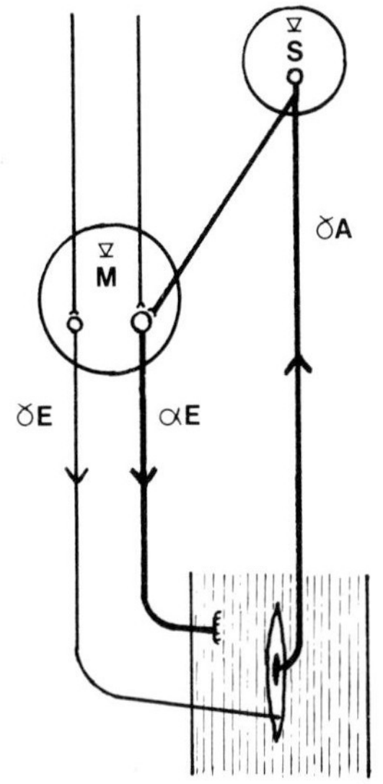

Fig. 272 Diagram of the proprioceptive control of a masticatory muscle. V M, Trigeminal motor nucleus; V S, Trigeminal mesencephalic sensory nucleus; αE, thick alpha efferent fibre; γE, thin gamma efferent fibre; γA, thick gamma afferent fibre from the nuclear region of a muscle spindle. Connections from higher centres are shown synapsing with the alpha and gamma motor cells in the Trigeminal motor nucleus.

the muscles concerned show isotonic contraction or relaxation whereas in the occlusal phase the elevating muscles show isometric contraction. During the occlusal phase the teeth are either in contact or may be separated from each other by hard foodstuff. The periodontal feed-back of information takes place during the occlusal phase. It has been estimated that the masticatory cycle takes about 0·8–1·0 sec.

Apart from the neural activity involved in strictly masticatory movements of the jaw all the other kinds of jaw movement and posture are similarly controlled. Throughout each day a constant stream of information on jaw movement and tooth contact is passed to centres in the brain stem during swallowing and various other momentary contacts of the teeth. In this way a memory pattern of various jaw postures such as physiological rest position and normal (centric) occlusion is built up and maintained. The certainty with which centric occlusion can be attained on sudden closure of the teeth is a demonstration of the exactitude of the neural control of jaw movement and posture.

A distinction can be made between morphological occlusion and physiological occlusion. Physiological occlusion means an occlusion suitable for the performance of mastication with efficiency and a biting force applied to each tooth which is within physiological limits. A physiological occlusion can exist where judged on morphological criteria alone the occlusion is imperfect.

Gland secretions. During mastication the secretions of the parotid salivary glands, opening into the vestibule, and of the sublingual and submandibular glands, opening into the floor of the mouth, moisten the food, partly digest it and, assisted by the secretions of the various mucous glands situated in the lips, cheeks, palate, and floor of the mouth, hold its particles together to form a soft bolus which is carried to the dorsum of the tongue in preparation for the act of swallowing. A certain amount of mastication takes place between the dorsum of the tongue and the hard palate and in the case of modern soft foodstuffs the teeth may play very little part in the process.

The amount and the nature of the mouth secretions vary according to the food present in the mouth. It is greater for dry substances. The sensation of thirst is produced by a drying of the mouth cavity following a marked reduction in the resting salivary secretions as a result of body dehydration. Saliva secreted when the mouth is empty of food keeps the tissues moist and fresh. It is swallowed at intervals, and during the swallowing process slight pressures are exerted upon the teeth by the cheeks, lips, and tongue which some orthodontists consider play a major part in determining and maintaining the normal form of the dental arches.

Saliva also assists in taste sensation by acting as a solvent; it digests starch and, by facilitating the movements of the tongue and lips, aids in speech. It contains some substances which inhibit bacterial growth and activity. About 1 litre is produced every day. The chief constituents are the enzyme ptyalin, mucin, albumins and globulins, and inorganic substances such as potassium, sodium, calcium, phosphates and chlorides. It has a slightly acid reaction (pH 6·3–6·8). Only when the mouth acidity falls to about pH 5·5 does decalcification of tooth surfaces commence. If the pH rises calcium carbonate and calcium phosphate are deposited on the teeth as tartar and may also form salivary calculi in the salivary glands and their ducts. Saliva reduces the clotting time of blood. This in association with its cleansing and antibacterial action is possibly related to the widespread instinct for animals to lick their wounds.

Oral sensation and reflexes. All parts of the oral cavity are sensitive to pain, heat, cold, touch and pressure. The lips are especially rich in touch and pressure end organs as is also the tip of the tongue. Heat and cold are best appreciated by the lips and tongue. The tongue and gums are fairly sensitive to pain especially towards the front of the mouth. Exposed dental pulps are extremely sensitive, the slightest stimulation producing acute pain. Light touch at the back of the mouth and soft palate may initiate the vomiting reflex. The presence of saliva determines a swallowing reflex at intervals independently of the presence of food. Stimulation of the taste buds determines the acceptance or rejection of the food and determines also the amount and nature of the salivary secretions.

Stimulation of the end organs of the periodontal membranes by the pressure exerted on the teeth determines the amount and direction of the masticatory force necessary to deal with various articles of food. Sensory impulses from the mucosa of the vestibule, tongue, and floor of the mouth control the action of the muscles, which keep the food between the grinding surfaces of the teeth. Hence in biting an apple or cracking a nut quite different relations between the jaws and teeth are required; the combinations of the muscles of mastication are quite different, as are the amount and direction of the forces used. There is also a difference in the mechanism of rejecting the shell fragments of a nut and the pips of an apple. Whereas swallowing is a mass reflex movement, mastication is a controlled, complex, integrated series of movements which have a different pattern to meet the needs of different foodstuffs.

The secretion of saliva following the introduction of food into the mouth cavity is an inborn or unconditioned reflex. This reflex was the basis of Pavlov's famous experiments in which he was able to produce salivation in dogs by replacing the normal effective stimulus by a process such as ringing a bell. This was done at first simultaneously with the presentation of food, but later without food, so as to bring about salivation through the establishment of a conditioned or acquired reflex. Other reflex activities involving the oral cavity which can be 'conditioned', or partly conditioned, include nervous swallowing, tooth grinding and thumb sucking.

Tongue movements. As well as being concerned in mastication, swallowing, and speech, the tongue plays an important role in maintaining mouth hygiene. The tip of the tongue can sweep over the vestibular surfaces of both upper and lower dental arches as well as their lingual and occlusal surfaces. It can also explore and cleanse the vestibule and the retro-molar areas. The muscles used in these movements are:

1. The genioglossi which protrude the tongue and can produce considerable pressure against the lingual surfaces of the incisor teeth.
2. The hyoglossi which depress the tongue to provide space between it and the palate for the food bolus prior to swallowing.
3. The styloglossi which draw the tongue upwards and backwards against the hard and soft palate assisted by the palatoglossi.

The tongue cannot be said to have any definite standard shape and adapts itself readily to the form and contents of the oral cavity. Changes in tongue shape are produced by the intrinsic muscle fibres which run in transverse, vertical and antero-posterior directions between the fibres of the extrinsic muscles (Fig. 273).

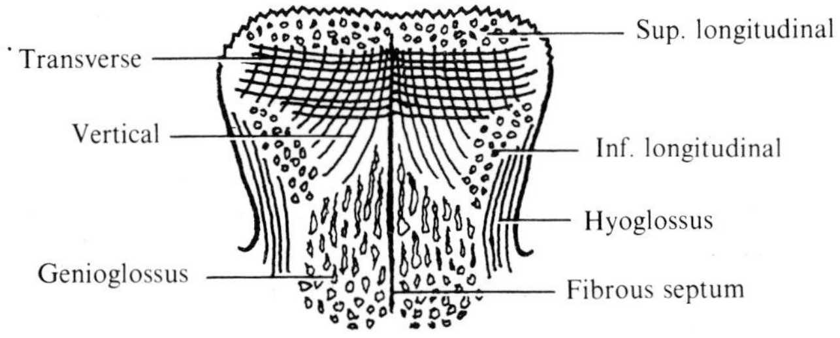

Fig. 273 Diagrammatic representation of a coronal section through the tongue showing the arrangement of the four groups of intrinsic muscle fibres; the hyoglossus and genioglossus muscles are also depicted.

Swallowing. There are considerable differences between the pattern of activity associated with swallowing in the infant as compared with that which is normally found in the adult. In the infant the large tongue is thrust forward between the gum pads and the mandible is positioned mainly by the action of the muscles which are innervated by the seventh cranial nerve. With the transition from the infantile state there is a change to semi-solid or solid food, the eruption and establishment of a functioning dentition, and a relative diminution in the size of the tongue. As a result the adult pattern of swallowing shows a minimal activity of the lip muscles, the tongue no longer thrusts forward but lies within the oral cavity proper with the tip placed against the anterior part of the palate behind the upper incisor teeth, the teeth usually come momentarily into contact and the mandible is positioned by the action of the muscles innervated by the fifth cranial nerve.

When the mastication of a mouthful of food is complete it is gathered together on the dorsum of the tongue as a bolus and is ready to be carried to the commencement of the oesophagus by the complex act of swallowing. The act of swallowing projects the food across the gap in the pharynx where the food passage from the mouth to the oesophagus crosses the air passage from the nose to the larynx. During swallowing the air passages are temporarily sealed off while the food is rapidly passed from the mouth to the oesophagus.

Although swallowing is a rapidly occurring uninterrupted process, it is usual to divide it into three stages for descriptive purposes.

1. The first stage is a voluntary one and consists of the passage of the bolus of food from the oral cavity through the oro-pharyngeal opening into the pharynx.

2. In the second stage the bolus of food passes through the pharynx to the beginning of the oesophagus. During this stage there is a suspension of respiration and closure of the naso-pharynx by the elevation of the soft palate. The larynx is elevated towards the epiglottis and this seals off the laryngeal opening together with the contraction of the muscles around the laryngeal opening.

3. In the third stage the food passes through the oesophagus to the stomach.

In swallowing the following muscle groups come into action:

1. The mylohyoid assisted by the anterior and posterior bellies of the digastrics with the stylohyoid, styloglossus, and palatoglossus muscles, lift the tongue against the under surface of the hard and soft palates.

2. The soft palate is elevated and made tense by the levator and tensor palati muscles forming a closed diaphragm between the nasopharynx and oral pharynx. The sealing off of the nasopharynx may be aided by contraction of a circular band of fibres at the upper margin of the superior constrictor.

3. The larynx is lifted up against the epiglottis and the opening reduced by the sphincter-like contraction of the thyro-arytenoid and arytenoid muscles. Elevation of the hyoid bone and the larynx takes place early in the act of swallowing, and before the descent of the bolus.

4. The sphincter muscles of the pharynx contract from above downward.

The food passes rapidly through the pharynx. A solid bolus usually passes over the posterior edge of the epiglottis, which lies like a lid above the elevated larynx, but liquids pass on either side of the epiglottis and through the piriform recesses between the pharyngeal wall and the side walls of the larynx. During normal swallowing the lips are closed, the teeth are in occlusion, and the tip of the tongue rests against the hard palate behind the upper incisors. If there is an open bite in the incisor region the tongue may protrude between the teeth. The hyoid bone is lifted upwards and forwards by the action of the digastrics, the mylohyoid, and the geniohyoids. The cricoid and thyroid cartilages ascend with the elevation of the larynx so that the upper margin of the thyroid cartilage comes to lie close to the hyoid bone.

Investigations with cinefluorography have shown that the bolus of food is not so much shot from the oral cavity into the pharynx as propelled by a squeezing action produced by the combined action of the muscles of the tongue, soft palate and pharynx. A smooth action is produced by a high degree of integrated reflex control. This coordinated muscular action is probably of more importance in the swallowing of solids than liquids in which gravity must play an important part.

Suckling. The nipple is taken into the mouth between the gum pads and above the tongue. Lips and tongue form a seal around the base of the nipple and against the breast. The baby forms an elongated teat from the nipple drawing it well back into the mouth cavity. Pressure is exerted between the upper and lower gum pads; the tongue is applied from before backwards pressing the elongated nipple against the palate. The jaw is then lowered, a vacuum is created between tongue and palate into which the milk flows, and the nipple returns to its normal size and the cycle is repeated. As soon as the mouth is filled with milk the posterior (palato-lingual) seal is opened and the milk is swallowed. Apart from the opening and closing movements the mandible appears to be protruded and drawn backwards during the suckling cycles; the lower lip maintaining contact with the breast by becoming more horizontal in position.

During the greater part of the suckling process the vestibule of the mouth is in open communication with the main oral cavity. Contraction of the buccinator muscles and the supporting action of the buccal pad of fat in the substance of the cheeks prevents them from being drawn inwards between the gum pads.

In the fetus and infant the lips show an outer smooth zone, the pars glabra, and an inner zone, the pars villosa which is studded with numerous villi. This inner zone is of advantage in suckling.

The stimulation of the nipple during suckling sets up a milk ejection reflex which is regulated by a combined neuro-hormonal mechanism whereby milk is expelled from the breast.

If the rate of suckling is too rapid or the lip-breast seal is broken, air may be swallowed with the milk producing stomach pain, belching or vomiting of milk.

Suckling is a complex muscular action involving the muscles of mastication, the muscles of the cheeks and lips with those used in swallowing. From the mass reflex activity of suckling develop the closely co-ordinated but separate activities of mastication and swallowing. Suckling and swallowing are both closely related with respiration in that respiratory activity is suspended during the act of swallowing and suckling. The complex co-ordination of the various muscles is carried out in the brain stem and involves numerous reflex arcs related to the fifth, seventh, ninth, tenth, eleventh, and twelfth cranial nerves.

These reflexes are fully established before birth so that the newborn baby, even if premature, can immediately take to the breast. The relationships of the various oral structures are also established during fetal life in such a manner as to facilitate the activity of suckling. These include the space between the anterior segments of the upper and lower gum pads, the resting position of the tongue and the form, mobility and relationship between the upper and lower lips (Fig. 274).

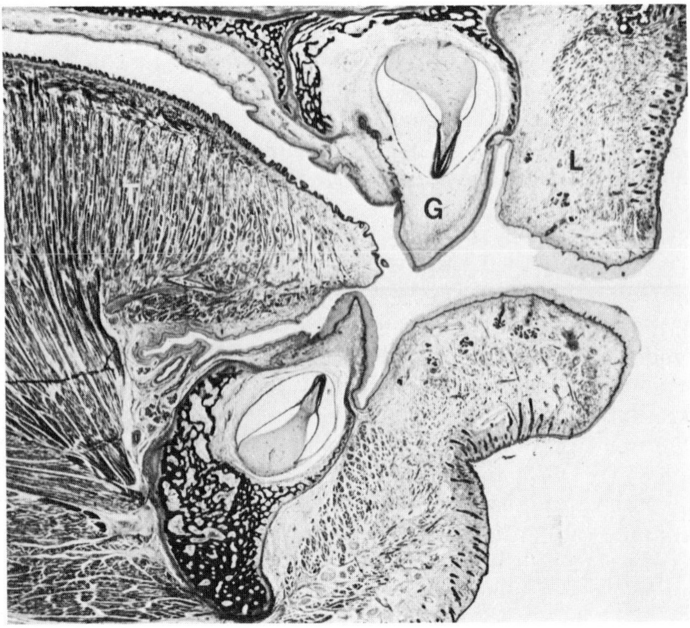

Fig. 274 The characteristic relationship of lips, gum pads, and tongue during fetal life. Human fetus of five months. 160 mm C.R. length. G, gum pad; L, lip.

Speech. In the production of speech the muscles of the tongue, lips, and soft palate co-operate with those of the larynx. The sounds produced by the larynx are modified according to whether the expired air passes through the nasal cavity, the oral cavity, or through both, and this depends on whether the soft palate is raised or lowered and on whether the lips are open or closed. Temporary obstruction to the escape of air is produced by the palate, lips, teeth, or tongue, and is responsible for the majority of consonant sounds, whereas in the production of vowel sounds there is little if any obstruction but various modifications in the form of the oral passage produced by the action of the muscles of the jaws, cheeks, lips, and tongue.

In patients with a cleft palate, suckling, swallowing and speech are interfered with to various degrees. The essential functional defect is the failure of the mutilated soft palate to seal off the nasopharynx. Therefore during suckling and swallowing food may pass into the nose, and the oro-pharyngeal vacuum, which is necessary in suckling and enables the process of transferring the food through the lower pharynx to take place with extreme rapidity in normal function, is incomplete. Speech is interfered with, especially in those sounds which require the use of the oral cavity alone.

Muscle balance and dental arch form. The teeth erupt and the alveolar arches develop between the muscles of the cheeks and lips which are related to their outer (vestibular) surfaces, and the tongue, which is related to their lingual surfaces. Under normal conditions the pressures exerted by these muscles probably play only a minor role in determining the form of the dental arches. Although the dental arches of Australian aborigines are much larger than those of persons of European descent, the tongue pressures exerted at rest and in swallowing are less in Australian aborigines. In a certain number of children, however, habits such as tongue thrusting and sucking of the thumb or fingers become established and persist. As a result the incisor and canine teeth and their supporting alveolar bone are displaced and deformed, producing conditions such as open bite, protrusion (forward displacement) of the upper teeth, and retrusion (backward displacement) of the lower teeth. Such conditions require a discontinuation of the habit and in many cases call for orthodontic treatment.

BIBLIOGRAPHY

Adatia, A. K. & Gehring, E. N. (1971). Proprioceptive innervation of the tongue. *J. Anat. Lond.* **110**, 215.

Anderson, D. J. & Matthews, B. (Eds.) (1976). *Mastication*. Bristol: Wright.

Ardran, G. M. & Kemp, F. H. (1951). The mechanism of swallowing. *Proc. R. Soc. Med.* **44**, 1037.

Ardran, G. M., Kemp, F. H. and Lind, J. (1958). A cineradiographic study of breast feeding. *Brit. J. Radiol.* **31**, 156.

Berry, D. C. & Yemm, R. (1976). Muscle functions and the occlusion of the teeth. In *Scientific Foundations of Dentistry*. Eds. Cohen, B. & Kramer, I. R. H. London: Heinemann.

Greenfield, B. E. & Wyke, B. D. (1956). Electromyographic studies of some of the muscles of mastication. *Brit. dent. J.* **100**, 129.

Kawamura, Y. (1967). Neurophysiologic background of occlusion. *Periodontics.* **5**, 175.

Matthews, B. (1975). Mastication. In *Applied Physiology of the Mouth*. Ed. Lavelle, C. L. B. Bristol: Wright.

Moller, E. (1966). The chewing apparatus—an electron-myographic study. *Acta physiol. Scand.* **69**, Supplement, 280.

Moyers, R. E. (1971). Postnatal development of the orofacial musculature, in *Patterns of Orofacial Growth and Development*. Washington: American Speech and Hearing Association.

Parfitt, G. J. (1960). Measurement of the physiological mobility of individual teeth. *J. dent. Res.* **39**, 608.

Picton, D. C. A. (1962). Distortion of the jaws during biting. *Arch. oral Biol.* **7**, 573.

Proffit, W. R., McGlone, R. E. & Barrett, M. J. (1975). Lip and tongue pressures related to dental arch and oral cavity size in Australian aborigines. *J. dent. Res.* **54**, 1161.

Rees, L. A. (1954). The structure and function of the mandibular joint. *Brit. dent. J.* **96**, 125.

Sarnat, B. G. (1964). *The Temporomandibular Joint.* 2nd ed. Springfield: Thomas.

Tulley, W. J. (1953). Methods of recording patterns of behaviour of the oro-facial muscles using the electromyograph. *Dent. Rec.* **73**, 741.

Wildman, A. J., Fletcher, S. G. & Cox, B. (1964). Patterns of deglutition. *Angle Orthodont.* **34**, 271.

Winders, R. V. (1958). Forces exerted on the dentition by the perioral and lingual musculature during swallowing. *Angle Orthodont.* **28**, 226.

19. A Summary of the Age Changes in the Teeth and the Jaws

Teeth usually become somewhat darker with age. This may be due to increasing pigmentation of the organic material in enamel and also to an increased thickness of the underlying dentine.

Enamel. The enamel gradually becomes less permeable, the change being confined to the outer layer of old enamel. The change is due to an alteration of the organic part of the enamel, this being the path along which the enamel is permeable. In the deciduous dentition, once resorption has begun, the permeability of the enamel rapidly decreases until it becomes practically impermeable. As a result of wear (attrition) there is a gradual loss of enamel over the cusps and incisive edges of the teeth. This loss of enamel also occurs on the interstitial surfaces of the teeth, with reduction in the total length of the dental arches. With increasing age the transverse ridges on the enamel surfaces (perikymata) become progressively flattened until the enamel surface becomes smooth.

Dentine. Throughout the life of the tooth there tends to be a slow formation of dentine (regular secondary dentine), which reduces the size of the pulp cavity. The rate of deposition is faster in the early years and slows down with age. The pronounced pulpal cornua of young teeth are gradually obliterated. This physiological deposition of regular secondary dentine varies in amount in different teeth and only takes place while the pulp is free from senile changes. In adult teeth many of the dentinal tubules become completely calcified, producing areas or tracts of translucent dentine. If attrition is severe the dentine is eventually exposed and the odontoblast processes in the tubules thus opened up degenerate and disappear, so producing a dead tract in the dentine. At the pulp end of the affected tubules a deposition of irregular secondary dentine occurs, further reducing the size of the pulp cavity until it may become almost entirely obliterated. The deposition of secondary dentine also changes the root canals from a simple to a complex pattern.

With advancing age the dentine in the region of the root apex becomes translucent and this process gradually spreads in a crownward direction. It is produced by occlusion of the dentinal tubules with calcified material.

Pulp. With increasing age the pulp tissue shows a reduction in the number of the cellular elements and an increase in the fibrous tissue. This occurs regularly in the pulp tissue of all teeth. Further changes may result in a loss of the connections of the fibroblasts with one another so that they no longer form a syncytium; individual odontoblasts atrophy so that the odontoblast layer becomes discontinuous. The collagen fibres increase in number and density so as to produce an actual fibrosis, the pulp tissue then resembling scar tissue. Calcification, either as discrete granules or as pulp stones, is common in such fibrosed pulps. The delicate capillary plexus of the periphery of the pulp is reduced and the whole tissue becomes less vascular; there is also a loss of sensitivity. As the pulp ages it loses its function of being the nutritive organ of the dentine, which becomes dehydrated and tends to shrink. This shrinkage weakens the support for the overlying enamel, which may crack. These changes of the pulp tissue, though degenerative, occur so frequently as to be almost considered a normal occurrence. They are senile changes.

Cement. Since there is a continued slow deposition of cement throughout the life of a tooth, the thickness of the cement gradually increases, and especially at the root apex. In older teeth the number of apical foramina may be increased as a result of cement deposition. The permeability of the cement, considered as a whole, gradually decreases. Permeability from the dentine side is soon lost, except in the apical region, whereas from the periodontal side, though permeability remains longer, it is eventually lost except in the most newly formed layers of the cement. The great majority of permanent teeth show small areas of resorption in the cement; many of these are repaired by the deposition of more cement.

Gingival tissue and periodontal membrane. With increasing age a continuous rootward migration of the gingival margin occurs leading to an exposure of more and more of the crown of the tooth in the mouth cavity, and sometimes eventually of the cement-covered root. In this way an increase in the amount of tooth substance exposed in the mouth cavity (clinical crown) may be brought about, though if attrition keeps pace with the rootward shift of the gingival margin the clinical crown may remain constant in size. In dentitions which are used in heavy mastication the reduction of the clinical crown by attrition protects the periodontal membrane by reducing the tooth leverage, especially in single-rooted teeth. To compensate for the shortening of the functional root area which follows on the migration of the epithelial attachment or cuff and the detachment of the cervical fibres of the periodontal membrane, the root is elongated at its apical end by the deposition of layers of cellular cement, which give further attachment to the periodontal membrane. The cement exposed in the mouth cavity becomes smooth and is often gradually worn away unless covered by a deposit of calculus.

General effects of attrition on the teeth. Where attrition progressively brings about a wearing down of the occlusal surfaces, the teeth erupt to the extent of the loss of tooth substance; as a result there is no diminution in height of the face. The loss of tooth substance caused by wear at the contact areas results in an increase in the area of contact between the teeth on their interstitial surfaces and a reduction of the interdental gingival tissue and of the depth and thickness of the alveolar septum between the roots of the adjacent teeth. The wearing at the contact areas also leads to a mesial drift of all the teeth with an associated reconstruction of the tooth sockets and periodontal membrane.

The wearing down of the cusps of the cheek teeth allows the lower jaw to move forward relative to the upper so that an edge to edge bite may develop between the incisors; this accelerates the process of attrition in those teeth. In the lower cheek teeth the buccal cusps are usually more worn than the lingual cusps, so that the occlusal surface no longer tilts lingually but slopes towards the buccal side (Fig. 275). In the upper cheek teeth the lingual cusps are usually more worn, so that their occlusal surfaces slope lingually.

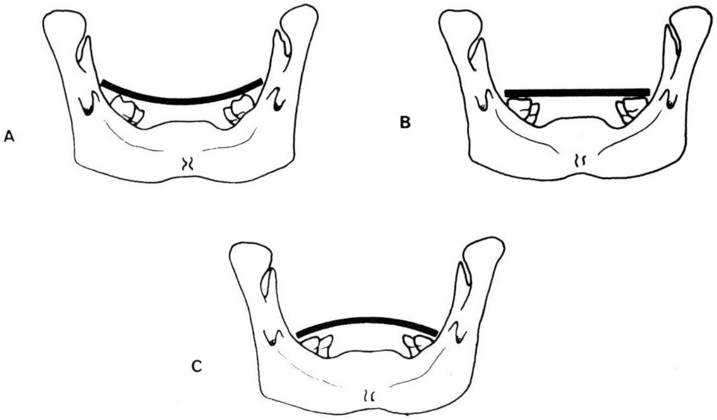

Fig. 275 Wear of the molar teeth. Mandibles viewed from behind: A, unworn; B, moderately worn; C, heavily worn. Occlusal plane (curve of Monson) represented by heavy line. (*Courtesy of Dr A. G. S. Lumsden and Prof. J. W. Osborn & the Journal of Dentistry*).

Attrition of the teeth is usually considered to be favourable since theoretically the cusps are made less pronounced and lateral thrusts on the teeth, during mastication, should thus be reduced. The form of the attrition and its effect depend, however, upon the patterns of movement established in each individual, and this can also result in a variation in tilting and migration of the teeth. Four kinds of movement pattern can be distinguished in adult dentitions which have been established for some time. These are:

1. Multi-directional gliding movements.
2. Predominating bilateral movements.
3. Predominating sagittal movements.
4. Predominating unilateral movements.

With (1) attrition is favourable as there is a reduction in overbite and in cusp inclination. This results in a more axial direction of the stresses on the teeth. With (2) attrition is somewhat unfavourable as steep mesial and distal facets are produced on the premolars, though the reduction of the cusps produced in a bucco-lingual direction is favourable. With (3) attrition and tilting are produced in the anterior segment of the dentition; the tilting is unfavourable because of the direction of the stress on these teeth. With (4) attrition is unfavourable, for it results in the formation of transversely arranged oblique planes on the molars and often on the premolars. The stresses on these teeth then deviate from the axial direction.

The degree of attrition can be estimated and recorded in the following stages. Stage 1: Wear of enamel on cusps and incisive edges without exposure of dentine. Stage 2: Wear of enamel and exposure of a thin strip of dentine on incisive edges and of isolated areas over individual cusps. Stage 3: Wear of enamel forming a broad strip on incisive edges and the confluence of two or more areas of wear over adjacent cusps. Stage 4: Wear of enamel and dentine on incisors to form a plateau and on the cheek teeth to form a central area of dentine surrounded by a peripheral rim of enamel. A marked degree of attrition is not often found in civilised communities, but it is generally present in primitive races and in prehistoric man. In dentitions showing attrition the incisors and molars show the greatest amount of wear in the lower jaw and the premolars in the upper jaw.

The jaws and temporo-mandibular joint. Microradiographic studies of the mandible show marked constructive activity in young bone, then a diminution of activity until early middle life followed by a comparative rise in bone resorption up to old age. With loss of teeth the supporting alveolar bone is resorbed, but this resorption is very much greater when a number of adjacent teeth are lost than when isolated teeth are lost. The controlling factor in the disappearance of the alveolar bone is probably pressure exerted upon the bone through the gums, and is therefore most evident when all the teeth are lost and the upper and lower gums are used as organs of mastication. When artificial dentures are worn the pressures exerted in mastication are partly transmitted, especially in the upper jaw, to regions other than the alveolar processes and resorption of the alveolar bone is less extensive and rapid.

As the alveolar processes are resorbed the height of the oral cavity is reduced, leading to characteristic changes in the profile. For some time after the extraction of all the teeth the upper and lower gums cannot be brought into contact, but in time this may be rendered possible by a stretching of the ligaments and capsule of the temporo-mandibular joint. Other changes in the joint associated with loss of all the teeth or the posterior teeth, and a consequent closure of the mouth, are a flattening of the articular eminence and a more backward positioning of the head of the condyle in the glenoid cavity. This abnormal position of the condyle produces structural and degenerative changes in the articular surfaces and the articular disc, which may lead to ear symptoms and pain referred reflexly to the vertex of the head.

In the upper jaw after the loss of the teeth the floor of the maxillary sinus may come very close to the mouth cavity with only a very thin plate of bone separating the mucous membrane of the sinus from that of the mouth. In the mandible loss of the teeth is usually associated with some atrophy of the muscles of mastication and the muscular processes of that bone. This leads to the typical narrow-pointed coronoid process and the wide mandibular angle of the senile edentulous mandible. The mental foramen comes to be closer to the upper border and may in extreme cases open on the upper border and beneath the gum, so producing a sensitive area where the mental nerve lies close to the surface of the oral mucous membrane. In old people the oral mucosa often appears thin and parchment-like.

Determination of age from teeth and jaws. For medico-legal and archaeological purposes it is often important to estimate the age of a skull, jaw bones, or isolated teeth. The state of closure of the skull sutures, including the synchondrosis of the cranial base between the occipital and sphenoid bones, and the thickness of the cranial and facial bones, provide a certain amount of evidence, but the state of development of the dentition is usually the most reliable evidence available.

If jaw bones or parts of the jaw bones containing teeth are available the evidence includes:

1. The development of the dentition. Up to about twelve to fourteen years the position and degree of formation of developing and erupting teeth, the number and the amount of wear of deciduous teeth, the occlusal relations and condition of the apices of erupted teeth, together provide information which usually renders it possible to calculate the age to within two or three years or less.

Between twelve to fourteen years and approximately twenty-five years of age the state of development, eruption, and occlusal relations of the third permanent molars (if present) in association with the state of development of the maxillary tuberosity and the evidence of wear of the remaining teeth when taken together usually enable the age to be estimated to within three to five years.

2. Other evidence of age up to about twenty-five years is provided by the condition of the openings of the gubernacular canals and the condition of the alveolar bulbs, which become replaced by the maxillary tuberosities in the upper jaw; the relation of the teeth to the zygomatic process (key ridge) of the maxilla; and the condition of the mandibular growth cartilage. After twenty-five years the age can be estimated with less accuracy by the degree of attrition of the permanent teeth; the progressive reduction in the thickness of the interdental septa associated with wear at the interstitial surfaces of teeth and mesial drift of the dentition; the relationship of the floor of the maxillary sinus to the root apices of the upper cheek teeth and the maxillary tuberosity; the condition of muscular processes such as the coronoid process, the angle of the

mandible, the zygomatic arches, and the lateral pterygoid plates. As these depend on muscle activity for their full development, the use to which the muscles are put as well as age changes must be taken into consideration.

The evidence provided by isolated teeth includes:

1. The degree of attrition on occlusal surfaces, incisive edges, and contact areas. As attrition depends on the amount of use of the dental apparatus, the nature of the diet, the hardness of enamel, and the presence of opposing teeth, it is not in itself a reliable guide to age. If, however, a number of teeth are available, and especially if the three permanent molars are present, the degree of attrition in relation to their times of appearance in the mouth (functional life) can give useful information.

2. The condition of the apical foramen or foramina. In young teeth these are open and funnel shaped (Fig. 97); with increasing age there is an increase in cement deposition in the apical region, but the rate at which cement is deposited shows a considerable individual variation.

3. The size of the pulp cavities. These are largest during and immediately after eruption. They gradually become reduced by the deposition of secondary dentine. If the three permanent molars are available the comparative size of the pulp cavities may provide useful evidence.

4. The transparency of the roots of teeth. With age the dentine becomes more highly calcified and translucent. This process of increasing translucency commences in the apical region and with age spreads towards the crown.

BIBLIOGRAPHY

Atkinson, H. F. & Matthews, E. (1949). An investigation into the permeability of human deciduous enamel. *Brit. dent. J.* **86**, 142.

Atkinson, J. P. & Woodhead, C. (1968). Changes in human mandibular structure with age. *Archs. oral Biol.* **13**, 1453.

Beyron, H. L. (1954). Occlusal changes in adult dentition. *J. Amer. dent. Ass.* **48**, 674.

Davis, T. G. H. & Pedersen, P. O. (1955). The degree of attrition of the deciduous teeth and first permanent molars of primitive and urbanised Greenland natives. *Brit. dent. J.* **99**, 35.

Gustafson, G. (1950). Age determinations on teeth. *J. Amer. dent. Ass.* **41**, 45.

Manson, J. D. & Lucas, R. B. (1962). A microradiographic study of age changes in the human mandible. *Arch. oral Biol.* **7**, 761.

Miles, A. E. W. (1963). The dentition in the assessment of individual age in skeletal material. In *Dental Anthropology*, ed. Brothwell, D. R. Oxford: Pergamon Press.

Miles, A. E. W. (1976). Age changes in dental tissues. In *Scientific Foundations of Dentistry*. Eds. Cohen, B. & Kramer, I. R. H. London: Heinemann.

Nalbandian, J., Gonzales, F. & Sognnaes, R. F. (1960). Sclerotic age changes in root dentine of human teeth as observed by optical, electron, and X-ray microscopy. *J. dent. Res.* **39**, 598.

Philippas, G. (1961). Influence of occlusal wear and age on formation of dentine and size of pulp chamber. *J. dent. Res.* **40**, 1186.

Phillipas, G. E. & Applebaum, E. (1966). Age factor in secondary dentine formation. *J. dent. Res.* **45**, 778.

SECTION V

Comparative dental anatomy

20. Classification of Vertebrates and Vertebrate Dentitions

The basic hierarchy of living creatures is:

Kingdom—The Vegetable Kingdom and the Animal Kingdom.
Phylum—*e.g.*, the Phylum Chordata.
Class—*e.g.*, the class Mammalia.
Order—*e.g.*, the order Primates.
Family—*e.g.*, the family Hominidae.
Genus—*e.g.*, the genus Homo.
Species—*e.g.*, the species *Homo sapiens.*

The genus name and species name go together in naming any species.

The Fishes, Amphibians, Reptiles, Birds, and Mammals which together make up the Vertebrate group of animals are similar to one another in that they all possess a vertebral column and teeth, unless the latter have been lost as a secondary process of degeneration or specialisation. They are all members of the Phylum Chordata, which are alike in the possession, during some period of development, of a notochord.

In the more detailed classification of animals intermediate groupings such as subphylum, superclass and subclass, subgenus and subspecies, are used. Modern classifications attempt to include not only living animals but also extinct animals. The latter are placed in their proper place as far as possible on the evidence provided by fossilised bones and teeth; and as teeth are less easily destroyed than bones, preserve their form better, and show more minute differentiating characteristics of form and dimensions, they play a most important part in the classification of vertebrates.

Apart from the fishes which fall into two or more classes according to which classification is used, but which can be divided into two great groups, the cartilaginous fishes (including the Elasmobranchs) and the bony fishes (of which the dominant modern forms are known as Teleosts), the classes of the vertebrate animals are:

Amphibia—frogs, toads, newts.
Reptilia—lizards, snakes, crocodiles.
Aves—birds.
Mammalia—mammals.

These four classes together are sometimes referred to as tetrapods. The class Mammalia is composed of the following subclasses:

Allotheria—order Multituberculata.
Triconodonta.

Symmetrodonta.
Pantotheria.
Prototheria—order Monotremata.
Metatheria—order Marsupialia.
Eutheria—of which the more important orders are:
- Primates—tree shrews, lemurs, tarsius, monkeys, apes, man.
- Insectivora—hedgehogs, moles.
- Chiroptera—bats.
- Carnivora—cats, dogs, bears, seals, walrus.
- Cetacea—whales, porpoises, dolphins.
- Perissodactyla (odd-toed ungulates)—horses, tapirs, rhinoceroses.
- Artiodactyla (even-toed ungulates)—pigs, sheep, oxen, deer, camels.
- Condylarthra—primitive ungulates (extinct).
- Proboscidea—elephants.
- Hyracoidea—hyrax.
- Sirenia—manatee, dugong.
- Rodentia—rats, guinea-pigs, squirrels, beavers.
- Lagomorpha—hares, rabbits.
- Edentata—armadillos, sloths.

The subclasses Allotheria, Triconodonta, Symmetrodonta, and Pantotheria are grouped together as the primitive mammals and are all extinct. It is generally held that all the modern mammals evolved from members of the subclass Pantotheria before these became extinct. The Prototheria and Metatheria which are limited almost entirely to Australia and Tasmania are in many ways more 'primitive' than the members of the subclass Eutheria. The order Condylarthra, which in some respects is intermediate between the primitive Carnivores (Creodonts) and Ungulates, together with some other Eutherian orders not included in the list given above, are extinct. Of the Eutherian orders still in existence the Insectivores are probably the most ancient, and it is possible that the Primates are derived from them. Little is known as yet of the phylogenetic relationship between the various orders.

THE SUBDIVISIONS OF TIME

Living creatures, for which there is a fossil record, have existed on earth for some 500 million years. For purposes of subdivision this great reach of time has been divided into Eras, Periods, and Epochs according to the nature of the sedimentary rocks deposited at different periods of the earth's history. The eras are:

1. The Palaeozoic era—the era of ancient life which has been divided into six great periods:

   1. The Cambrian.
   2. The Ordovician.
   3. The Silurian.

4. The Devonian.
5. The Carboniferous.
6. The Permian.

The Cambrian period began some 550 million years ago and the Permian period ended some 200 million years ago.

Fossil fishes first appear in the rocks of the Silurian period.

Fossil amphibians first appear in rocks of the Devonian period.

Fossil reptiles first appear in rocks of the Carboniferous period.

2. The Palaeozoic era was succeeded by the Mesozoic era—the era of 'middle life,' which has been subdivided into three periods:

a. The Triassic, with a duration of some 50 million years.
b. The Jurassic, with a duration of some 30 million years.
c. The Cretaceous, with a duration of some 50 million years.

TABLE 3 Geological Time Scale

Era	Period	Epoch	Time	First Appearance of
Cainozoic	Quaternary	Holocene		
		Pleistocene	1–2 million years ago	Man
	Tertiary	Pliocene		
		Miocene		
		Oligocene		Anthropoid Apes
		Eocene		
		Palaeocene	70 million years ago	Primates
Mesozoic	Cretaceous		120 million years ago	Modern Mammals
	Jurassic			Early Mammals
	Triassic		200 million years ago	
Palaeozoic	Permian			
	Carboniferous			Reptiles
	Devonian			Amphibians
	Silurian			Fishes
	Ordovician			
	Cambrian		550 million years ago	

The Mesozoic era was dominated by the reptiles and is sometimes known as the Age of Reptiles, but in the Triassic period the fossils of the first of the primitive mammals appear in the rocks and later those of the first birds. During the Cretaceous period the fossils of the first modern mammals appear; by the end of the era the primitive mammals became extinct except for the Multituberculates which have had the longest life-span of any Mammalian order to date.

3. The Mesozoic era was succeeded by the present Cainozoic era, which began some 70 million years ago and which is subdivided into two periods:

1. The Tertiary.
2. The Quaternary.

The Tertiary period has been divided into five epochs:

a. The Palaeocene.
b. The Eocene.
c. The Oligocene.
d. The Miocene.
e. The Pliocene.

And the Quaternary period into two epochs:

a. The Pleistocene.
b. The Holocene—since the last Ice Age.

It is approximately 1–2 million years since the beginning of the Pleistocene epoch and 70 million years since the beginning of the Palaeocene epoch and of the Tertiary period of the Cainozoic era.

Fossil primates first appear in the rocks of the Palaeocene epoch.

Fossil anthropoid apes appear in rocks of the Oligocene epoch; the Australopithecinae fossils are from the upper Pliocene and lower Pleistocene and the earliest human fossils discovered to date are from the Pleistocene epoch.

METHODS OF DATING THE PAST

Radioactive methods. These are based on the fact that radioactive minerals disintegrate at a constant and determinable rate. For example, uranium with an atomic weight of 238 disintegrates in a series of steps to uranium lead with an atomic weight of 206. At each step in the process an atom of helium gas is given off. The time taken for each step varies enormously from nearly 5000 million years for the first of the series from uranium 1 to uranium X, to 3 minutes for the step from radium A to radium B. By the use of such methods the age of the rocks with which fossils are associated can be ascertained.

Radioactive carbon. All organic tissues take up a certain amount of the radioactive isotope of carbon (C^{14}) from the atmosphere. After death no further uptake is possible and the radioactive carbon disintegrates to ordinary carbon at a constant rate. This method gives a direct determination of the age of a fossil within the approximate time range of 1000–30 000 years from the present.

Fluorine method. Fossil bones and teeth take up fluorine from the adjacent soil water at a rate which is fairly constant relative to the availability of this mineral. It is most useful in establishing whether two or more fossils found in the same strata are contemporaneous. It was the application of the method of fluorine analysis which first cast serious doubt on the genuineness of the 'forged' Piltdown skull.

These modern methods supplement the older classical methods of dating fossils such as determining the rate of deposition of sedimentary rocks and the oscillating movements of ice caps.

GENERAL CHARACTERISTICS OF VERTEBRATE DENTITIONS

Tooth attachment. Teeth are attached to the epithelium of the mouth, to the adjacent mesoderm, and to the jaw bones. The epithelial attachment is provided by the continuity between the gum epithelium and the enamel epithelium. It represents the union of the mouth epithelium with the epithelial derivative enamel; it is of little mechanical significance. Through its pulp, which provides the matrix for the growth and calcification of dentine, the tooth is in continuity with the adjacent mesodermal tissues at the apical foramen. This attachment, through which the tooth receives its nutrition and sensitivity, is also of little mechanical significance.

The attachment of the teeth to the jaws may be by means of a specialised ligament continuous with the substance of the dentine or with a special bone-like tissue, cement, or by a continuity between dentine and jaw bone known as bony anchylosis. The latter provides a firm but somewhat brittle attachment, and such teeth are often shed as a result of fracture of the bony attachment. In mammals the teeth are attached through a specialised ligament to the walls of a socket in the alveolar bone. This provides firm attachment with a limited degree of mobility, permitting the tooth to withstand the shocks produced by mastication. In some animals the teeth are specialised in the method of their attachment to allow of a wide range of movement. The elasticity necessary to allow such mobile teeth to return to their resting position is provided by a variety of interesting mechanisms.

Tooth succession. The problem of establishing a functional correlation between the life history of individual teeth and that of the animal is solved in the lower vertebrates by a process of continual tooth succession. This involves a complex interaction of mechanical and developmental processes to ensure that tooth loss is correlated with tooth succession, and all the factors involved are not yet understoood. Among the mammals tooth replacement occurs at the most only once in the animal's life time. In order that the life history of the second, final, or 'permanent' dentition should coincide with that of the animal, a firm but flexible method of attachment has been evolved (gomphosis) and in some animals tooth growth continues throughout life. In such animals a process of continual replacement of the dental tissues takes the place of a continual replacement of dental units.

It has generally been held that a continuous succession of teeth allows for the replacement of teeth that have become worn or possibly broken. However, since many of the shed teeth show little signs of wear the basic function of this arrangement may rather be the supply of successively larger teeth to furnish the jaws which continue to grow throughout life.

Fishes. Some fishes are without teeth, but in the majority teeth are present. In the elasmobranch fishes the teeth are attached by fibrous tissue to the upper and lower jaws (Meckel's cartilage and the pterygoquadrate bar). In bony fishes they may be attached to a number of bones including the premaxilla, maxilla, palatine, vomer, and parasphenoid in the upper jaw, the dentale in the lower jaw, and to bones of the branchial arches. They may be attached by bony anchylosis or by a fibrous ligament. In a very few cases they are implanted in sockets. The teeth in most fishes are small conical recurved structures whose function is to hold the prey. In some deep-sea fishes, however, the teeth are immense structures. Other types of teeth found in fishes are plate-like slicing teeth and blunt crushing teeth. In a few the dentition is heterodont; that is, different forms of teeth are found in different parts of the mouth cavity. Since the teeth show a continual succession the dentition is described as polyphyodont.

Amphibians. In some amphibians (*i.e.*, the toad) teeth are absent. In others they are present in one jaw only. Sometimes there are two rows in the upper jaw between which the teeth of the lower jaw bite. The teeth of amphibians are usually small conical structures attached by bony anchylosis and undergo a process of continual replacement.

Reptiles. Teeth are absent in turtles and are replaced by horny plates. The typical reptilian dentition consists of a row of conical teeth of varying sizes in each jaw, attached by bony anchylosis and undergoing a process of continual succession. However, in some cases the dentition is much more complex with piercing, cutting, and crushing teeth. In some reptiles the cheek teeth have a number of cusps usually arranged around a principal cusp. From such a dentition the teeth of primitive mammals were probably derived. In certain reptiles such as the crocodile, the teeth are attached by a periodontal membrane to bony sockets. Multi-rooted teeth are not found among living reptiles. In some snakes certain teeth are modified to form poison fangs. These contain a canal or a groove which conducts the venom from the base of the tooth to just below the tip in a manner similar to a hypodermic needle.

Primitive mammals. The earliest known mammals are fossils from the rocks of the late Triassic and early Jurassic periods of the Mesozoic era and are about 150 million years old. The fossil material at present available falls into four groups:

1. The order Multituberculata (subclass Allotheria) which lasted through the Mesozoic era to the Palaeocene epoch of the Tertiary period, when they became extinct without giving rise to any modern orders.

2. The subclass Triconodonta which existed through the Jurassic period and became extinct in the early Cretaceous period of the Mesozoic.

3. The subclass Symmetrodonta which had a similar history to that of the Triconodonta.

4. The subclass Pantotheria which was limited as far as is known to the Jurassic period. It is believed that this order gave origin to primitive Marsupials and Eutherian (modern mammalian) orders before becoming extinct.

The earliest fossils attributable to an order (Insectivora) of the modern mammals come from rocks of the late Cretaceous period. It is as yet uncertain whether these four early mammalian groups arose from a common stem or whether each evolved independently from different orders of the mammal-like reptiles in the Triassic period. It would seem probable that the Multituberculates at least arose from a reptilian ancestor independent of the other three groups.

Pantotheria. In this subclass the incisors, canines, and premolars were of a simple pattern. The upper molars were triangular shaped teeth, with two main cusps, an outer (buccal) amphicone, and an inner (lingual) protocone. The lower molars consisted of two parts, an anterior trigonid made up of three cusps, an outer protoconid and two inner (lingual) cusps, the paraconid in front (mesial) and the metaconid behind (distal); and behind the trigonid with its pointed cusps came the lower basin-like talonid (Fig. 276A).

In occlusion the disto-lingual surface of the upper first molars sliced down against the mesio-buccal surface of the lower second molars and the protocone of the first upper molar occluded with the talonid element of the first lower molar. There was a similar relationship between all the molar teeth of the series, which numbered eight or more on each side of each jaw. In the Pantotherian dentition, therefore, all three basic dental functions were performed by the molar teeth:

1. Piercing and holding the pointed cusps of the upper teeth (amphicones) and lower teeth (trigonid cusps).

2. Slicing and cutting by the shearing edges and surfaces of the upper and lower molars.

3. Grinding and crushing by the occlusion of the upper protocone elements with the lower talonid elements.

From such a dental mechanism all the higher dentitions, specialised as in the carnassial apparatus of the Carnivores, generalised as in the human dentition or secondarily degenerated as in the dentition of the seal or porpoise, could be derived and, according to the Cope–Osborne Tritubercular theory as modified by Gregory and Simpson, it was from the Pantotherian type of dentition that all higher mammalian dentitions evolved.

The fossil *Deltatheridium* from the late Cretaceous geological level shows a dentition similar in basic pattern to that of the later Pantotherians. The number of molars is, however, reduced to three on each side of each jaw, and the summit of the amphicone of the upper molars is split to form two subsidiary cusps, the anterior paracone and the posterior metacone, producing an upper tooth with three principal cusps arranged in a triangle of cusps (Fig. 276B).

Later a talon developed at the back of the tricuspid upper molars to form a fourth cusp (hypocone) and the lower talonid gave origin to three cusps, the hypoconid (buccal), the entoconid (lingual), and the hypoconulid (distal), so that a six-cusped lower molar was produced (Fig. 276C). Such four-cusped upper molars and six-cusped lower molars are characteristic of the lower primates and are found in the living *Tarsius*. In man the paraconid of the lower molars is lost in the first lower molars, producing a five-cusped tooth; and usually the hypoconulid (distal cusp) is also lost in the second molars, producing a four-cusped tooth.

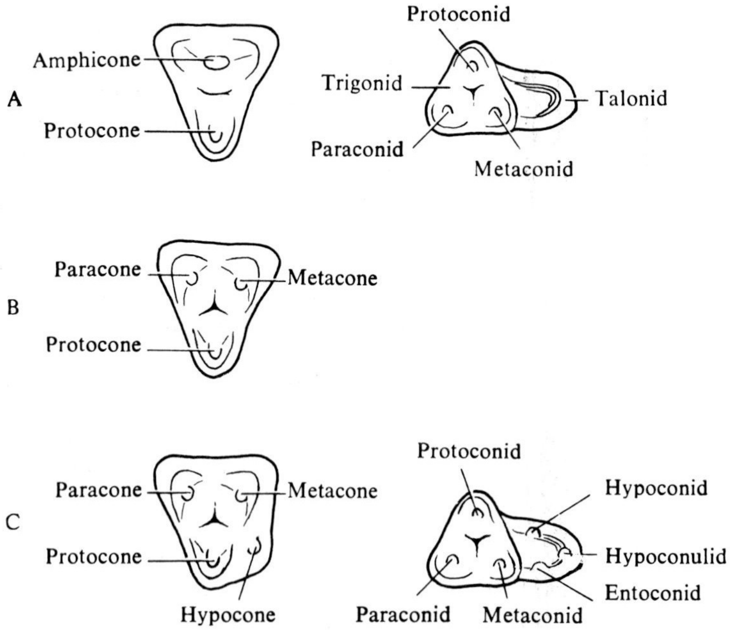

Fig. 276 Diagram illustrating the evolution of the typical mammalian molar according to the Tritubercular Theory. (A) Upper and lower molar of a Pantothere. (B) Upper molar of primitive insectivore. (C) Upper and lower molar of a lower primate.

Modern mammals. The characteristic dentition of Eutherian mammals is heterodont; that is, the teeth vary in form in different parts of the mouth. In the non-mammalian vertebrates the dentitions are generally homodont, since the teeth are similar in form in different parts of the month. The typical mammalian dentition is generally considered to have the following dental formula:

$$I\tfrac{3}{3}C\tfrac{1}{1}P\tfrac{4}{4}M\tfrac{3}{3}$$

There are, however, a great number of variations from this formula.

The teeth are attached by a periodontal membrane to the walls of a bony socket in the mandible, premaxilla, and maxilla. There are usually two dentitions, the deciduous and permanent; a diphyodont arrangement. Of the permanent dentition certain members replace deciduous teeth (successional teeth); these are usually the incisors, canines, and premolars, whereas others, the permanent molars, come into place behind the deciduous teeth (accessional teeth). The cheek teeth have usually more than one root and in many cases their crowns carry a number of cusps, which may be modified to form ridges. In the majority of mammals the teeth consist of dentine, cement, and enamel. However, enamel may be absent, and in some animals cement contributes to the structure of the crown part of the tooth as well as acting as the means whereby the periodontal membrane is attached to the root. Sometimes teeth continue to grow and erupt for the greater part of the animal's life. A characteristic feature of mammalian dentitions is the specialisation of certain individual teeth or groups of teeth to meet the requirements of specialised functions. Sometimes these function are not related to the mastication of food but to activities such as fighting, defence, manipulation, and holding. Within each of the mammalian orders there is usually a wide range of dentitions, but the characteristic features of the chief orders are as follows.

Marsupials. Apart from the opossums, which are also found on the American continent, the members of this order are at the present time limited to Australia. Among the various groups which make up this order of ancient mammals most of the features characteristic of the dentitions of the more modern mammalian orders, carnivores, rodents, and ungulates, are reproduced in their general form by a process of parallel evolution. A classical example is the 'rodent' dentition of the wombat. There are, however, certain unique and typical features not found in other mammals. The number of incisors is often increased beyond that found in the Eutheria as are the number of 'permanent' molars. As, however, there is often only one dentition, or else the number of teeth with successors is very limited, there is some difficulty in classifying the teeth into 'deciduous' and 'permanent.'

Insectivores. These animals as their name indicates feed largely on insects. The order includes shrews, moles, and the hedgehog. In the typical dentition the cheek teeth carry a number of pointed cusps which occlude between those of similar teeth in the opposite jaw. Such teeth are well adapted for holding and piercing the bodies of insects. The incisors are often modified for picking up and rooting out insects, and other small animals such as worms and grubs and snails.

Most of the insectivores are small, rather defenceless animals, but the order to which they belong is probably the most ancient among the mammals, and from the early members of the order it is probable that the majority of the other orders have evolved.

Rodents. Of all the mammalian orders the rodents have the most constant type of dentition: at the front of the mouth are the specialised chisel-shaped, continually erupting, incisor teeth used in the typical gnawing action, and at the back of the mouth a series of cheek teeth which are usually similar to one another in their form. They sometimes carry cusps, but more often a pattern of transversely directed ridges. There are no canines, and a characteristic feature is the natural tooth-free space (diastema) between the incisors and anterior members of the cheek tooth series. The muscles of mastication are complex, especially the masseter muscles, which as well as closing the jaw work with the pterygoids and temporal muscles in producing the characteristic backward and forward movement of the lower jaw.

Carnivores. Among the carnivores there is a wide variety of dentitions, from the specialised flesh-eating dentition of the great and little cats to the specialised fish-eating dentition of seals and sea-lions and the extraordinary dentition of the walrus. The dog with its well-marked dental departmentalisation occupies a central position and is adapted to a more omnivorous diet. Badgers, bears, and racoons are also adapted in their dentition to a generalised diet. A characteristic feature of the dentition of the carnivores, especially in the flesh-eating and in the majority of omnivorous forms, is the specialisation of one of the cheek teeth in each half of each jaw (the carnassial tooth). The blade-like upper tooth slices against the buccal surface of a similar lower tooth in a scissors-like action. Another characteristic feature which is present in all members of the order is the large size of the canine tooth. In some forms, especially among extinct members of the cat family, these are huge tusks which are used as weapons of offence and defence.

Ungulates. These are now divided into two orders: the perissodactyl ungulates, which include the horses, rhinoceroses, and tapirs among living forms; and the artiodactyl ungulates, which include two large subgroups, one made up of the pigs and hippopotami, and the ruminantia, which include oxen, deer, antelopes, camels, and giraffes. The pigs have a dentition adapted to an omnivorous diet, and in them the canines, especially in male animals, are well-developed tusk-like structures. Horses and the ruminantia are adapted to a vegetable diet, especially that of grass, which because of its high silica content is a very tooth-destroying substance. However, the adaptation which the two groups have made for this diet is quite different. If numbers living at the present time is a criterion of success the more successful adaptation has been made by the ruminantia. Among the ruminantia canines are poorly developed or absent as a rule, but in certain hornless deer the upper canines form long sharp-pointed tusks which take the place of horns in defence and attack.

Cetaceans. This order contains the whales, dolphins, and porpoises, mammals which have returned to a life in the sea. As the variety of available food is very much less than on land, their dentitions have either undergone a specialised reversion towards a simple set of teeth, usually conical in shape and similar to one another (homodont dentition), or their teeth have been lost altogether. In some whales teeth develop, calcify, but never erupt. Cetaceans with teeth (suborder Odontoceti) include the porpoises, dolphins, the killer whale, the sperm whale, and the bottle-nosed whale. In the narwhal there is a specialised development of one of the upper incisors to form a long spear-like tusk. Cetaceans without teeth (suborder Mystacoceti) develop a series of baleen plates suspended from the upper jaw. These act as sieves which catch the vegetable matter and small animals (plankton) on which the animals live. These 'whalebone' whales include the blue whale, the fin whale, and the right whale. 'Whalebone' (baleen) is not composed of bone but is developed from the epithelium of the hard palate.

Primates. This order contains the tree shrews, lemurs, *Tarsius*, New World and Old World monkeys, the anthropoid apes, and man. Apart from the peculiar specialisation of the lower incisors found in lemurs, the dentitions of primates have many features in common. Incisors are often spatulate, canines are usually well developed; in some primates (monkeys and apes) they form large tusks. In man, however, they do not project beyond the level of the adjacent teeth. The cheek teeth (premolars and molars) have two or three roots and two or more cusps. In man there is a tendency towards reduction both in the number of roots and cusps. In the Old World monkeys the molar teeth are specialised being lophodont. The upper and lower teeth usually carry four cusps which are connected by transverse ridges, the ridges of the upper teeth occluding with the corresponding grooves of the lower teeth and vice versa. This type of ridge and groove occlusion is quite distinct from the more primitive cusp and fossa occlusion found in the New World monkeys, anthropoid apes, and man. The crowns of the teeth are covered with enamel and cement is limited to the roots. There are two sets of teeth, deciduous and permanent.

Three main theories have been produced to explain how the polyphyodont condition found in the sub-mammalian vertebrates has evolved into the limited, diphyodont, succession of mammalian teeth; these are the Odontostichos Theory of Bolk, the Zahnreihe Theory and the Tooth Family Theory (Fig. 277). Among the mammals a deciduous dentition is usually replaced by a permanent dentition.

According to the Odontostichos Theory all the deciduous teeth are made up of the sole surviving members of the tooth families which developed at a higher (more superficial) level on the dental lamina (exostichos or parietal teeth). The permanent teeth are made up of the sole surviving members of the tooth families which developed at a lower (deeper) level on the dental lamina (endostichos or terminal teeth). Owing to a crowding of the teeth, so that (apart from regional diastemata) the teeth are usually in contact, the permanent teeth cannot erupt between the deciduous teeth while these are still in place; they come up in the place occupied by the deciduous teeth after the deciduous teeth are shed and therefore appear to belong to the same tooth family.

The Odontostichos theory has been abandoned generally since it is unsupported by the actual sequences of tooth initiation and eruption in reptiles and mammals. The Zahnreihe theory has sought to explain these features on a wave replacement of teeth from front to back of the reptilian jaw and on the supposition that mammalian dentitions are equal to two reptilian Zahnreihen. However, the sequence of tooth

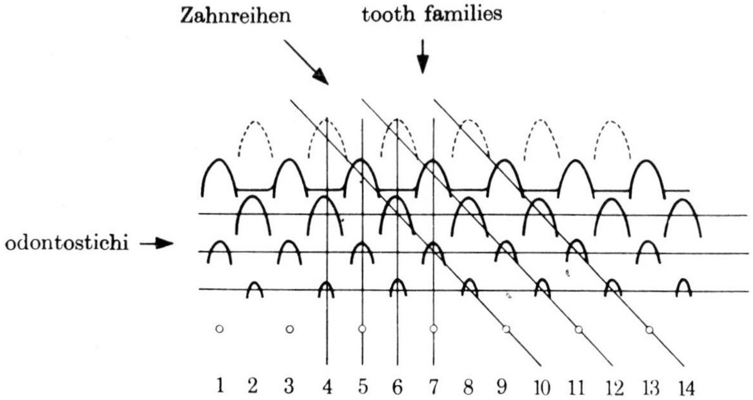

Fig. 277 A diagram of a dentition in which alternate teeth are replaced at the same time. The interrupted lines represent teeth that have been lost. The size of developing teeth is proportional to their stage of development. The lines connect rows of teeth called odontostichi, tooth families and Zahnreihen. (*Reproduced with kind permission of Prof J. W. Osborn and Proc. R. Soc. Lond.*)

development and eruption in mammals does not show such a front to back sequence. The most recent theory to account for the evolution of mammalian dentitions from those of reptiles is the Tooth Family theory. According to this theory the vertical row of teeth, the Tooth Family, is the important feature, the rate of tooth replacement being vertically controlled. In addition there appear to be several developmental regions in mammalian dentitions, the incisor, the canine and molar regions each with its own determinant. The teeth in each developmental region arise in orderly sequence but this is disguised by the combined sequence of the total dentition in which the four developmental regions appear over the same period.

BIBLIOGRAPHY

Bolk, L. (1922). Odontological essays—fifth essay. *J. Anat. Lond.* **57,** 55.

Edmund, A. G. (1960). Tooth replacement phenomena in the lower Vertebrates. *Contr. Life Sci. Div. R. Ont. Mus.* **52,** 1.

Osborn, J. W. (1973). The evolution of dentitions. *Amer. Scientist.* **61,** 548.

Romer, A. S. (1966). *Vertebrate Paleontology.* 3rd ed. Chicago University Press.

Young, J. Z. (1950). *The Life of Vertebrates.* Oxford University Press.

Zeuner, F. (1952). *Dating the Past.* 3rd ed. London: Methuen.

21. Evolution of the Jaws and of the Mandibular Joint

The skull and jaws of elasmobranch fishes (sharks and rays) are composed of calcified cartilage throughout life. In higher vertebrates the base of the skull, the nasal capsules, and the skeleton of the lower jaw develop first in cartilage. With development three further processes take place (Fig. 278).

1. Parts of the primordial cartilaginous skeleton are replaced by bone. This takes place at the base of the skull; at the front of Meckel's

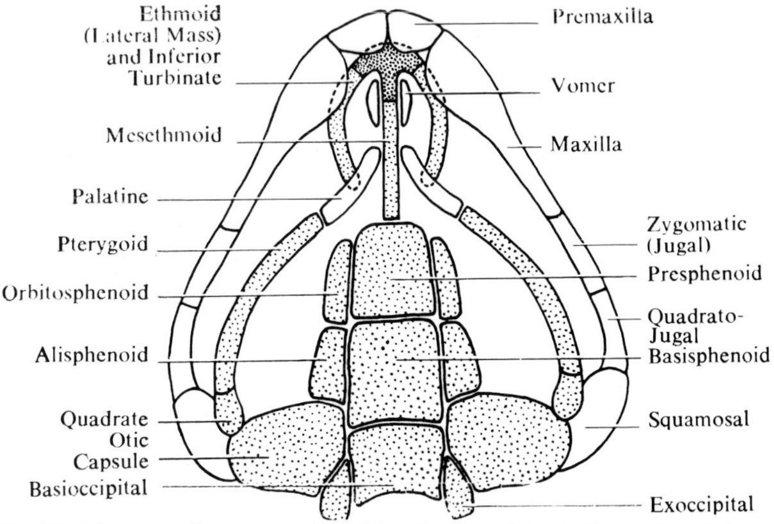

Fig. 278 Diagrammatic representation of the elements of the skull seen from below. Chondrocranium shaded, dermal elements unshaded. Cartilage, heavy stippling; cartilage bones, light stippling; membrane bones, unshaded. (Modified from Kingsley.)

cartilage, which becomes incorporated in the mandible; at the back of Meckel's cartilage, where the malleus of the middle ear develops; at the back of the palato-quadrate bar, where the incus of the middle ear develops; and in the face, where the lateral masses of the ethmoid and inferior turbinates replace parts of the nasal capsule.

2. Over the vault of the skull membrane bones develop in regions where the cartilaginous skeleton was incomplete. Such membrane bones (dermal bones) include the frontal bones, the parietals, the inter-

parietal part of the occipital, the squamous parts of the temporal bones, and the greater part of the great wings of the sphenoid.

3. Membrane bones apply themselves around parts of the cartilaginous skeleton which later atrophies. The replacement of the greater part of Meckel's cartilage by the mandible; the lateral walls of the nasal capsule by the premaxillary, maxillary, lacrimal, and palatine bones; and the replacement of part of the nasal septum by the vomer are examples in human ontogeny.

Primary and secondary jaws. In elasmobranch fishes the upper jaw is the palato-quadrate bar which is attached to the cranial part of the skull in front by ligaments and behind through the intermediary of the hyomandibular cartilage. The lower jaw skeleton is Meckel's cartilage which articulates with the back of the palato-quadrate bar (Fig. 279)

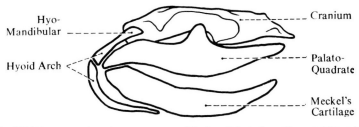

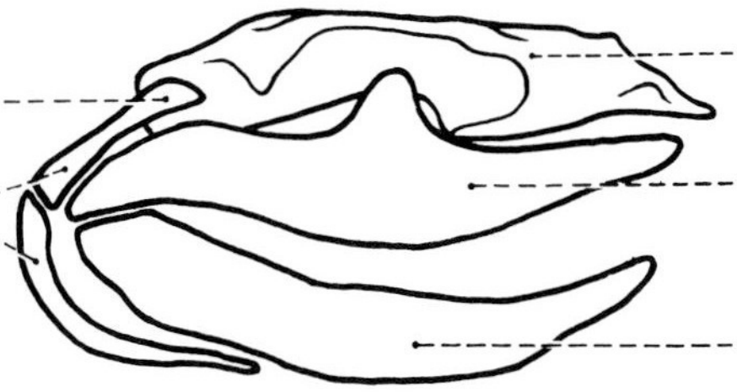

Fig. 279 Diagram to show the arrangement of the jaws (Meckel's cartilage and the palato-quadrate) and the associated cartilages in an elasmobranch.

Hence, according to functional requirements, in different species, varying degrees of movement could take place between the upper and lower jaws and between the upper jaw and the cranial part of the skull.

In bony fishes, amphibians and reptiles, a series of dermal bones are laid down around these cartilaginous primary jaw elements. Around the palato-quadrate bar develop the palatine and transverse bones which in some species carry teeth. Around Meckel's cartilage develops a complex series of bones of which the most important are the dentary, splenial, angulare, surangulare, coronoid, and goniale. Of these the first two may carry teeth. In all bony fishes and tetrapods other than mammals, the back parts of the palato-quadrate and Meckel's cartilage ossify to form the quadrate and articulare bones and between these two is the primitive jaw joint.

In modern fishes and in the tetrapods a new upper jaw develops outside the old palato-quadrate jaw and its associated dermal bones. The new jaw is made up of a series of dermal bones which include from before backward the premaxilla, the maxilla, the jugal, and the quadrato-jugal. The first two of these are associated with teeth. In many animals the teeth of the lower jaw, carried by the dentary, bite between an outer row of upper teeth carried on the premaxilla and maxilla and an inner row carried on the palatine and pterygoids. The prevomer and vomer bones which are dermal bones applied to the base of the nasal capsule and cranial part of the skull and forming the roof of the mouth and pharynx may also carry teeth.

Primary and secondary jaw joints. In the evolution of the reptiles, the number of dermal elements in the lower jaw becomes gradually reduced until the dentary comes to make up the greater part of the jaw with the angulare, surangulare, and goniale much reduced in size. The articulare, a bone which has replaced the back part of Meckel's cartilage, still forms the hindmost element of the jaw and articulates with the quadrate. This is the condition found in the mammal-like reptiles. In these creatures, moreover, the back of the dentary has grown upwards to come into close relation with the squamosal part of the temporal.

In mammals a new joint (mandibular joint) has been created between the dentary, which is now the only bone remaining in the lower jaw, and the squamosal part of the temporal. The articulare in mammals is quite separate from the mandible and forms the malleus of the middle ear. Its articulation with the quadrate (incus) remains as the malleolar-incudal joint of the middle ear. The angulare becomes the tympanic plate of the temporal.

In the early human embryo Meckel's cartilage, articulating behind with the cartilage for the incus (quadrate), makes up the skeleton of the lower jaw. The mandible (dentary) commences to develop in the 18 mm embryo and the mandibular joint when the fetus is about 57 mm (C.R.) in length. For some time before the development of the mandibular joint the early spasmodic gasping movements of the fetus involve the articulare-quadrate (primitive) jaw joint at the back of Meckel's cartilage. After the mandibular joint becomes established there is a period when both it and the primitive joint work together on each side as Meckel's cartilage remains continuous for some time before its intermediate part becomes converted into fibrous tissue (spheno-mandibular ligament) and its posterior part becomes isolated in the developing middle-ear region as the malleus.

In the submammalian vertebrates Meckel's cartilage, in virtue of its close relation to the inner ear apparatus (otocyst), acts not only as the primitive jaw joint but also, in resting upon the ground in amphibians and reptiles and in relation to water vibration in fishes, as part of the hearing apparatus. The mammalian jaw is not at all concerned with hearing, but the dorsal end of Meckel's cartilage maintains in a new setting this primordial premammalian function.

The history of the primitive jaw joint illustrates very well two characteristic features of phylogenetic development:

1. When a new organ develops the old organ is not lost immediately but continues to function for a period while its successor is in the early period of its functional activity.
2. Later, when the new organ is well established the old organ may take on some other function.

22. Comparative Anatomy of the Dental Tissues

Enamel. The criteria used to distinguish the three calcified dental tissues in the mammals are frequently of little value in the other vertebrate classes, and this is particularly true in the case of the enamel. The characteristics of mammalian enamel are taken to be that: (1) it forms an outer layer covering the whole or part of the tooth exposed in the mouth cavity; (2) it is highly calcified, and disappears with ordinary methods of decalcification; (3) it is of ectodermal origin; and (4) it shows a prismatic structure.

In Reptilia the corresponding outer layer on the crowns of the teeth, though fulfilling the first three of the above conditions, does not show a prismatic structure; it is, however, considered to be enamel. The absence of a prism pattern in reptilian enamel is related to its development in which there is a relatively flat mineralising front with perpendicular crystallite orientation throughout (see pp. 185–187).

In Amphibia and in the fishes the position is much more difficult. The outer layer on the teeth though highly calcified and disappearing with decalcification does not show any prismatic structure and may not be of ectodermal origin. Moreover, it is frequently difficult to distinguish from the underlying dentine. In some fishes the outer layer is structureless; in others it shows a system of tubules. It is on account of these difficulties that the outer layer in fishes, though sometimes called enamel, has at times been given a variety of names such as vitro-dentine, duro-dentine, or ganoin (particularly in elasmobranch and ganoid fishes). Very often the outer layer on the teeth of fishes does not form a complete investment to the exposed part of the teeth and is only found as a cap covering the tip.

It has been widely held that the outer layer in amphibian and piscine teeth is formed by the mesodermal tissue of the dental papilla as it is deposited before dentine appears, has a collagen containing matrix and develops in contact with not only internal enamel epithelium but also the cells of the dental papilla. On these grounds this layer had been described as mesodermal enamel to distinguish it from the true ectodermal enamel of Reptilia and Mammalia. However more recent work has shown that amino-acids are secreted in this layer by the cells of the internal enamel epithelium and that these cells show organelles typical of protein synthesis and secretion. It may be that the outer layer of the teeth of Amphibians and fishes is partly of ectodermal and partly of mesodermal origin and it has been suggested that it should be called

Enameloid to distinguish it from the true enamel of reptiles and mammals. Enameloid is also distinguished from enamel in that its organic basis is laid down in its full extent before calcification begins, and it is the first part of the tooth to show calcification.

Prismatic enamel. There is considerable variation in the pattern of

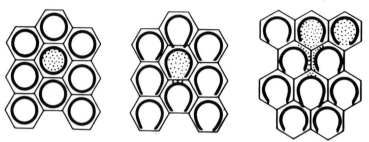

Fig. 280 Schematic representation of prism patterns in the enamel of mammals. The curved heavy lines represent the prism outlines, prism sheaths, in cross-section, that is planes where abrupt changes in crystallite orientation occur. The hexagonal outlines represent the areas of enamel produced by single ameloblasts. The stippled areas show the full extent of 'prisms'; thus 'interprismatic regions' can be distinguished in Patterns a and b, though not generally in Pattern c. This may depend on the extent of the prism sheath. (*By courtesy of Dr A. Boyde and Third Symposium on Calcified Tissues.*)

the prisms in the enamel of mammalian teeth (Fig. 280). The pattern is produced by the orientation of the crystallites which may be arranged in bundles, as in prisms, or in sheets as in interprismatic regions. The boundaries of the prisms are planes at which there is an abrupt change in the orientation of the long c-axes of the crystallites. This orientation is determined at the mineralising front during the deposition of the enamel (see pp. 185–187).

a. In Sirenia, Cheiroptera, Insectivora, and Odontoceti the usual arrangement is one of cylindrical prisms (circular in cross section) surrounded by interprismatic substance. This is also found in the cuspal areas of human teeth.

b. The prisms are horse-shoe shaped in cross-section and arranged in rows so that the 'open' side of each prism abuts on to the convex 'closed' side of the adjacent prism. The rows of prisms are separated from each other by sheets of parallel-orientated crystallites forming an interprismatic substance. This arrangement is found especially in Ungulata, Lagomorpha and Macropodidae (Marsupialia), but also occurs in the Rhesus monkey.

c. In human and elephant enamel the most commonly found arrangement is that the 'open' side of each prism faces the gap between two adjacent prisms. With this pattern there is no region which can be described as interprismatic.

In rodent enamel there are two zones distinguishable by the prism arrangement (Fig. 281). In the inner part of the enamel there is a decussa-

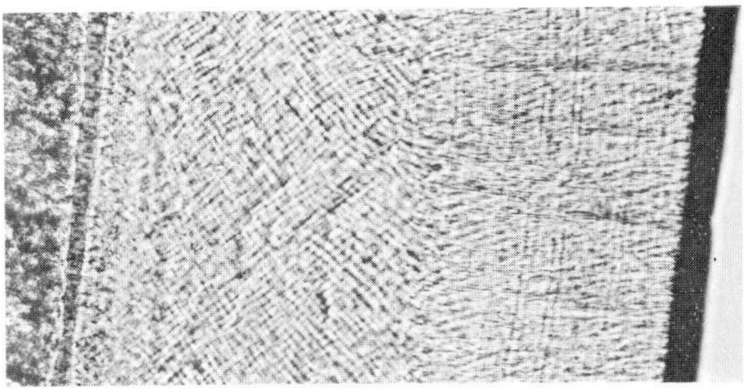

Fig. 281 Enamel of the beaver (*Castor canadensis*) showing the typical rodent arrangement of the prisms into two layers according to their direction. Ground section. × 250.

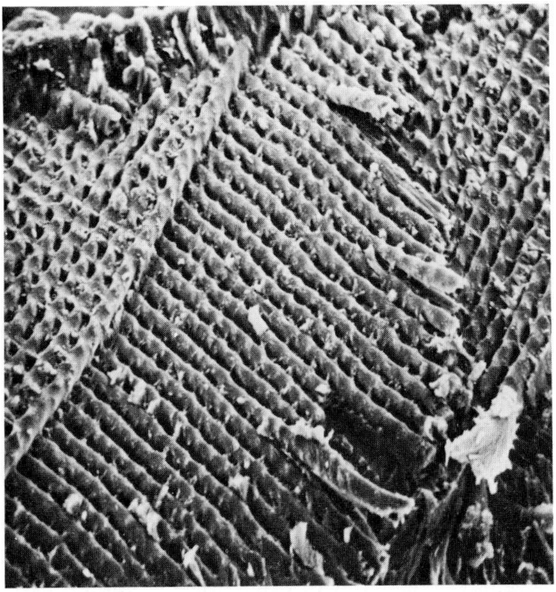

Fig. 282 Fractured surface of rat enamel showing the arrangement of the prisms in alternate layers which gives the decussation of the prisms. Original magnification × 1800. (*By courtesy of Dr A. Boyde.*)

tion of alternate transverse rows of prisms (Fig. 282). There is no interprismatic substance. In the outer part of the enamel all the prisms pass in a more or less similar direction towards the surface.

Tubular enamel. Since 1849 it has been accepted that among the members of the marsupial order (with the exception of the rodent-like wombat) the enamel is tubular in structure (Fig. 283). Recently it had been suggested that the apparently tubular nature of marsupial enamel is in fact due to the presence of uncalcified organic matrix, derived from non-mineralised enamel prisms. Observations made with the electron microscope, however, support the classical concept of tubules in marsupial enamel, and have shown that during the early stages of enamel formation the tubules are occupied by cytoplasmic extensions of the ameloblasts. Among the rodents the jerboa has tubular enamel, and tubular enamel has been found also among a few members of the order insectivora. Tubular enamel has been described among the lemurs and in *Tarsius* (Primates) and the extinct Multituberculates and also among certain members of the Sparidae family of fishes where the extent of penetration varies from partial to complete.

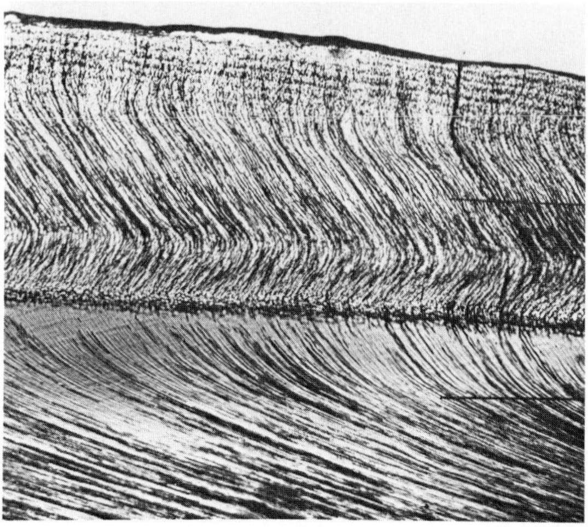

Fig. 283 Tooth of marsupial (*Hypsiprymnus*) showing the tubules in the enamel. Ground section. × 80.

Dentine. Dentine in some form makes up the bulk of all teeth, and is the fundamental tissue without which a tooth cannot exist. Tubular dentine (ortho-dentine) as found in human teeth and among the great majority of mammalian teeth is a very primitive tissue which is also present among the elasmobranch fishes (sharks, etc.). In certain fishes and reptiles the dentine is not built up around a simple pulp chamber but thrown into a series of complicated horizontal or longitudinal folds. The name plici-dentine has been given to the dentine of these creatures (*e.g.*, *Lepidosteus*, *Pristis*, and *Myliobatis* among fishes, and *Varanus* and *Labyrinthodon* among reptiles). The dentine is, however, essentially tubular in structure; the complexity is one of the pulp rather than of dentine (Fig. 284).

Among members of the cod family (hake, flounder, etc.) part of the

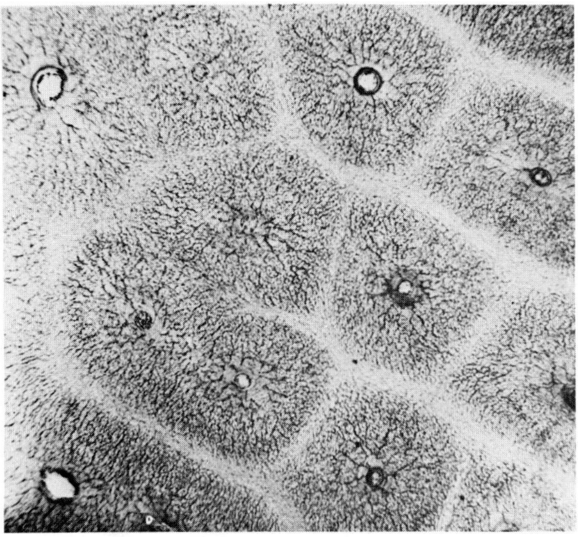

Fig. 284 Transverse section of a tooth from *Myliobatis*. Note the branches of the pulp each surrounded by a radiating system of dentinal tubules. Decalcified section. × 90.

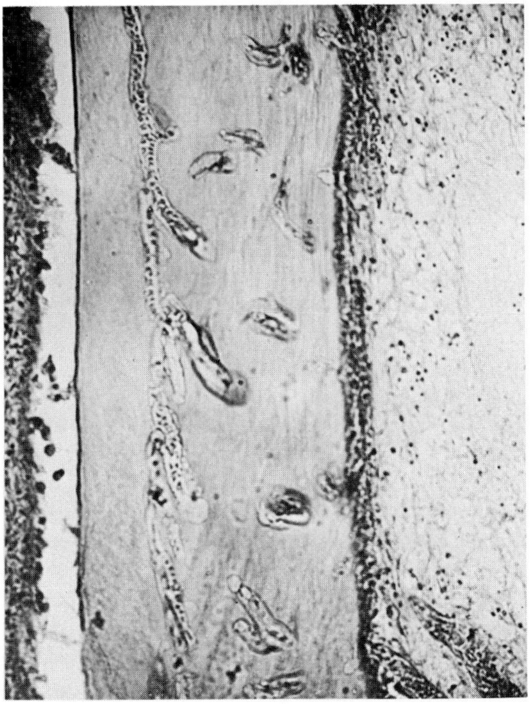

Fig. 285 Longitudinal section of the tooth of a hake (*Merlucius vulgaris*) showing the vascular canals in the dentine (vasodentine). Decalcified section. × 150.

dentine has a quite distinctive structure. There are no dentinal tubules, but in their place and subserving the function of nutrition is a series of blood capillaries passing from the pulp through the dentine and forming within the dentine a series of anastomotic loops (Fig. 285). The endothelial walls of the capillaries alone separate the circulating blood from the substance of the dentine. In the flounder the enamel-covered dentine forming the tip of the tooth is tubular dentine, whereas the remainder of the dentine is vascular dentine (vaso-dentine) without tubules.

Occasionally in human teeth an isolated capillary loop becomes incorporated in the forming dentine, but in the great majority of cases it loses connection with the pulp and there is then, of course, no blood circulation. In the manatee and some other mammals such isolated capillary loops are more numerous.

In a shark (*Lamna*) and in the anchylosed teeth of the pike the surface dentine is tubular in structure (ortho-dentine), but the pulp chamber becomes filled up with a bone-like tissue which has been called osteo-dentine (Fig. 286). By means of this tissue the tooth structure becomes continuous with the bone of the jaw, so that the tissue is a tissue of tooth attachment and probably homologous with cement. Cases have been described in which layers of cement-like tissue have been deposited on the inner (pulpal) surface of human teeth.

Two distinct forms of dentine have therefore been evolved among the vertebrates:

1. Vaso-dentine in which the blood is separated from the dentine only by the endothelium of the capillaries; such a form of dentine is rather soft in structure.
2. Tubular dentine (ortho-dentine), including plici-dentine, in which the tissue fluids have to pass through the endothelium of the superficial capillaries of the pulp and across (or into) the odontoblast layer before it can enter the dentinal tubules along which it slowly circulates by capillary attraction. This is from the nutritional standpoint much less efficient than the circulation found in vaso-dentine.

Weidenreich has attempted to show that throughout the whole range of the vertebrates the dentine in each tooth is made up of two different elements. These he calls mantle dentine and circumpulpal dentine. The former composes the outermost, usually narrow, layer next the enamel and its matrix is composed of relatively thick fibres. The circumpulpal dentine forms the main mass of the dentine and has a matrix showing very fine fibres with a different orientation to those in the mantle dentine. The proportions of the two elements can vary; in mammals it is as described, whereas in the pike the mantle dentine has assumed considerable bulk and the circumpulpal dentine has become reduced. Weidenreich admits that in the pike the relative positions of the mantle and circumpulpal dentine have become altered. There is no doubt that in human teeth the organic matrix of the very narrow zone between

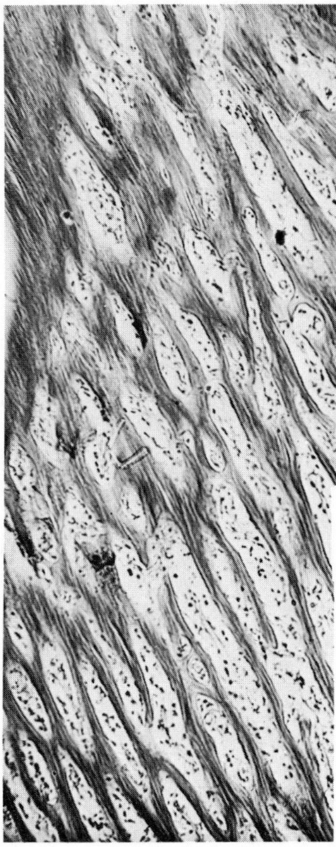

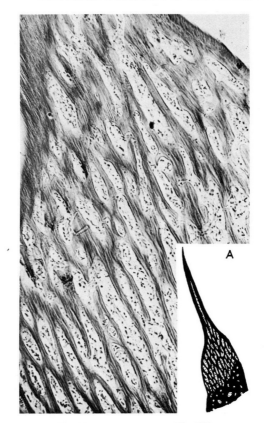

Fig. 286 Fig. 286A

Fig. 286 Longitudinal section of an ankylosed tooth of a pike (*Esox lucius*) showing the trabeculae of osteo-dentine passing through the pulp. Decalcified section. × 100.
Fig. 286A Diagrammatic illustration of an ankylosed tooth of a pike showing its attachment to the jaw.

the enamel and the commencement of the dentinal tubules does show coarser fibres with a different arrangement compared with those of the bulk of the dentine.

The distribution of the mammalian dental tissues. Dentine forms the greater part of each tooth, contributing to both its crown and root portions. It is always built around the dental pulp and is the only dental tissue directly related to the pulp in normal tooth development.

Cement is the tissue of tooth attachment and is always found in relation to some part of the implanted root part of mammalian teeth. In human teeth it covers the whole of the roots of the teeth, ending at the enamel-cement junction. In the incisors of rodents, however, cement covers only one surface of the implanted part of the tooth (the lingual or root surface), and only this part of the tooth is attached to the alveolar bone through the periodontal membrane (Fig. 287). In these incisors, moreover, the cement continues on to the lingual surface of the 'crowns' of the teeth. In the cheek teeth of the horse, or certain rodents, the elephant, and the wart-hog a modified form of cement contributes to the crown part of the teeth covering the enamel of newly erupted teeth and, being worn away from the occlusal surface with use, exposes enamel, and with wear of the enamel, dentine. The unequal rate of wear of the three dental tissues gives a rough occlusal surface which is useful in the mastication of a vegetable diet.

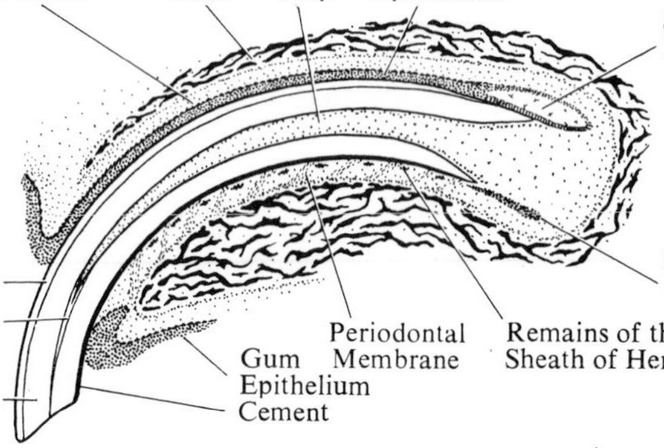

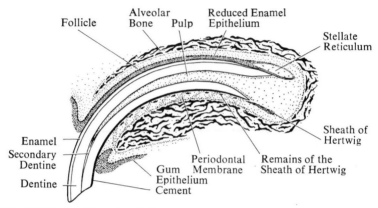

Fig. 287 Diagram illustrating the form, structure, and growth of a rodent incisor (upper jaw).

In human teeth, and in most other mammalian teeth, enamel covers the crown (oral) part of each tooth. In teeth of persistent growth, however, the enamel is found not only on the part exposed in the mouth but also on the part within the bony socket, reaching to the growing base of the tooth. In the rodent incisor it covers the whole labial surface of the tooth, and the relationship of the three dental tissues and their unequal rate of wear maintains the chisel-like incisive edges of these teeth as they continue to erupt (Fig. 288). In the elephant and hippopotamus the incisor tusks have only a cap of enamel. The canines of pigs and wart-hogs have one or more strips of enamel covering the whole length of the teeth. Among the members of the order Edentata (armadillos and sloths) enamel is absent and the teeth consist of dentine and cement only.

THE STRUCTURE OF THE RODENT INCISOR

The development of the rodent incisor illustrates a number of interesting features in the formation of the dental tissues as well as characteristics peculiar to teeth of continual eruption. For research purposes the

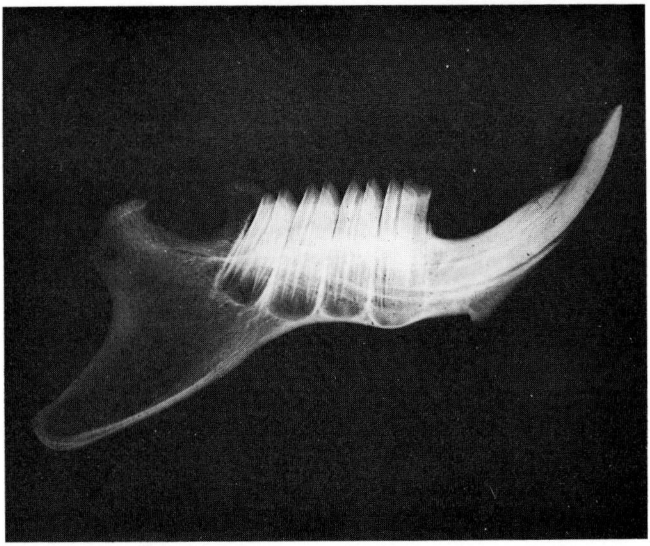

Fig. 288 Radiograph of one half of the lower jaw of a guinea-pig (*Cavia porcellus*) to show the shape, size, and arrangement of the incisor. × 1·5.

rodent incisor is invaluable as all stages in the formation of the dental tissues may be observed in the same tooth and at any time in the life of the animal.

Microscopical examination of the rodent incisor and its associated structures shows the following features (Fig. 287).

1. Over the enamel-covered labial surface of the implanted part of the tooth the enamel epithelium is complete from the gingival trough where it is continuous with the gum epithelium, to the growing apical region of the tooth. Over the completed enamel the epithelium is in the form of a reduced enamel epithelium; there is here no stellate reticulum. In the apical region where enamel formation is taking place the enamel epithelium shows full differentiation into external enamel epithelium, stellate reticulum, stratum intermedium, and ameloblast layer. The complete covering afforded to the enamel by the epithelium separates it from the adjacent tissue of the follicle.

2. Over the lingual surface of the implanted tooth the epithelium can be divided into three regions:

a. The region of the epithelial attachment where the gum epithelium is attached to the cement-covered surface of the tooth as the tooth passes into the mouth cavity.

b. Over the greater part of the implanted lingual surface of the tooth the epithelium is broken up and allows of attachment of the fibres of the periodontal membrane to the cement-covered tooth surface.

c. In the apical region the epithelium is complete as a two-layered sheath of Hertwig, inducing the deposition of dentine.

3. On the labial surface of the implanted part of the tooth a true periodontal membrane does not develop between the alveolar bone and the tooth. The enamel-covered tooth surface with its protecting epithelium is quite free of any attachment to the alveolar bone. The orientation of the fibrous tissue between the epithelial-covered enamel and the bone is the same as in the follicular stage of development; the fibres run in longitudinal bundles outside the enamel epithelium.

On the lingual side of the implanted part of the tooth where the epithelium becomes broken up the follicle becomes a true periodontal membrane. Hence in rodent incisors the periodontal membrane is attached to the lingual (concave) surface of the tooth and in part to the sides of the tooth, but not to the labial (convex) surface. The periodontal membrane shows a well developed intermediate plexus where the fibres from the cement of the tooth and from the bony socket intermingle. This arrangement is probably related to the process of continual tooth eruption, the necessary adjustments between the fibre bundles being allowed.

4. At the apical region of the tooth the enamel epithelium undergoes continual growth. On the labial side the full differentiation of the parts of the enamel organ takes place so that both dentine and enamel are formed. On the lingual surface and over the sides of the tooth only the two layers of Hertwig's sheath are formed and there dentine, but not enamel, is produced. In the apical region the basal part of the follicle grows backwards excavating the bone and permitting a backward migration of the tooth apex up to adult life.

5. During the functional life of the erupted tooth the incisive edge is being continuously worn away. This process would in time open up the front end of the pulp cavity, but the deposition of dentine within the pulp cavity continues throughout life so that exposure of the pulp never takes place. The secondary dentine deposited in this way is quite regular and there is no interruption in the direction of the dentinal tubules.

6. A characteristic feature of the incisors of many rodents is the bright pigmentation of the enamel. In rats this has been shown to be an iron derivative very similar to the blood pigment haemosiderin. Rats fed on a diet poor in iron fail to form pigment. The colour varies in different species from shades of yellow and orange to shades of red.

BIBLIOGRAPHY

Adams, D. (1962). The blood supply to the enamel organ of the rodent incisor. *Arch. oral Biol.* **7**, 279.

Appelbaum, E. (1942). Enamel of shark's teeth. *J. dent. Res.* **21**, 251.

Boyde, A. (1965). The structure of developing mammalian dental enamel. In *Tooth Enamel*, eds. Stack, M. V. & Fearnhead, R. W. Bristol: Wright.

Carter, J. T. (1922). On the structure of enamel in primates and some other mammals. *Proc. zool. Soc. Lond.* 599.

Eda, S. & Takuma, S. (1965). Microstructure of the peritubular matrix in horse dentine. *Bull. Tokyo dent. Coll.* **6**, 1.

Herold, R. C. (1970). Vasodentine and mantle dentine is teleost fish teeth. *Archs. oral Biol.* **15**, 71.

Kerr, T. (1955). Development and structure of the teeth in the dogfish. *Proc. zool. Soc. Lond.* **125**, 95.

——— (1960). Development and structure of some actinopterygian and urodele teeth. *Proc. zool. Soc. Lond.* **133**, 401.

Kvam, T. (1950). *The Development of Mesodermal Enamel on Piscine Teeth.* Aktietrykkeriet I. Trondhjem.

Lawson, R. (1965). Tooth structure in the Amphibia. *Proc. zool. Soc. Lond.* **145**, 321.

Lester, K. S. (1970). On the nature of 'fibrils' and tubules in developing enamel of the Opossum, *Didelphis marsupialis. J. Ultrastruct. Res.* **30**, 64.

Listgarten, M. A. (1968). A light and electron microscopic study of coronal cementogenesis. *Archs. oral Biol.* **13**, 93.

Moss, M. L. & Appelbaum, E. (1963). The fibrillar matrix of marsupial enamel. *Acta anat.* **53**, 289.

Ockerse, T. (1961). Tubular enamel in some sea fishes in Southern Africa. *J. dent. Res.* **40**, 1170.

Parsons, T. S. & Williams, E. E. (1962). The teeth of Amphibia and their relation to Amphibian phylogeny. *J. Morph.* **110**, 375.

Poole, D. F. G. (1971). An introduction to the phylogeny of calcified tissues, in *Dental Morphology and Evolution.* (Ed. A. A. Dahlberg). University of Chicago.

Reith, E. J. (1959). The enamel organ of the rat's incisor, its histology and pigment. *Anat. Rec.* **133**, 75.

Tims, H. W. M. & Henry, C. B. (Editors) (1923). *A Manual of Dental Anatomy.* By C. S. Tomes. 8th ed. London: Churchill.

23. Dental Adaptations to the Demands of Function

Animals in the wild state depend upon their teeth for their existence almost to the same extent as upon sight, hearing, and swiftness of movement.

In fishes, amphibians, and reptiles, in which tooth succession continues throughout life, teeth, often with specialised methods of attachment, are developed and are replaced as soon as they have lost their edge or point or other speciality of form. In mammals, however, in which at the most there is only a single change of dentitions, the teeth, and especially those of the permanent dentition, must develop structural adaptations to meet the requirements of use extending over a period of many years. Of the various methods in which various animals have solved this vital problem the following examples illustrate the intimate correlation of form, structure, and function which is the essential response of living things to the environment in which they live.

1. **Teeth of continual eruption.** Teeth may continue to grow and to erupt throughout the life of the animal. As the teeth are worn away by use at their occlusal surfaces and incisive edges they maintain their normal length and occlusal relationships by a delicate correlation of tooth formation, rate of eruption, and rate of wear. Examples of this method of adaptation to the needs of function are seen in the incisors of rodents, the tusks of elephants, the canines of wild pigs, and the cheek teeth of many rodents, such as the beaver and guinea-pig. In the cheek teeth of the sheep and the horse the teeth continue to grow and erupt for a considerable period after they first cut the gum, but ultimately, at the end of the period of skeletal growth, when the demands upon food supplies become less intense, these teeth form roots and cease to undergo active eruption (Fig. 289).

In many teeth undergoing continuous eruption enamel continues to cover some part of the tooth throughout the life of the tooth. In such teeth, illustrated by the incisors of rodents and the canines of wild pigs, the periodontal membrane is attached only to a limited surface of the implanted part of the tooth, the root surface, there being no attachment between enamel and alveolar bone (see section on the Structure of the Rodent Incisor). In other cases, as in the horse and elephant, cement covers the whole surface of the tooth, enamel as well as dentine, but

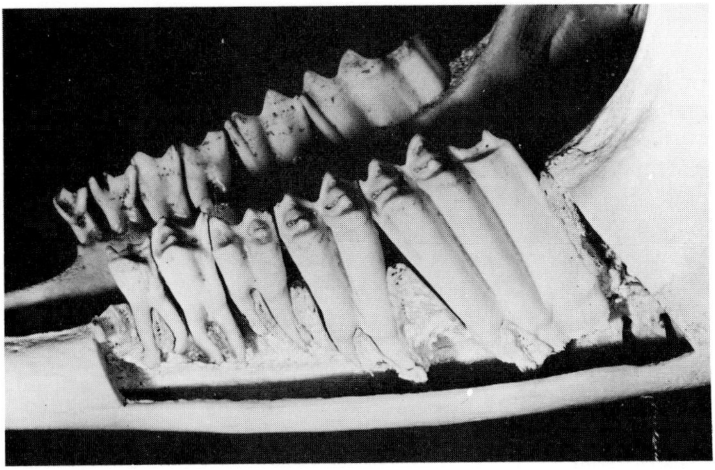

Fig. 289 Profile view of the permanent lower cheek teeth of the sheep. Bone has been cut away to show the hypsodont form of these teeth. The small first premolar has been lost on the left side.

the union of cement and enamel is much less intimate than that between cement and dentine.

2. **Increase in size.** The teeth may increase their size by extension in the mesio-distal or bucco-lingual diameters. In the wart-hog, and to a less extent in the pig, the third permanent molars are very much longer teeth than are the other molars. The third molar of the wart-hog is as large as the other molars together. In the elephant the crowns of the cheek teeth are built up of a series of plates held together by cement (Fig. 290), and come into occlusion by a rotary movement so that the front of each tooth is well worn while the back of the tooth is still

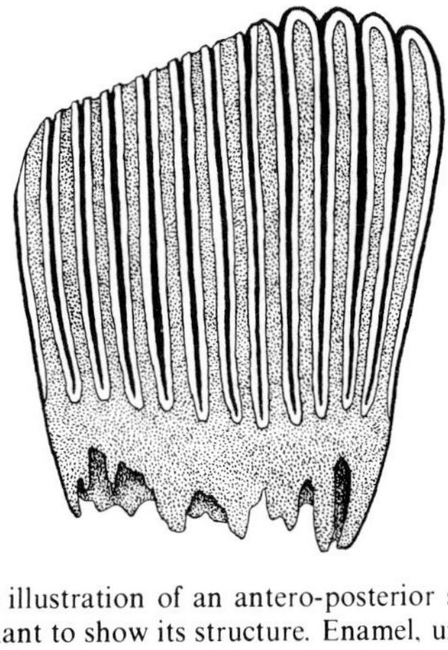

Fig. 290 Diagrammatic illustration of an antero-posterior section through the molar tooth of an Indian elephant to show its structure. Enamel, unshaded; dentine, stippled; cement, solid black. The anterior part of the occlusal surface is worn.

erupting. In the badger one molar tooth on each side of each jaw is greatly widened in the bucco-lingual direction by the development of the lingual portion of the cingulum.

3. **Horizontal succession.** The site of maximum masticatory stress falls upon the teeth below the zygomatic process of the maxilla. In many animals there is a horizontal succession of the teeth from behind so that one after another the cheek teeth occupy the position of maximum stress. This form of horizontal succession is most developed in the elephant, where only one cheek tooth is in use on each side of each jaw at a time and the six cheek teeth succeed one another from behind as the anterior members of the series are worn down and shed. In the manatee as many as eleven molar teeth develop on each side of each jaw, and move forward through the alveolar bone from the elongated tube-like alveolar bulbs in which they develop, to be shed as they are worn by use. A similar condition is found in the kangaroo. In old animals the solitary terminal molar lies beneath the zygomatic process, while the alveolar bulb in which it developed is empty and collapsed. In the pig each of the three permanent molars lies in turn beneath the zygomatic process until in old animals the position is occupied by the large third molar and the worn first molar is well forward of this position. To a limited extent the same conditions occurs in man and the antrhopoid apes.

4. **Molarisation of premolars.** In the modern horse the extent of the masticatory surface of the cheek tooth series has been increased by a process of 'molarisation' of the premolars which, except for the first, are similar in form and size to the permanent molars (Fig. 291). A similar change has taken place in certain rodent dentitions, in lemurs and in *Tarsius*.

5. **Elongation of cusps.** Animals such as the horse have cusps which

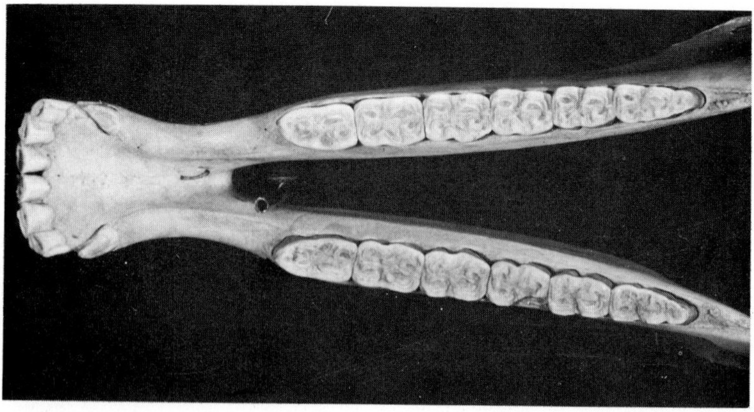

Fig. 291 Lower teeth of horse. Note the similar shape of the premolars and molars. The first premolars have already been lost.

are greatly elongated and the areas between the cusps may be filled in by a modified form of cement. As a result a complex arrangement of all the dental tissues is produced. The occlusal pattern is thus maintained throughout the life of the animal in spite of the loss of tooth substance (Fig. 292).

It will be seen that some animals use more than one of these methods to adapt the teeth to the requirements of use. In the pig extension in tooth size is associated with a modified horizontal succession; in the horse molarisation of the premolars is associated with the development of high-crowned (hypsodont) teeth, whereas in the elephant horizontal succession is associated with a rotatory eruption and elongation of each tooth from before backward.

Certain specialisations of tooth form, such as the carnassial mechanism of the carnivores, by their nature reduce the liability of the dental tissues to wear. The greatest destruction of dental tissues is produced by grinding and chewing movements at wide occlusal surfaces or at incisive edges used in gnawing. Grass is probably the most destructive of foodstuffs and a diet of meat the least destructive. Man, however, in finding how to reduce the demands of function upon his teeth, has acquired dental caries and parodontal disease. The removal of function tends always to the destruction of structure or its failure to reach its full development, and undermines the resistance of tissues to disease.

Sexual dimorphism. Among some animals certain teeth, usually incisor or canine tusks, are better developed and are often very much larger in the male than in the female. Examples include the canine tusks of wild boars, the incisor of the narwhal, the tusks of elephants, the canines of certain hornless deer, and the canines in the anthropoid apes. In the gorilla the difference in size is especially well marked in the canines, but all the permanent teeth are larger in the male animal. In

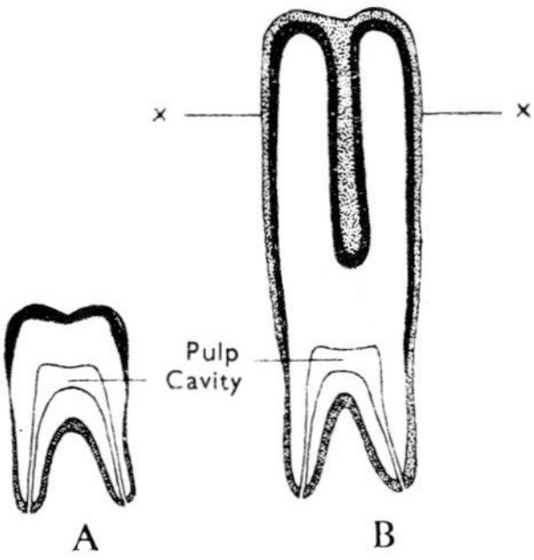

Fig. 292 Diagram to show the modifications leading to a hypsodont tooth. The white areas represent dentine, the enamel is black, and the cement is stippled. (A) Low-crowned tooth, as in man. (B) Hypsodont tooth as in the horse; the cusps are elevated and the whole tooth covered by cement. As a tooth of this kind wears down to any level, such as that indicated at x–x, no less than nine layers of contrasting materials are present in cross-section [*After Romer.*]

the deciduous dentition there is in the gorilla a slight difference in tooth size, but this is not found in the chimpanzee. These differences are in part under the control of the hormones of the individual animal, but there would also appear to be a genetic mechanism involved in these differences in size and form which acts during the formation of the enamel organs.

24. Characteristics of the Human Dentition in the light of Comparative Anatomy

Number of teeth. The total number of teeth which develop and erupt in man is fifty-two. Of these, twenty are deciduous and thirty-two are permanent. Of the permanent set twenty have deciduous predecessors.

Unlike such animals as the pig, the dog, and the horse, there are no permanent teeth (in these animals the first premolars) which have lost their deciduous predecessors. As compared with the typical mammalian number, the human dentition has lost four incisors in each dentition and eight premolars in the permanent dentition. The corresponding deciduous molars may also have been lost, or alternatively the first and second 'permanent' molars may represent 'deciduous' molars which have lost their permanent successors, in which case eight permanent molars have been lost at the back of the dentition. There is evidence suggesting that the next units to be lost in the human dentition are the upper lateral (second) incisors, the lower second premolars (leaving the second deciduous molar without a successor), and the third molars.

Teeth above the usual number are known as supernumerary teeth. They can be divided into those which are abnormal in form, usually peg-shaped or with crowns in the form of a peripheral ridge around a central fossa, and found most frequently in the upper incisor region or alongside the permanent molars (paramolar teeth); and those which are normal in form (sometimes known as supplemental teeth). The latter are most frequent in the premolar region and behind the third permanent molar as fourth molars which are in line with the dental arch. Supernumerary teeth of normal form are sometimes interpreted as examples of evolutionary recession towards the full mammalian dentition. They may exceed this number, however.

Form of the teeth. The most specialised members of the human dentition are the spade-like cutting incisors which are even further developed in the other higher primates. In primitive human dentitions the incisors usually met at an edge-to-edge bite. The comparative rarity of this functional development among modern races is possibly due to lack of use of the dentition. The cusps of the cheek teeth are not worn away, with the result that there does not take place the relative forward movement of the mandible which permits the overlapping of the lower incisors by the upper incisors to be converted into the edge-to-edge type of occlusion. The human incisors show a high degree of adaptation to an omnivorous diet. They can be used for tearing meat off bones as the carnivores use their incisors for biting into articles of diet held in the hands such as fruits, vegetables, and roots and so determining the amount of such substances which can be dealt with by the molars at a time. Furthermore, owing to the free side-to-side movement (permitted by the absence of interlocking canines), a lateral gnawing action can be used. In rodents the gnawing action is produced by a backward and forward movement and entails a quite different use of the muscles of mastication.

The human canines are quite unlike those of any other living primate (Figs. 293, 294). It is uncertain whether their lack of specialisation is

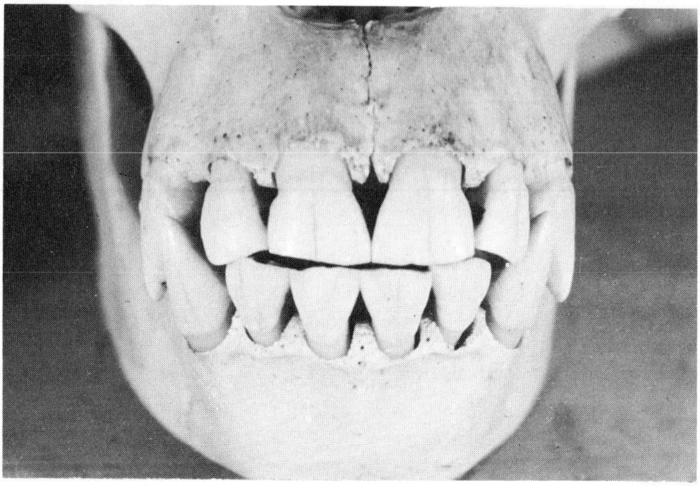

Fig. 293 Anterior permanent teeth of the chimpanzee. (*By courtesy of Prof S. Friel.*)

primary and has been maintained throughout the human stock since its origin, or whether it is secondary and is the result of a reduction in size during evolution. Newly erupted unworn deciduous canines, however, usually project slightly beyond the occlusal level and in their form are more similar to those of anthropoid apes.

Human premolars and molars are primitive in form. The lower first premolars do not show the specialised form of those of the anthropoid apes and most monkeys associated with the large projecting canines of these creatures. The human molars, like those of the great apes and some of the New World monkeys, do not show the lophodont ridges characteristic of the more specialised molars of the Old World monkeys. The human upper molars are in fact very primitive, showing the outline of the trigone and usually the additional hypocone. The latter is often reduced in the second molars and in third molars may be absent, so that in these teeth the tooth has reverted to a more primitive three-cusped form. In the lower molars the paraconid is lost as in all higher

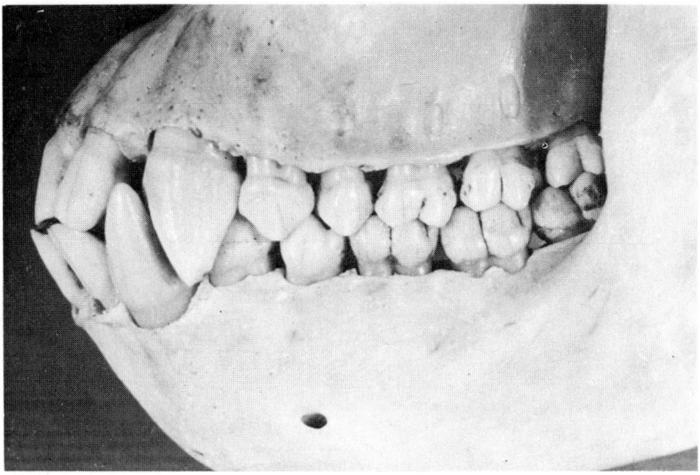

Fig. 294 Profile view of the permanent dentition of the chimpanzee. (*By courtesy of Prof S. Friel.*)

primates, and one of the cusps of the talon (the hypoconulid) is usually lost in second molars and often in third molars. The loss of this cusp, like the loss of the upper hypocone, is a secondary reduction more often found in modern than in primitive and prehistoric human dentitions.

The differences in form between the deciduous molars, premolars, and permanent molars present some interesting morphological and developmental problems. The deciduous molars and permanent molars present a more gradual and harmonious series both in regard to size and form than does that of the premolars and permanent molars in which there is a very definite break between the second premolar and the first molar. The human dentition shares this feature with the anthropoid apes and New World monkeys, but in *Tarsius* and the lemurs the cheek teeth of the permanent dentition make up a more harmonious series. They have an extra premolar, but this is also true of the New World monkeys in which there is a break in the series between the third premolar and first permanent molar. It is difficult to interpret these differences in terms of variations in diet or function.

There is also in the human dentition a sharp break in form continuity between the incisors and the canines and between the canines and premolars or deciduous molars. In the anthropoid apes both the first deciduous molar and first premolar are more 'caniniform,' especially in the lower jaw (Fig. 295). Here there is a closer correlation between form change and function, but these serial changes in tooth form along the dental arches would appear to depend on factors which determine functional differences rather than upon the direct effects of function. The problems involved require further investigation.

It is usually held that tooth form is closely related to tooth function,

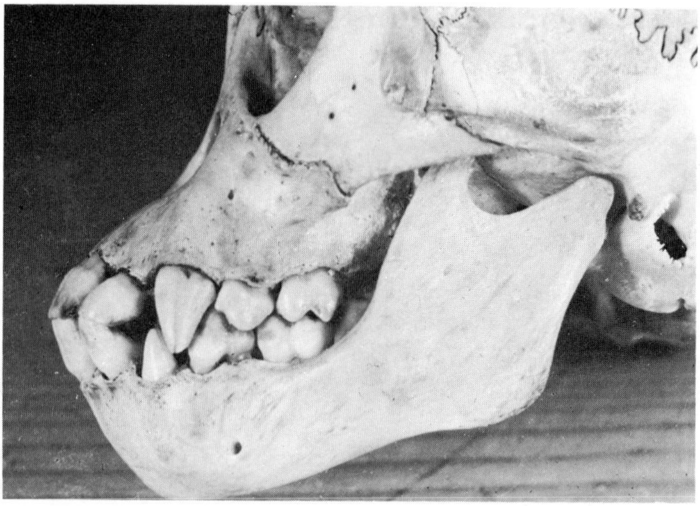

Fig. 295 Profile view of the deciduous dentition of the chimpanzee. The lower canine is in the process of erupting. (*By courtesy of Prof S. Fried.*)

and by tooth function is meant the use of the teeth in mastication. As far as is known the diet of New World monkeys, the Old World monkeys, and the anthropoid apes consists largely of fruit and other forms of vegetation. These creatures are not usually meat eaters and have certainly not the variety of diet even of primitive human races. It is, moreover, difficult to understand the molar specialisation found among Old World monkeys in terms of any specialised diet in comparison with either the New World monkeys or the anthropoid apes, which have a more primitive molar crown pattern. Furthermore, in primitive and prehistoric human dentitions the occlusal surfaces of the molar teeth soon become worn flat and lose all their cusp to fossa articulations. It is therefore difficult to see any strict masticatory significance in cusp relationships. It may be, however, that relationship between the cusps and fossae of upper and lower molars is of more importance in the establishment and maintenance of occlusal relations between the jaws during the period of facial growth and in determining the type of masticatory movement pattern to be established by the muscles of mastication. Hence the lophodont ridge and groove type of occlusion found in the Old World monkeys produces a more stable type of occlusion with a more fixed pattern of movements at the mandibular joint. The first step in this fixation of the masticatory movements has already been taken in both the New World monkeys and the anthropoid apes but not at all in man, or if so it has been lost before the molar specialisation could occur. This first step is the overgrowth and interlocking of the canines.

It would appear, therefore, that the pattern of the cheek teeth is related not only to the type of diet but also to the pattern of jaw movements established at the mandibular joint by the muscles of mastication under the influence of occlusal relations established early in development. By the time these relations are lost by tooth wear the adult functional pattern has been established.

In the human dentition sexual dimorphism is poorly developed. In females the difference in size between the upper central and lateral incisors tends to be greater, the canines narrower and more pointed, and the bucco-lingual width of the cheek teeth is relatively narrower. It has already been pointed out that in girls the teeth tend to calcify and erupt earlier. Sexual dimorphism was much more marked in certain human fossils, such as *Pithecanthropus*.

Tooth succession. It is characteristic of the human dentition that the time of eruption of the permanent molar series is spread out over a long period of time (twelve years or more). This is seen not only in the actual time of eruption of the teeth, but in the fact that all the permanent molars have their crowns fully formed and are ready for eruption three years or more before eruption in fact commences. This delay in molar eruption is related to the slow long-drawn-out growth of the human face, which is in turn related to the slow continuous growth of the general skeleton which is not complete until between twenty and twenty-five years of age. The fact that the teeth are ready to erupt at a much earlier date would seem to indicate that more primitive human forms underwent their skeletal maturity at least three years earlier and that tooth development is quite independent of bone growth. In support of this we have the evidence of the history of tooth development and the very common clinical fact that disorders of bone growth do not affect the teeth.

Growth of the modern human face is not only more drawn out in time, but it is less in amount. The reduction is largely a reduction in length, and is in part a reduction of the length of the whole face and in part a reduction of the tooth-bearing part of the face (the alveolar bone). Reduction of the face as a whole is not altogether dependent on the masticatory apparatus and may be related to other factors such as the blood-cooling function of the nasal mucous membrane. Reduction of the length of the alveolar bone must to some extent follow any reduction of the length of the face as a whole, but the reduction in alveolar prognathism which has taken place in modern man indicates that there has been superimposed on the reduction of the basal skeleton a reduction in the length of the alveolar processes of both jaws.

In man space for the permanent canines depends on growth in width of the arches rather than on growth in length. Associated with the reduction in the length of the alveolar bone there has been a failure in the forward movement of the permanent molar teeth. In the pig and also in the long-faced baboon, the permanent molars replace one another beneath the zygomatic process (key ridge) of the maxilla during growth of the face. In the pig the last deciduous molar and in turn each of the three permanent molars, lies below the 'key ridge' and the tooth occupying this position takes the maximum masticatory stress. The last tooth to occupy this position, the third permanent molar, is the largest and strongest of the cheek teeth. In modern man only the second deciduous molar and the first permanent molar occupy this position in turn. In some primitive and prehistoric human skulls and in the anthropoid apes the second permanent molar usually succeeds the first molar, but among the higher primates the third molar never comes so far forward.

Whereas the third upper molar is often reduced in size in the dentition of the higher primates, the third lower molar is smaller than the first only in modern man. Even in primitive and prehistoric human dentitions it is sometimes the largest of the lower molar teeth as it is in the orang-utan and gorilla.

A characteristic feature of modern human dentitions is the fact that though the occlusal length of the lower molars is reduced, the width of the ascending ramus of the mandible is even more reduced so that the ramus width is often less than the occlusal length of the lower molars. This does not occur in primitive human skulls or in the anthropoid apes. The index, mesio-distal length of the permanent molars × 100/minimum width of the ramus gives a useful indication of the reduction of the functional activity of the muscles of mastication. It is highest in modern urbanised races.

Sequence of tooth eruption. This shows considerable variability among the primates. In the tree shrew the order is $M_1M_2M_3I_1I_2CP_1P_2$. In *Aotes*, a New World monkey, the premolars erupt before the canines. In *Pigathrix*, an Old World monkey, the order is $M_1M_2I_1I_2M_3P_1P_2C$ which is the same as in the Lemurs. In *Tarsius* the order is $M_1M_2I_1I_2CP_1P_2M_3$. In the Colobus monkey it is $M_1I_1M_2I_2P_1P_2CM_3$; among anthropoid apes $M_1I_1I_2M_2P_1P_2CM_3$, and in man usually $M_1I_1I_2(CP_1P_2)M_2M_3$ although in some cases the central incisors may erupt before the first permanent molars. The tendency for the time of the eruption of the second and third molars to move from the beginning to the end of the sequence, a process completed in human dentitions, is possibly related to the long drawn out period of facial growth.

Tooth function. Human teeth are fully developed one to three years after eruption. There is some evidence that root development was delayed among some prehistoric humans, *i.e.*, the so-called 'taurodont' molars of some Neanderthal skulls, but the matter requires further investigation. In primitive and prehistoric dentitions the enamel covering the incisive edges and occlusal surfaces of the teeth becomes worn away from the permanent teeth in young adult life, exposing the dentine. In the teeth of old adults the secondary dentine filling the cornua and roof portions of the pulp chambers was usually exposed and the teeth were worn down to or close to the gum margins. This excessive wear of the teeth was in part the result of more effective use of the muscles of mastication and in part due to the rough nature of the uncooked and unprepared food which made up the diet of early man. It would be interesting to know if among primitive human dentitions used in this manner there was any evidence of the formation of teeth with higher enamel-covered crowns and delayed root formation as occurred among the early horses. Mankind, however, finally solved the problem not by any radical change in dental anatomy but by a revolution in food habits. It is interesting to notice that tooth wear is much less marked among the non-human primates than in prehistoric humans. The vegetable and fruit diet of these creatures is much less destructive of dental tissue than was that of early man.

THE DENTITIONS OF FOSSILS OF IMPORTANCE IN DETERMINING THE ANTIQUITY OF MAN

The Australopithecinae. The first fossil of this group of creatures was described by Dart in 1925 and was the skull of a young individual in which the deciduous dentition was complete and the first permanent molars had erupted. Since 1925 many other fossils of the same general type have been found in South Africa (Fig. 297).

The molars are intermediate in size between those of the orang and gorilla and considerably larger than those of any living known human races. The increase in size from before backward among the lower molars is also characteristic of *Pithecanthropus* and some of the *Neanderthal* specimens. The third molar is also the longest tooth of the series in *Dryopithecus* and *Proconsul africanus*, but in modern man the molar series usually decreases in size from before backward. Except in the male gorilla and orang-utan, the lower third molar is smaller than the second but larger than the first molar among the living anthropoid apes. All the lower molars in the Australopithecinae show the primitive *Dryopithecus* pattern of five cusps; the molars sometimes show six cusps as in some primitive human dentitions. They show the flat even type of occlusal wear characteristic of human dentitions. The upper premolars have two roots, the first lower premolar is a rounded bicuspid tooth as in modern man and not conical and sectorial as in living anthropoid apes. The second premolar is larger than the first and its dimensions exceed those of many human first molars. The canines are spatulate in form with a blunt cusp which does not rise more than a slight degree above the common occlusal level. The incisors and canines are much less massive than the cheek teeth.

In the deciduous dentition the canines are also human in form and the lower first deciduous molar has two well-separated and well-developed cusps (metaconid and protoconid) as distinct from the sectorial form found in the living apes.

The skull has a massive facial skeleton and a cranial capacity of about the same dimension as that of the gorilla. The face is somewhat less prognathous than that of the living anthropoid apes. There is no chin. The angle of the cranial base is intermediate between that found in the great apes and modern man. The form of the pelvis is much closer to that of man than to that of the anthropoid apes. Australopithecinae had probably acquired the power to run upright on the lower limbs.

The dental arches are evenly curved as in man as compared with the parallel or converging tooth rows characteristic of the living anthropoid apes: there is no diastema in relation to the canines. The order of eruption of the permanent teeth appears to have been similar to that of modern man.

A more recently discovered member of the Australopithecinae is *Australopithecus boisei* (*Zinjanthropus*), discovered in 1959. The skull is nearly complete except for the lower jaw. The third molars had just erupted. It shows strong brow ridges, a massive palate and large teeth. The cranium carries large muscular crests.

The Australopithecinae fossils probably extend from late Pliocene to early Pleistocene times. They appear to have consisted of a genus divided into two species. The less specialised group, *Australopithecus africanus*, may have evolved towards *Homo erectus* whereas the other, *Australopithecus boisei*, became extinct. The latter was characterised by the presence of large post-canine teeth developed in relation to a primarily herbivorous diet. Ancestors of the Australopithecinae may have included *Ramapithecus*.

Homo habilis. This species of fossil man, established in 1964, was discovered in the Olduvian gorge in Tanzania. The type specimen consists of the greater part of the lower jaw with teeth, an upper molar, and parts of the parietal bones. In their general features the teeth and bones are intermediate in form between those of the Australopithecinae and *Homo erectus* (*Pithecanthropus* and *Sinanthropus*).

The earlier discovered *Telanthropus* fossil jaw probably belongs to this group.

Homo erectus. *Pithecanthropus* (Fig. 296). The dental elements of the original *Pithecanthropus* (Dubois, 1891–92) fossil material consist of two upper molar teeth. One is considered to be a third molar and the other

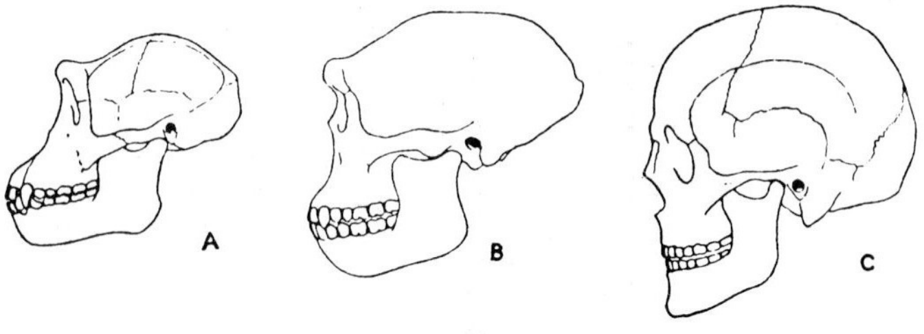

Fig. 296 Side view of the skull of (A) chimpanzee. (B) Homo erectus [Pithecanthropus] (as reconstructed by the late Dr Weidenreich), and (C) Homo sapiens. (*By courtesy of Sir Wilfred Le Gros Clark and the Trustees of the British Museum.*)

either a second or third molar. Its crown is badly worn. In both teeth the roots are strong and widely divergent. Isolated third molars are unsatisfactory evidence owing to their wide individual variation of form.

Further finds from Java (von Koenigswald) include parts of the jaws with teeth.

The teeth are smaller than in *Australopithecus boisei* but show the same primitive characteristic of increase in size from the first to the third molar. All the lower molars have the primitive five-cusped *Dryopithecus* pattern. The canines are human in form but project farther above the common occlusal level than in other human dentitions; in one specimen there is a well-developed precanine diastema in the upper jaw which is not found in other human dentitions. The upper incisors are shovel-shaped. The dental arch is slightly convex outwards in the cheek tooth region but less than is usual in human dentitions. The palatal area is large; alveolar prognathism is well developed; the 'chin' is absent; and there is no 'simian shelf'. Cranial capacity is considerably less than in modern man; the cranial vault is low and long with a large area for the attachment of powerful neck muscles; supraorbital ridges are well developed and are already prominent in the skull of a two-year-old child.

Sinanthropus. Black first described this in 1927 from the evidence of three teeth. Since that time many fossil skulls and parts of skulls have been found. In many respects the skull and material resemble that of the Pithecanthropus group but the average cranial capacity is greater in *Sinanthropus.*

In *Sinanthropus* the second lower molar may be smaller than the first or equal in size with the third molar which is the smallest of the series, as in modern man. In this respect the dentition is less primitive than that of *Pithecanthropus* and the Australopithecinae. The teeth are also smaller in size with dimensions which are reached occasionally in modern human dentitions. The incisors and canines of *Sinanthropus*, however, are larger than in *Pithecanthropus* and as in the latter the canines project above the occlusal level to a greater extent than in modern man although they are not at all ape-like in form. The incisors are shovel-shaped as in living mongoloid races. There is in *Sinanthropus* no precanine diastema. In the *Sinanthropus* canines a well-developed basal cingulum is present on the lingual surface, a feature also found in Neanderthal teeth. In the *Sinanthropus* dentitions the typical human outward convexity of the dental arch in the cheek tooth series is more marked than in *Pithecanthropus* of Java. The area of the palate is less extensive than in *Pithecanthropus.* There is no chin; a characteristic finding is the presence of multiple mental foramina, a primitive feature. The glenoid fossa is deep with a well-developed articular eminence. Cranial capacity is greater than in the Java fossils; the cranial vault is higher and more convex in outline.

Both the *Pithecanthropus* and *Sinanthropus* fossil material is probably of early (Mindel–Riss interglacial) Pleistocene antiquity. The two groups of fossils are now grouped together in the species *Homo erectus*. Recently *Homo erectus*-like fragments have been found in Africa.

The Heidelberg mandible. The lower jaw with the complete dentition, except for the crowns of the left premolars and first two molars, was discovered in a sandpit at Mauer in 1907. The outstanding characteristic of this fossil is the massive build and size of the jaw bone. The minimum width of the ascending ramus is 51 mm on one side and 50 mm on the other, which is almost twice the width of an average European mandible (28·30 mm) and only approached by the jaw of an Eskimo with a width of 49·5 mm.

There is no 'chin' as the alveolar element projects beyond the level of the lower border of the body of the bone. The lingual surface of the symphyseal region is human rather than ape-like; there is no indication of any 'simian shelf' as found in the anthropoid apes, and in the *Dryopithecus* fossils.

The teeth are large, but relative to the jaw the dental arch length of 57 mm is not great.

As in many Neanderthal jaws and in *Sinanthropus*, but unlike the condition found in modern man or in *Pithecanthropus* and the Australopithecinae, the second molars are the largest teeth and the third molars although larger than the first are smaller than the second. A similar condition is common in living anthropoid apes. The molars show five cusps but the distal cusp is not very large. The pulp cavities of all the teeth are large; the canine is completely human in form and does not extend above the common occlusal level. The occlusal surfaces and incisive edges are worn to expose the dentine, but wear is less extensive on the third molars, indicating the jaw was probably that of a young adult. The bicondylar width of 130 mm indicates that the skull base was large.

The Heidelberg jaw is considered to be at least as old as the second (Mindel–Riss) interglacial period of the Pleistocene and is the oldest human fossil found in Europe. Its relationship to other early human fossils is still uncertain.

Neanderthal man. The number of fossils belonging to the Neanderthal group is now quite large. The majority come from sites in western Europe and northern Africa, but an important series has been found in Palestine (Mount Carmel) and isolated material from Asia.

The skull of typical late Neanderthal type is long, low, and wide with a large cranial base, large cranial capacity, and a well-developed occipital and supraorbital torus as in *Pithecanthropus* and *Sinanthropus*. The face is large, prognathous, chinless as in all primitive human fossils, with large orbital cavities and a wide nasal opening. Earlier Neanderthal skulls appear to have been less specialised in form except for the size of the supraorbital torus.

The teeth are larger than the average for modern man with strong and well-developed roots, but individuals living to-day have teeth with dimensions within the Neanderthal range.

It is usual in Neanderthal dentitions for the second lower molar to be as large as or larger than the first molar. The third molar is sometimes the largest tooth of the lower molar series. The upper incisors are usually 'shovel-shaped' with well-marked mesial and distal marginal ridges lingually. The lingual cingulum of the upper incisors and canines is usually well developed and sometimes large enough to merit the name of a lingual cusp. A characteristic feature of some Neanderthal molar teeth is the elongation of the unbifurcated region of the root. With this is associated a large deep pulp chamber (taurodontism). The lower molars usually carry five cusps, but the fifth cusp is sometimes reduced in size, especially on the second molar. The hard palate is usually wide; a characteristic primitive feature is the relative large width between the canines.

The width of the mandibular ramus is 46·5 mm in the La Chapelle skull, 47 mm in the La Quina skull, and 36 mm in the adolescent Le Moustier skull. These measurements exceed the modern average and are only exceeded by the Heidelberg jaw and among the living Eskimo. The glenoid fossa is somewhat flattened and the tympanic plate more tube-like than in modern skulls. Neanderthal man (*Homo sapiens neanderthalensis*) lived during the third interglacial period (Riss-Würm) of the Pleistocene and became extinct as a special branch of the human family during the last glacial period (50 000 years ago). His exact relationship to modern man (*Homo sapiens*) is uncertain.

There is as yet no agreement on the classification of the various human fossils. Coon suggests two species; *Homo erectus* including *Pithecanthropus* and *Sinathropus*, and *Homo sapiens* including Neanderthal and modern man. It is possible however that all human fossils from *Pithecanthropus* to modern man make up a single highly variable polytypical species.

The earliest fossil skulls considered to be typically *Homo sapiens* are from Swanscombe in England and Fontechevade in France. These coexisted with Neanderthal man. Unfortunately the only material available consists of portions of the cranial vault.

CHANGES OF DENTAL INTEREST DURING HUMAN EVOLUTION

In comparing modern man, *Homo habilis*, *Homo erectus* and Neanderthal man the chief dento-facial changes include:

1. A reduction in the size of the teeth but little change in tooth form apart from a tendency to a reduction in the number of cusps in the permanent molars.

2. A greater reduction in the size of the alveolar processes with a loss

of facial (alveolar) prognathism and an increasing tendency for crowding of the teeth in the jaws.

3. A reduction in the facial buttress system, in the supraorbital torus and general robustness of the facial skeleton, especially in those parts concerned with giving attachment to the muscles of mastication (Fig. 296).

4. The development of the characteristic chin of modern man.

Many of the facial skeletal changes are probably the result of a reduction in masticatory function as the consequence not only of a change in the nature of the diet but the time taken in chewing food. This reduction of functional activity probably results in a failure of certain genetically determined features to reach their full development and growth rather than their complete suppression.

THE EVOLUTION OF THE HUMAN FACE

In a typical non-primate such as the dog, sheep or hedgehog the facial skeleton projects in front of the cranial region of the skull. During primate evolution the facial skeleton becomes gradually more bent downwards until in man it lies below the overhanging frontal region of the cranium. This change is associated both with the increasing relative predominance of the brain and a bending of the axis of the cranial base in the region of the pituitary gland. This alteration appears to be associated with the gradual attainment of the upright posture, first in the sitting posture of the sub-human aboreal primates, and later with the upright standing position of the whole skeleton already attained in the Australopithecinae and perfected in modern man.

Throughout primate evolution there has been a gradual reduction of the importance of the sense of smell with a reduction in the size and complexity of the nasal cavities and of the snout. This also reduces the space available for the teeth but in the anthropoid apes this deficiency is made good by a secondary compensatory development of the alveolar processes, leading to the characteristic alveolar prognathism still evident in primitive human types such as *Pithecanthropus*.

The forward migration of the eyes from the sub-mammalian lateral position to the anterior forward-looking position associated with stereoscopic vision also reduces the size of the upper (olfactory) portion of the nasal cavities. As a consequence a typical nasal bone such as the facial ethmoid comes to contribute to the medial wall of the orbital cavity of the human skull.

The reduction of the elongated primitive facial skeleton reduces the space available for the tongue. This in part is compensated for by a remodelling of the chin area, the anterior supporting internal strut—the simian shelf—being replaced by the external chin.

In the anthropoid apes, living on a vegetable diet, mastication is an almost continuous daytime activity and the whole masticatory apparatus, dental, skeletal and muscular is highly developed. This shows itself, especially in male animals, in which teeth are also weapons, in superimposed cranial crests for muscle attachment and a massive facial buttress system including well developed supraorbital ridges. With growth of brain and cranium in man the crests are no longer necessary. With change in eating habits the dentition is less developed and what remains of the supraorbital crests becomes submerged in the development of a forward placed vertical forehead.

The direction of facial growth throughout the primate series, and especially in man, becomes more vertical. In the latter the vertical component of facial growth is greater than the forward component. This is especially noticeable in the alveolar processes associated with an increasing frequency of crowded misplaced teeth.

One of the secondary consequences of this predominance of vertical growth is disengagement of the larynx from the nasal cavity, an important factor in the development of speech.

TEETH AND JAWS AS EVIDENCE OF EVOLUTION

Because of their relatively indestructible nature teeth play an important part in the attempt to establish the relationship between living and extinct forms of mammalian and submammalian life. Certain features of the human dentition are similar to those found among the anthropoid apes. These features include the total number of the teeth, deciduous and permanent, their general form and relationship to one another, and in particular the form of the incisors and permanent molars. There are, however, differences which make it quite easy to distinguish a typical human from a typical anthropoid ape dentition. These include the size of the teeth, the characteristic tusk-like form of the ape canines and the associated diastema and modifications in the form of the first lower premolars (Figs. 293, 294), the number of roots possessed by the cheek teeth, the type of wear of the occlusal surfaces, and the order of tooth eruption. It is uncertain whether the human canines are primitive and the ape canines specialisations of this primitive form, or whether the human canines are derived from the ape type of tooth by a process of reduction.

It is sometimes stated that the length of the root of the human canine indicates the previous presence of a larger crown, but this is a classical example of the dangerous application of verbal logic to the complex question of morphological origins. All canines have long roots; some canines have long crowns; there is no correlation adequate to answer the question. If the present anthropoid apes were known only by their fossilised teeth, arguments could be used for and against their possible 'humanity.' The form of their molars and incisors could be used as evidence for their close human affinities, their canines and lower first premolars against. Teeth can give useful evidence for the general affinities between related species; they cannot answer such questions as whether a certain fossil was 'human' or 'sub-human.' The answer to that question depends not upon structural relationships but on evidence for the presence or absence of human behaviour. In the absence of direct experience of how a primitive creature with possible human characteristics behaved in everyday life we can only rely with any confidence on the evidence of the ability to make instruments and objects of cultural or utilitarian significance. There is some evidence that *Sinanthropus* knew the use of fire and that certain of the Australopithecinae were hunters who used bones as weapons and ran in the upright posture. The teeth of *Sinanthropus* were much more like those of modern man than like those of any known anthropoid ape.

The teeth of the various Australopithecine fossils from South Africa have been described as human in certain of their characteristics (Fig. 297); some of them have canines and lower premolars of more or less

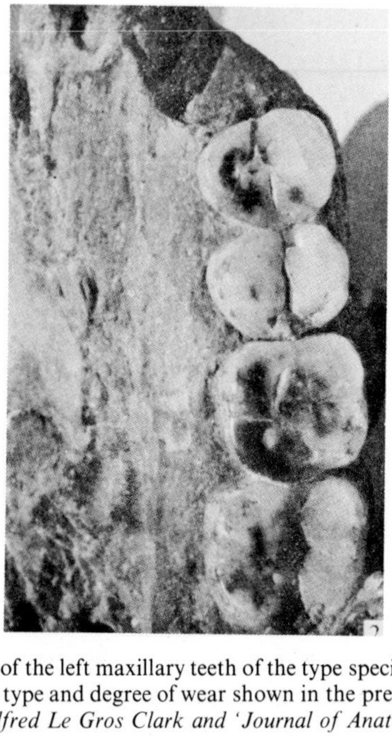

Fig. 297 Occlusal view of the left maxillary teeth of the type specimen of *Plesianthropus*. × 5/4 approx. Note the type and degree of wear shown in the premolar and molar teeth. (*By courtesy of Sir Wilfred Le Gros Clark and 'Journal of Anatomy.'*)

human form. Their pelvic structure is more human-like than that of any living ape, but their brain size is but slightly larger than that of the gorilla. They were, in fact, creatures with certain features resembling humans and certain others resembling anthropoid apes. It is probable that they were neither one nor the other, and there is as yet no convincing evidence that human beings evolved directly from them, although it is quite possible that during evolution the human stem passed through a stage showing a similar dental or skeletal morphology.

When we limit our survey to fossils associated with evidence of human abilities, that is, to *Pithecanthropus*, *Sinanthropus*, Neanderthal man and early modern man, we find that there has been no very great change in the dentition. The difference between the earliest human fossils and modern man is much less than the difference found between different breeds of dog. Modern teeth show less wear, are somewhat reduced in size as also are modern jaws, are more liable to malocclusion, dental decay, and gingival disease, but the same could be said of the dentition of the Pekinese as compared with that of the wolfhound. The conditions under which prehistoric man existed did not encourage the appearance and persistence of types which were less than perfectly adapted to their harsh environment. When man began to master his environment he began to permit the establishment of genetic variations which had previously been kept in check.

The dental apparatus should be considered as a functional organ or system and not as a series of isolated units. Within each species there is a range of variation in the dental apparatus, and in some species this range is greater than in others. Furthermore, when a new species arises in the course of evolution certain organs such as the dentition may show little change. The human type of dentition, which is relatively unspecialised, may have been established very early in the evolution of the higher primates and have persisted with little change in the human line of evolution over a period during which dramatic changes were occurring in brain size, locomotion, and cranio-facial morphology. Great care must be exercised in attempting a reconstruction of the morphology or habits of an animal or fossil when only the teeth are available.

The basic postulate of evolution is that there is continual genetic variation within each species. Geographical or other forms of partial or complete isolation result in a section of the total population of a species becoming separated from the other members of the species. Within this localised environment those genetic variations, which, as a result of natural selection, render the group more adaptable to the new environment produce over a period of time a change in the genetic constitution of the isolated group and therefore in its appearance, behaviour, and morphology. These changes enable the isolated group to be classified first as a subspecies and then, if the process continues, as a new species. This interpretation of the mechanism of evolution depends upon the occurrence of a gradual change within a population. It should be remembered, however, that while genetic variations are random events, animals often deliberately choose certain environments in which to live and that to this extent choice is superimposed on chance. The weakness in this so-called Neo-Darwinian interpretation of the evolutionary process is that while isolation and the accumulation of numerous small variations account for the variability which is found in many species and for the origin of categories such as the subspecies, it does not provide altogether convincing evidence that new species or categories above the species level arise in this manner. The appearance of these higher categories may involve much more dramatic changes in the genetic constitution, which may take place suddenly (saltations) either in a random manner or as a result of predetermined alterations in the genetic constitution of the species.

It is well known that drastic genetic changes can be produced by the use of X-rays, radiations, and certain chemicals and although the majority of such changes are harmful, this may be because of the rather crude nature of our present experimental methods. In nature massive changes of the genetic constitution may occur as a result of cytological influences acting upon the germ plasm, or changes occurring in the germ plasm itself. Such changes may show themselves suddenly in a single individual, or in a small group of individuals, or even as a 'genetic crisis' involving many members of the species at a certain period in its life history. It would be difficult, however, to find evidence for such rapid changes within a species in the fossil record, and as yet there is little experimental evidence for such a theory of evolution.

Apart from these more general questions regarding evolution, there are many problems relating to the evolution of tooth form which remain to be solved. Certain types of dentition which are related in their functional adaptations to certain kinds of diet or other behaviour patterns involving the use of the teeth have appeared and reappeared throughout the phylogenetic history of the mammals. Among the incisor teeth, for example, the range of morphological variation extends from the simple peg-shaped tooth with an enamel covered crown and a closed root as found, for example, in seals, to the continually erupting tooth as exemplified by the rodent incisor in which there is a more specialised arrangement of the dental tissues and a complex growth mechanism correlating tooth formation with tooth wear. Even when such specialised teeth as the hook-like incisors of certain bats or the comb-like incisors of *Galeopithecus* are taken into consideration, the pattern of incisor variation is not unlimited and certain basic types appear and reappear many times during evolution. This relative fixity of the range of fundamental dental patterns would appear inexplicable on a theory of chance variations occurring entirely at random. In the case of structures such as the teeth, random variations if they occurred would express themselves in the form of the calcified crowns of the teeth even prior to their use and should appear in large numbers in the fossil records. They do not. The relative stability of the repertoire of tooth form and the structural and functional correlation of the morphology of the teeth making up the incisor, canine, and premolar-molar regions in any dentition seems to indicate a limitation to the number of patterns within which living creatures can experiment in the development of tooth form. Furthermore, within each basic pattern there often appears to be a predetermined direction of evolution. Within its environment organic life repeats itself as it improves upon itself, but the amount of variation which is possible on the theme of dental morphology is limited.

Neuroblasts, not odontoblasts and ameloblasts, contain the possibilities which enabled humanity to raise itself into a category apart from the rest of the animal kingdom. Those who are interested in the theme of the functional possibilities of mind as opposed to mastication should read the famous seventh chapter of Sherrington's great book, *Man on His Nature.*

BIBLIOGRAPHY

Brothwell, D. R. (1963). *Dental Anthropology.* Oxford: Pergamon Press.

Clark, W. E. Le Gros (1955). *The Fossil Evidence for Human Evolution.* University of Chicago Press.

Coon, C. S. (1963). *The Origin of Races.* London: Cape.

Dart, R. A. (1957). The osteodontokeratic culture of *Australopithecus prometheus. Transvaal Museum Memoir* No. 10. Pretoria.

Frisch, J. E. (1965). *Trends in the Evolution of the Hominid Dentition.* Basel: Karger.

Howells, W. W. (1966). Homo erectus. *Scientific American.* **215**, 46.

von Koenigswald, G. H. R. (1956). *Meeting Prehistoric Man.* London: Thames & Hudson.

Korenhof, C. A. W. (1960). *Morphogenetical aspects of the human upper molar* Utrecht: Druk.

Koski, K. & Garn, S. M. (1957). Tooth eruption sequence in fossil and modern man. *Amer. J. phys. Anthrop.* **15** (N.S.), 470.

Laughlin, W. S. & Osborne, R. A. (1967). In *Human Variation and Origins.* Ed. Freeman, W. H.

Robinson, J. T. (1956). The dentition of the Australopithecinae. *Transvaal Museum Memoir* No. 9. Pretoria.

Straus, W. L. (1949). The riddle of man's ancestry. *Quart. Rev. Biol.* **24**, 200.

Weidenreich, F. (1937). The dentition of *Sinanthropus Pekinensis.* A comparative odontography of the hominids. *Paleont. sinica* (N.S.) D. No. 1.

Appendices

1. Dental Measurements

MESIO-DISTAL LENGTH OF PERMANENT TEETH IN HUMAN RACES (in millimetres)

	American Whites (Black)	*Lapps* (Selmer-Olsen)	*Eskimos* (Pedersen)	*Pecos Indians* (Nelson)	*Javanese* (Mijsberg)	*Australian Aboriginals* (Campbell)	*Bantus* (Shaw)	*Bushmen* (Drennan)
Upper Teeth:								
1st incisor	9·0	8·4	8·4	8·7	8·6	9·4	8·9	8·3
2nd ,,	6·4	6·8	7·0	7·1	7·0	7·7	7·2	6·7
Canine	7·6	7·7	7·8	8·0	8·0	8·4	7·6	7·5
1st premolar	7·2	6·8	7·5	7·4	7·5	7·8	7·2	6·8
2nd ,,	6·8	6·5	6·8	7·0	7·0	7·2	7·0	6·5
1st molar	10·7	10·2	10·7	10·7	10·8	11·4	10·3	9·9
2nd ,,	9·2	9·3	10·2	9·9	10·0	10·9	10·0	9·7
3rd ,,	8·6	8·0	9·6	9·4	9·2	10·0	9·5	8·2
Lower Teeth:								
1st incisor	5·4	5·4		5·5	5·5	6·0	5·9	5·0
2nd ,,	5·9	6·0		6·1	6·2	6·7	6·0	5·6
Canine	6·9	6·8	7·1	7·3	7·2	7·6	7·3	6·8
1st premolar	6·9	6·7	7·1	7·1	7·3	7·6	7·1	6·9
2nd ,,	7·1	6·7	7·1	7·4	7·3	7·7	7·2	7·0
1st molar	11·2	11·0	11·8	12·0	11·5	12·3	11·0	10·9
2nd ,,	10·7	10·5	11·4	11·4	10·9	12·5	11·0	10·6
3rd ,,	10·7	9·9	11·4	11·1	10·9	11·9	11·1	9·9

The Lapp and Javanese teeth are male; the others are mixed.

REFERENCES

BLACK, G. V. (1902). *Descriptive Anatomy of the Human Teeth*, 4th ed. Philadelphia: White.

CAMPBELL, T. D. (1925). *Dentition and Palate of the Australian Aboriginal.* Adelaide.

DRENNAN, M. R. (1928). The Dentition of a Bushman Tribe. *Ann. S. Afr. Mus.* **24.**

MIJSBERG, W. A. (1931). On sexual differences in the teeth in Javanese. (Quoted in Selmer-Olsen.)

NELSON, C. T. (1938). The teeth of the Indians of Pecos Pueblo. *Amer. J. phys. Anthrop.* **23**, 261.

PEDERSEN, P. O. (1949). *The East Greenland Eskimo Dentition.* Copenhagen: Reitzels Forlag.

SELMER-OLSEN, R. (1949). *An Odontometrical Study on the Norwegian Lapps.* Oslo: Dybwad.

SHAW, J. C. M. (1931). *The Teeth, the Bony Palate, and the Mandible in Bantu Races.* London: Bale.

2. Correlation of Dento-facial Development

(*Modified from Arey.*)

Age in Weeks	*Size (C.R. length in mm.)*	*Head and Neck*	*Mouth Cavity*	*Skeletal System*	*Dentition*	*Other Regions*
$3\frac{1}{2}$	2·5	First two visceral arches defined in neck region	Oral membrane rupturing	Notochord present		Thyroid gland commencing to develop
4	4–5	Visceral arches completed. Eye and otocyst present. Olfactory placodes forming	Rathke's pouch forming Tongue primordia present	Somites complete		Trachea and lung buds developing. Neural tube closed. Nerves forming. Heart commences to beat
5	6–8	Nasal pits and fronto-nasal process formed	Tongue primordia uniting			Parathyroid glands developing
6	10–14	Maxillary process united with fronto-nasal process. Olfactory pits open into stomodeum	Nasal septum developing. Palatal folds at side of tongue. Parotid gland developing followed by submandibular gland.	Chondro-cranium and Meckel's cartilage developing	Primary epithelial lamina developing	Jacobson's organ developing. Naso-lacrimal duct developing
7	16–20	Face acquires characteristic human form. Eyelids developing	Tongue musculature differentiating	Ossification of maxilla, premaxilla and mandible	Dental lamina and vestibular band developing	Voluntary muscles differentiating

Age in Weeks	*Size (C.R. length in mm.)*	*Head and Neck*	*Mouth Cavity*	*Skeletal System*	*Dentition*	*Other Regions*
8	20–30	Epithelial union of eyelids	Palatal process uniting. Sublingual gland developing	Ossification of palatine bones	Enamel organs and tooth germs forming for incisors, canines and first deciduous molars	First contractions in facial and jaw muscles. Smooth muscle differentiating in alimentary canal
10	40–50		Palatal and nasal processes fully united. Lips separating from jaws. Tongue papillae developing	Secondary cartilage appears in mandibular condyle. Full development of chondro-cranium	Enamel organs of second deciduous molars developing. Mesodermal niches in anterior enamel organs	First peristaltic movements in gut
12	55–65		Muscles developing in soft palate	Mandibular joint cavities developing	Laminae of successional permanent teeth appearing	Blood vessels fully differentiated
16	90–120			Maxillary sinus developing. Secondary cartilage in coronoid process	Full differentiation of deciduous enamel organs. Enamel organs of first permanent molars forming	Body hair developing

Glossary

Abrasion: The wear of teeth by physical agencies other than the friction of one tooth against another.

Alveolar bulb: A backward projection of the alveolar process of the jaws in which the most distal (posterior) members of the cheek teeth develop before eruption.

Alveolar process: That portion of the maxilla, premaxilla, and mandible which contains the sockets of erupted teeth and the alveoli or crypts of developing teeth.

Alveolus: A cavity in the alveolar process containing the developing tooth germ of a deciduous tooth.

Ameloblast: A specialised cell of epithelial origin concerned in the formation of enamel.

Amelogenesis: The process of enamel formation.

Anchylosis: The direct union of tooth and bone by continuity of calcified tissue.

Anlage: The first rudimentary appearance of a structure during development.

Argyrophil fibres: Connective tissue elements which stain readily with silver stains.

Attrition: The wear of teeth in mastication and produced by the friction of one tooth against another.

Basal bone: A term sometimes used for that part of the facial skeleton which supports the alveolar processes of the jaws.

Brachyodont: referring to teeth with low crowns.

Carabelli, tubercle of: A supernumerary cusp sometimes present on the lingual surface of upper second deciduous molars and upper first permanent molars.

Carnassial: Referring to teeth specialised for cutting—characteristic of certain carnivores (also known as sectorial teeth).

Cheek teeth: Used to describe collectively those teeth adjacent to the cheeks, *i.e.* premolars and molars.

Chondrocranium: The primary cartilaginous skeleton of the cranium and face around which and in which the later developing bony elements appear.

Cingulum: Marginal areas of the crown of a tooth at the cervical region.

Cribriform plate: The bone lining tooth sockets which is perforated by numerous vascular channels.

Crown, anatomical: That part of a tooth which is covered with enamel.

Crown, clinical: That part of a tooth appearing in the mouth cavity.

Crypt: A cavity in the alveolar process containing the developing tooth germ of a permanent tooth.

Dead tract: An area of dentine in which the processes of the odontoblasts have been destroyed.

Dental lamina: A downgrowth of the oral epithelium from which the enamel organs of the deciduous and permanent teeth develop.

Dental papilla: The principal mesodermal contribution to the formation of a tooth germ and from which the dentine and pulp of the tooth develop.

Dermal bone: Bone developing directly in membrane and usually close to the surface of skin or mucous membrane.

Dermis: The connective tissue layer of the skin or mucous membrane deep to the covering epithelium (epidermis).

Diastema: A morphological space between adjacent teeth in the same jaw, usually related to the canines.

Diphyodont: Referring to an animal which develops two sets of teeth, *i.e.* deciduous and permanent.

Diprotodont: Referring to members of the marsupial order which have two lower incisors.

Embrasure: The space produced, buccally, lingually and occlusally by the diverging interstitial surfaces of two adjacent teeth.

Enamel knot: A transient structure of the developing enamel organ which partly divides the dental papilla into buccal and lingual parts.

Enamel niche: A mesodermal invagination of the dental lamina appearing during the process of differentiation of the enamel organ.

Enamel organ: The epithelial contribution to the formation of a tooth germ. It is responsible for determining the form and size of the crown and gives origin to the enamel.

Enamel prism or rod: A unit of enamel structure.

Enamel septum: A transient structure which partly divides the developing enamel organ into two halves.

Eutheria: Modern mammals excluding monotremes and marsupials.

Fibres of von Korff: Collagenous fibres forming a part of the organic matrix of dentine.

Follicle: The fibrous tissue sac which surrounds the developing tooth germ and by which the germ is attached to the oral mucous membrane.

Gingival crevice: A shallow sulcus bounded by the gingival margin and the tooth surface.

Gomphosis: The union of tooth and alveolar bone by the periodontal membrane in a socket.

Gubernaculum: A fibrous cord uniting the tooth follicle to the lamina propria of the oral mucous membrane.

Hertwig's sheath: A two-layered epithelial sheath covering the developing root portion of teeth. It is later broken up allowing of the deposition of cement.

Heterodont: Referring to a dentition in which the teeth differ in form.

Homodont: Referring to a dentition in which all the teeth are alike in form.

Howship's lacunae: Shallow excavations on the surface of bone, dentine, or cement undergoing resorption and often containing osteoclasts or similar multinucleated giant cells.

Hypsodont: Referring to teeth with high crowns.

Key ridge: The root of the zygomatic process of the maxilla, so-called because it is through this ridge that the maximum stress of mastication is transmitted to the base of the skull.

Lacunae: Minute spaces containing isolated cells found in bone and cement.

Lamina dura: The bone lining tooth sockets (alveolar and dental bone).

Lamina propria: See Dermis.

Lophodont: Referring to teeth in which the occlusal surface shows a well-marked pattern of ridges.

Malassez, rests of: Epithelial strands derived from Hertwig's sheath found in the periodontal membrane.

Meckel's cartilage: The primary skeleton of the mandibular (first visceral) arch.

Monophyodont: Referring to an animal which develops only one set of teeth.

Odontoblast: A specialised cell concerned in the formation of dentine.

Ontogenetic: Referring to the developmental history of an individual.

Ortho-dentine: Dentine containing tubes radiating from a simple pulp cavity.

Orthogenesis: Evolution proceeding in a definite direction as a result of changes initiated within the organism.

Osteo-dentine: Dentine similar in structure to bone; usually occupying the pulp chamber.

PAS: The abbreviation commonly used for periodic acid-Schiff.

Pedestal bone (bone of attachment): Bone developing around the basal portion of the dental papilla and supporting the tooth.

Perikymata: Horizontal lines on the surface of enamel formed by outcropping of enamel prisms (imbrication lines of Pickerill).

Phylogenetic: Referring to the developmental (evolutionary) history of a group of animals.

Plici-dentine: Dentine in which tubules radiate from a pulp cavity rendered complex by folding or branching.

Polyphyodont: Referring to an animal which has a continuous succession of teeth throughout life.

Polyprotodont: Referring to members of the marsupial order which have more than two lower incisors.

Primary enamel organ: The enamel organ from which develops (*a*) the enamel organ of a deciduous tooth, (*b*) its permanent successor.

Primary epithelial band or lamina: An epithelial structure which gives origin to the dental lamina and vestibular band.

Prognathism: The degree of protrusion of the facial skeleton beyond the cranial base.

Reduced enamel epithelium: The remains of the epithelium of the enamel organ covering the enamel surface of the teeth prior to eruption.

RNA: The abbreviation commonly used for ribonucleic acid.

Secondary cartilages: Regions of modified cartilage which develop independently of and later than the primary cartilage skeleton.

Sharpey's fibres: The partly calcified portions of the collagenous fibres of the periodontal membrane which penetrate the cement covering the root or roots of the teeth and the alveolar bone. The term is also used to describe the penetrating fibres of periosteum entering bone.

Stomodeum: The primitive mouth cavity separated from the foregut by the oral membrane.

Talon (Talonid): The posterior (distal) part of the primitive molar tooth which usually carries two cusps (hypocone or hypoconid; entocone or entoconid).

Taurodont: Referring to teeth in which the pulp chamber extends well into the root area; found in Neanderthal man and ruminants.

Tetrapod: A vertebrate with four limbs; *i.e.* amphibians, reptiles, birds and mammals.

Tomes, granular layer of: A region of minute areas of interglobular dentine beneath the cement.

Tooth germ (Tooth bud): The formative structures making up the developing tooth and consisting of the enamel organ and dental papilla within the dental follicle.

Trigone (Trigonid): The anterior (mesial) part of the primitive molar tooth which usually carries three cusps (paracone or paraconid; metacone or metaconid; protocone or protoconid).

Vaso-dentine: Dentine containing blood vessels.

Vestibular band (Lip furrow band): The band of oral epithelium which develops to the buccal (outer) side of the dental lamina and gives origin to part of the vestibular region of the oral cavity.

Volkmann's canals: Vascular channels entering bone from its surface and joining the Haversian canals.

Index